BASIC
RESCUE AND
EMERGENCY
CARE

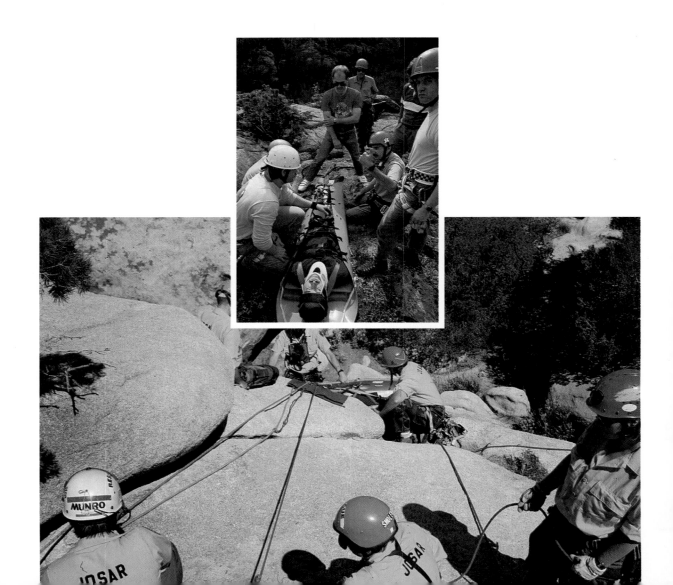

THE RESCUE
AND EMERGENCY
CARE SERIES

BASIC
RESCUE AND
EMERGENCY
CARE

By the American Academy
of Orthopaedic Surgeons
with the assistance
of the National Association
for Search and Rescue

Editor:
Robert A. Worsing, Jr., MD

Technical Editor:
Tom Vines, EMT

Contributors:
Paul Anderson,
Michael Brown,
Peter Goth, MD,
Ross Kinman,
James O'Brien,
Douglas Stutz

FIRST EDITION

Telephone 1–800–626–6726

ISBN 0-89203-040-2

Library of Congress Catalog Card Number 90-83796

10 9 8 7 6 5 4 3 2 1

Published and distributed by:

American Academy of Orthopaedic Surgeons
222 S. Prospect Ave., Park Ridge, IL 60068

Printed in the United States of America

This textbook is intended solely as a guide to the appropriate procedures to be employed when rendering emergency care to or transporting the sick or injured. It is not intended as a statement of the standards of care required in any particular situation, since circumstances and patients' physical condition can vary widely from one emergency to another. Nor is it intended that this textbook shall in any way advise emergency personnel concerning legal authority to perform the activities or procedures discussed. Such determinations should be made locally only with the aid of legal counsel.

The rescue series is written with the assumption that the reader has completed a basic EMT training course. The editors believe this level is the minimum level of medical training suitable for patient care in the rescue setting, but all rescue personnel are encouraged to attain the highest level of training available. Throughout this module, assessment and treatment skills are mentioned that require a higher level of training and licensure than are available to basic EMTs. In addition, there are wide variances throughout the United States in what rescue personnel are permitted by law to do. This text is intended for nationwide use, and we have sought to include various techniques that may be helpful in particular situations; it must fall to the instructor and the reader to determine what is acceptable within one's training and jurisdiction. Before using the advanced techniques presented in the text, the rescuer must review his or her scope of practice as well as the legal limits of his or her training and authorization, so as not to exceed the limits of the law and to ensure the provision of the highest possible patient care.

This book is dedicated to
the families at home whose support, solace, and sacrifice
enable our care in the field and allow lives to be saved and
family and friends to be reunited.

ACKNOWLEDGMENTS

Before I was asked to contribute to *Emergency Care and Transportation of the Sick and Injured,* (the Orange Book) eight years ago, I did not know that when Jim Heckman asks for a little help, the best option is to head for the hills. However, if I had given him a simple "No," I might have avoided "a couple of simple little projects," and missed a lot of opportunities and excitement.

I am indebted to Tom Vines for his constant commitment to this project and to the National Association for Search and Rescue for their participation and support.

Special thanks to Peter Goth, MD, director of Wilderness Medical Associates, for his contribution to the medical chapters of this book. I also thank Warren Bowman, MD, National Medical Advisor, National Ski Patrol System, for his medical review and input.

Fire services play a major role in rescue operations in many areas of the country. Deputy Chief Robert Zickler of the Indianapolis Fire Department has been this project's fire expert and resource person for the many urban rescue questions that arose. Although he has lent me his turnout gear, there is no way that I can ever fill it.

Law enforcement agencies were represented by Gregory Noose, now with the Montana Law Enforcement Academy, who provided the rural rescue perspective while he served as the Stillwater County, Montana, Sheriff. Michael Quinn from the Los Angeles County Sheriff's Department and his associates in the Medical Detachment of the Special Enforcement Bureau and the Harbor Patrol demonstrated aspects of urban law enforcement as they relate to rescue procedures.

Two individuals provided valued assistance as reference resources and for arranging the personnel, materials, and locations for many of the photographs used in the book. I appreciate the assistance provided by Steve Dewell, EMT-P, from Montana, and Tom Patterson who is with the National Park Service at Joshua Tree National Monument.

Others who have helped make this book possible by contributing their valuable time and expertise in reviewing the manuscript throughout its various stages are J. W. "Bill" Wade, Rod Dennison, William C. Wade, Bunny Johns, and John Toohey, MD.

Without the support of the American Academy of Orthopaedic Surgeons' Executive Director, Thomas C. Nelson, Deputy Executive Director, Fred V. Featherstone, MD, and the Academy's publications staff—particularly Mark W. Wieting, director; Marilyn L. Fox, PhD, assistant director; and Keith F. Levine, marketing manager—this project might never have become a reality. Their good counsel, understanding, and forbearance helped in completing this project.

Every author and editor of a major textbook needs a publications manager—part counselor, part teacher, and part tyrant (deadlines). Sally King Jessee is also a friend. Her editorial management and administrative skills have taken ideas, words, paper, and ink, and turned them into something of worth. Her assistant, Kathy Brouillette, has done an excellent job coordinating manuscripts and other details.

Finally, I thank Jim Heckman, for his counsel, support, and faith. I hope this book lives up to his expectations and, maybe, as we refine it in the future, it will match the example he has set with the Orange Book.

Robert A. Worsing, Jr., MD

FOREWORD

Search and rescue (SAR) community members who cut their teeth on the excellent books on mountain and wilderness rescue by Wastl Mariner, W. G. May, Tim Setnicka, Hamish MacInnes, and others will be pleased by *Basic Rescue and Emergency Care.* In this first of the American Academy of Orthopaedic Surgeons' Rescue and Emergency Care Series, the Academy has taken the commendable course of recognizing that, while high angle rescue in the mountains may be spectacular and a wilderness search for a lost child stirs the emotions, a large part of search and rescue takes place closer to home, and that most of it is plain hard work rather than high drama. These vital efforts will be more efficient and effective if performed by rescuers who have acquired the basic knowledge and skills common to all types of SAR operations. *Basic Rescue and Emergency Care* is the first book of its kind to present this basic information in a lucid format and logical progression, moving from preplanning into the four phases common to all types of SAR: location, access, stabilization, and transport. The next units of the series—vehicle rescue and agricultural rescue—will refine and modify the basic principles as they apply to special problems of context, site, and topography.

As a logical extension of the classic Orange Book—*Emergency Care and Transportation of the Sick and Injured*—this text continues to emphasize state-of-the-art emergency care as the *cornerstone* of modern search and rescue. The reader is presumed to be an emergency medical technician (EMT) trained to the basic level or equivalent. Moreover, in Section V on patient stabilization, the authors acknowledge what most experts in the field have realized for years: Current urban EMS protocols that assume rapid transportation to a medical facility and radio communication with a control physician may be impossible to follow. In the wilderness environment or in a disaster where the usual amenities of civilization do not exist, the environment may be unfriendly and difficulties in obtaining food, water, and shelter may be significant. Basic survival of both patient and rescuer may be a major problem. Definitive medical care may be many hours or days away because of distance, bad weather, lack of transportation, or lack of communication. Because of this delay, rescuers must learn the extended care of illnesses and injuries as they develop over time and are modified by the environment. The amount of equipment that can be carried by even a large SAR group with helicopter support is limited, so that innovation and improvisation may be necessary. Certain standard urban protocols, such as the requirement that CPR be started in all cases of cardiac arrest and continued until the patient arrives at the emergency department, may be unrealistic or even hazardous to rescuers. The Academy is to be congratulated for being willing to move ahead by building on and modifying its previous urban protocols and lending its considerable prestige to the development and legitimization of these urgently needed remote area protocols.

Warren D. Bowman, MD, FACP
National Medical Advisor,
National Ski Patrol System
Chairman, Medical Committee,
National Association for Search and Rescue

PREFACE

For 20 years, the American Academy of Orthopaedic Surgeons has actively published training materials for emergency medical services personnel. The development of the Rescue and Emergency Care Series is an extension of the Academy's commitment to the education of prehospital care providers. This series covers rescue techniques and medical care designed to supplement the basic EMT course outlined in the Academy's text, *Emergency Care and Transportation of the Sick and Injured* (the Orange Book).

The idea for this project originated in 1986 during one of the development meetings for the fourth edition of the Orange Book. One of the editors commented that a reasonable overview of rescue and extrication would far exceed the size constraints of the chapter. What followed was not just a "tongue-in-cheek" suggestion by one of the editors to double the size of the Orange Book, but a lengthy discussion of the need to bring emergency medical care one step closer to the patient with a text on the basics of rescue.

Following that discussion, the editorial board of the Orange Book and the Academy's Committee on Emergency Medical Services continued informal discussions on a basic rescue text. In July 1986, the Academy sponsored a formal meeting and invited representatives from the National Association for Search and Rescue (NASAR); the National Park Service; and the fields of EMS, law enforcement, and fire services. Two conclusions came out of the meeting: the existing rescue/extrication texts were outdated and ignored the principles of emergency medical care and, there was a definite need for a medically oriented, technically correct rescue text.

An ad hoc committee was formed consisting of Drs. James D. Heckman, Luther M. Strayer III, Richard L. Withington, and myself. Charged with the task of writing a proposal to the Academy's Board of Directors, we started by paring the initial list of 35 types of rescue down to five major areas—basic, agricultural, vehicle, high angle (vertical), and water. We also proposed an editorial approach that was new to the Academy—using outside expert technical editors to work in conjunction with physician medical editors appointed by the Academy. When the Board of Directors approved the initial outlines for the series, our committee began working with an in-house management team headed by Fred V. Featherstone, MD, deputy executive director of the Academy, to prepare the formal business plan. The initial phase of the project included the development of a basic text, to be followed by agriculture and vehicle rescue modules. In December 1987, the Board accepted the proposal. I was appointed the managing editor of the project, with Dr. Heckman, editorial board chairman of the third and fourth editions of the Orange Book, serving as consultant. Drs. Strayer and Withington agreed to serve on the editorial board.

Over the last three years, the rescue modules have evolved into documents that no longer remotely resemble the original outlines. With no standard rescue curriculum in existence, we relied heavily on technical reviews of our material and refined the outlines as questions and suggestions arose.

In the basic text, the rescue operation has been divided into five elements—preplanning, plus the four phases of rescue: locate, access, stabilize, and transport. Preplanning covers personal preparation and safety, as well as rescue administration and operations. The four phases of rescue offers concepts and explains techniques for *locating* the subject of the rescue operation; use of present skills and materials to *access* the subject safely; review of basic emergency medical care, with alterations that are useful in *stabilizing* patients during an extended incident; and selection of the appropriate modalities for properly packaging and *transporting* the patient safely.

I have learned that writing a book is a lot like helping my children with their LEGOs®. Many little pieces have to fit together in just the right way. The enthusiastic, intelligent, and helpful new friends and associates I acquired have become extremely important to me. I appreciate the wonderful education and delightful memories they have provided.

NASAR has been a strong supporter and contributor to this project since its inception. Its willingness to join the Academy on this project has helped to strengthen the goals and objectives of rescue and the emergency medical field. In addition to their work on the basic text, NASAR is developing an instructor's course with future plans to launch a formal course of classroom and skills instruction for basic training of rescuers. I am indebted to Greg McDonald, Peggy McDonald, Bill Wade, Jim O'Brien, and the Board of Directors of NASAR for their efforts, input, reviews, and suggestions.

In particular, *Basic Rescue and Emergency Care* is a tribute to the time, skills, and efforts of Tom Vines. Without his technical expertise and writing skill, I would have been lost and the project would never have made it to print. Tom is a respected, nationally recognized instructor on rescue techniques and writer from Red Lodge, Montana. He is currently chairman of the Technical Rescue Project of NASAR and serves as editor of *Response,* the official publication of NASAR.

Peter Goth, MD, director of Wilderness Medical Associates, has also made an enormous contribution by sharing information from the Wilderness EMT course which he developed. Peter's review, counsel, and permission to build on his original material have been a valuable asset.

Especially appreciated are the three people who perhaps gave the most, Linda, Kalli, and Ryan. They have had to endure three years of "Daddy's got to work on *The Book* tonight." In many ways, their sacrifices represent the families of all of us who have heard the siren call of rescue and EMS. While we wear our rescue/EMS hats, we receive the vicarious thrills and "warm fuzzies" of saving lives and helping others. Meanwhile our families endure the cold, late dinners, the phone calls in the wee hours of the morning, the beepers intruding on important occasions, the plans disrupted by extended operations, and the difficulties of planning around call and duty schedules. With that in mind, this book is dedicated to the families at home whose support, solace, and sacrifice enable our care in the field and allow lives to be saved and family and friends to be reunited.

Robert A. Worsing, Jr., MD
St. Paul, Minnesota

CONTENTS

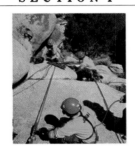

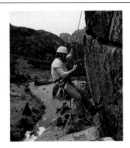

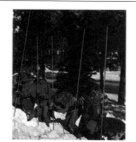

SECTION IV

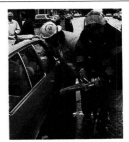

ACCESS   183

CHAPTER 11
Gaining Access in an Urban Setting   184

CHAPTER 12
Gaining Access in Remote Areas   200

SECTION V

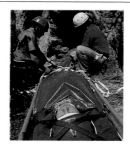

STABILIZE   209

CHAPTER 13
Medical Care in the Rescue Setting   210

CHAPTER 14
Patient Assessment in Rescue Medical Care   222

CHAPTER 15
Indications and Treatment of Common Medical
Conditions and Injuries   232

CHAPTER 16
Indications and Treatment of Environment-Specific
Medical Conditions and Injuries   266

SECTION VI

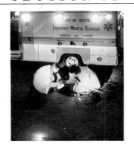

TRANSPORT   283

CHAPTER 17
Patient Packaging and Litter Evacuation   284

OVERVIEW

An emergency exists when an individual is unable to protect himself or herself from a threat to his health and well-being caused by mental and/or physical isolation or other threats. The goal of rescue is to *locate* and *access* that individual, *stabilize* the situation, and *transport* him or her to safety while managing any injuries and avoiding additional risk or injury to the patient or rescuer.

RESCUE TERMS

Standard terms were adopted during the development of this text to avoid confusion. These definitions and rationales are:

- *Subject:* The individual who needs to be rescued. When the subject is ill or injured, he or she is called a patient.
- *Victim:* An individual requiring rescue. Once a rescue operation begins, the victim is the subject of the operation, or is a patient if in need of medical care.
- *Patient:* A subject with injuries or illness requiring medical intervention.
- *Extended incident:* Any rescue incident lasting longer than two hours from the time of injury until the patient is delivered to definitive medical care. The delay may be the result of delayed notification, extended response or transport times, or difficult access problems that prolong the scene time. Such incidents may occur in urban, suburban, rural, or wilderness settings. Extended incident is a broader, more generic term than prolonged transport. It is a term preferable to delayed transport, which could imply that the rescue team is not working or cannot work in an efficient and timely fashion.

THE FOUR PHASES OF RESCUE

The four phases of rescue are known as the **LAST** sequence: *locating* the subjects at risk, *accessing* them to make an initial assessment of conditions and provide assistance, *stabilizing* them to prepare for transport, and finally, *transporting* them from the scene.

In all of these phases, preplanning helps select the quickest, easiest, and safest processes. Preplanning develops and maintains a plan for response to and management of a rescue. The preplan establishes who will be in charge and outlines the organization of the operation. In essence, preplanning defines procedures and makes decisions for conducting a rescue operation well before the incident occurs, when alternatives may be calmly discussed and logical decisions made.

Locate Phase

The first step of a rescue operation is to locate the individual at risk. This may simply require the dispatcher asking for the location of the incident, or it might be a complex operation involving several hundred searchers looking for a lost child.

A rescue response is activated on the **first notice**: relatives or friends report a person overdue; 911 is called about an abandoned vehicle or an accident; distress signals are reported; satellite relays detect aircraft emergency locator transmitters (ELTs) or vessel emergency position indicating radio beacons (EPIRBs). In any event, once the first notice is received, the name of the person reporting the emergency and a callback number must be obtained as part of the initial planning data.

Planning data are the pieces of information used to select the appropriate response for a rescue incident. Depending on the nature of the emergency, these might include such factors as the subject's physical and mental condition, last known location, and planned route of travel—information requested at the time of first notice of the incident. Other factors are the current and predicted weather, geographic information, structural diagrams or blueprints, available resources, access routes, and potential hazards. Knowing the current status of all factors that influence the rescue is critical for rescuers to determine their response. In addition, the history of previous rescues in the area can help responders predict where and how people get in trouble and how they behave in emergencies.

The person in charge then determines the urgency in responding to the incident by developing a priority system to rank such factors as age and condition of the subject, weather, and hazards. The **urgency** of the situation determines the speed, level, and nature of the response. An appropriate response may be as simple as reassuring the subject and talking him or her out of the situation. Or it may require a red lights and siren response to a critical incident. The most appropriate response generally lies between the two extremes.

As soon as possible, the person in charge initiates **scene confinement** both to ensure that the subject of the rescue does not leave the area without the rescue team's knowledge and to keep unauthorized persons out.

If the incident involves a search, you should begin making assumptions about the subject. A responsive subject may help to solve the location problem by reacting positively to offered assistance. Injured patients may welcome aid but be unable to assist in their rescue.

However, a lost subject may complicate the search operation by moving about, thus expanding the search area. Wandering or evasive subjects may fail to recognize problems they encounter and ignore or evade your attempts to locate them.

Rescuers often fail to follow-up on information they receive from people reporting an emergency. The individual in charge of the rescue operation should assign the investigation function early and maintain it throughout the incident. Investigators can uncover and compare disjointed pieces of information and lend important insight to solving the location problem.

Search Tactics At the beginning of an incident, rescue units may not know the subject's specific location. But the history of previous rescues in the area may indicate likely places to begin the search. **Tactics** are the specific actions you should use during the search and rescue operations.

Initial search tactics include using quick response resources to pinpoint probable rescue sites. The most efficient techniques provide the highest probability of locating the subject with the least time and effort. Examples of quick response resources in rural areas are air scenting dogs and trained human trackers. These resources work best in well-defined and identified search areas that are likely to contain the subject.

In urban areas rescue from fire follows the same principles. Fire in a building reduces the amount of time during which people must be located, accessed, and removed from danger. Search and rescue from a fire building works best when the rescue teams have preplanned the operation by inspecting the building and scrutinizing their tactics beforehand. This knowledge allows you to focus your efforts on specific, defined areas and thereby increase your chance of a successful rescue. The quick response resources in the urban fire scenario are often ladder truck or rescue companies assigned to the fire response to carry out the search and rescue mission.

More thorough tactics systematically examine all possible subject locations but are labor intensive and less efficient. Grid searching or a room by room building search is an example of a thorough, labor intensive tactic.

Searchers should diversify resources allocated to the incident to prepare for problems ahead. Duplication and backups will help ensure success if the initial approach fails.

Access Phase

After locating the subject of the search, you must access the individual to assess his or her condition and provide appropriate assistance. Access methods range from walking across the street to climbing up 900 feet of a sheer rock face.

The **size-up** of the rescue scene requires gathering information on the subject, weather, resource capabilities, and limitations. A critical part of the size-up is an evaluation of your hazards as well as your patient's.

Access techniques may change when patient and rescuer safety is threatened. Locations that unexpectedly become hazardous may require you to alter medical protocols and quickly remove patients without stabilization. A patient's deteriorating medical condition may also require accelerated rescue techniques. Such hazardous situations include:

- A surrounding atmosphere that is poisonous, flammable, explosive, or burning
- Unstable structures or ground
- Adverse weather that threatens the safety of you or the patient
- Natural conditions such as avalanche or rockfall areas that endanger the lives of persons in the area
- Civil disturbance or other hostile environment

Patient care begins as soon as you arrive and the scene is made as safe as possible. This involves eliminating as many environmental hazards as possible. This is an ongoing process, because environmental hazards may change. As part of their preplanning, many rescue units designate one member of the access team to initiate patient assessment and provide initial emergency medical care when reaching the patient. Other team members assist with patient management, packaging, and evacuation.

External influences may hinder all phases of the rescue effort, creating real hazards and obstacles during the access phase. Relatives, bystanders, media representatives, and government officials may interfere, particularly if they perceive insufficient action by the rescuers. Ways they may become involved vary, but include:

- Anxious relatives feeling compelled to contribute to the rescue effort
- Media representatives using aggressive reporting methods to "scoop" their competition
- Curious bystanders looking for excitement at the rescue scene; some people monitor rescue efforts on home scanners and frequently such people appear at rescue scenes
- Government officials seeking public exposure or trying to appear as if they are in charge of the rescue; officials may also react to pressures by relatives to "do more"

An information officer serving as a liaison to the family, media, or government officials may reduce problems caused by these external influences.

Stabilize Phase

Once the rescue team members locate and access the subject, they begin initial assessment and medical management. The initial assessment is an evaluation of the ABCs (airway, breathing, circulation) and, if necessary, initiation of basic life support—lifesaving procedures to manage failure of the respiratory or cardiovascular systems. If there are possible spinal injuries, you must carefully immobilize the patient.

After you complete the primary patient survey and initiate treatment of life-threatening conditions, begin the secondary survey. Take vital signs; determine the patient's level of consciousness; elicit a brief history; and examine the patient for other injuries, wounds, or fractures. Then stabilize the patient and package for transport. The patient must be reassessed frequently during packaging and transport. Treatment plans are adjusted as indicated by changes in the patient's condition.

Transport Phase

Transport is the fourth phase of rescue. It might be as simple as escorting a lost child to safety. Or it could be as complex as providing advanced life support to an injured climber during a backcountry evacuation that combines a litter carry, four-wheel drive vehicles, and an aeromedical helicopter.

Transportation involves several elements. **Packaging** is preparing the stabilized patient to be moved. It includes preparing the patient to allow necessary medical interventions during the transport phase, providing as much patient comfort as possible during the transport, and securing and protecting the patient to avoid additional injury. Appropriate packaging of the patient depends on the injuries present, the environment through which the transport will occur, the method (or type) of transport, and the time required for the transport.

The choice of specific transport method must be based on the patient's condition, the weather and terrain conditions, types of transportation available, and manpower resources. The person in charge must always have an alternative means of transportation available in case the primary means of transportation cannot be used or becomes unavailable.

If medical care is required, the transportation phase of rescue is also a continuation of the stabilization phase. You must continue to pay close attention to the ABCs and the patient's medical condition during transport, as well as to handle the patient carefully to avoid additional injury.

During transport, you must monitor the airway for blockage by the tongue, foreign objects, or vomitus. The patient must be packaged so that he or she may safely be placed on his or her side for airway management in the event of vomiting. In the unconscious patient, an artificial airway should be used so the tongue does not block the natural airway.

The patient must maintain sufficient respiratory function for adequate oxygenation. If the patient cannot maintain adequate oxygenation on his own, then you must consider such alternatives as supplemental oxygen and ventilatory support.

Effective cardiac circulation must also be maintained. This may mean that you use pressure dressings to control blood loss. If the patient is in a more serious condition, it could mean providing circulatory support using intravenous fluid therapy (IVs) or pneumatic antishock garments(PASGs). If circulation ceases,then you must employ cardiopulmonary resuscitation (CPR).

Throughout the rescue operation, you work with preplans that have been prepared in advance for each rescue phase. Using this process ensures that the rescue can be started, conducted, and completed in the most efficient, safe, and successful manner.

BASIC
RESCUE AND
EMERGENCY
CARE

S·E·C·T·I·O·N

I

PREPARING FOR THE RESCUE EFFORT

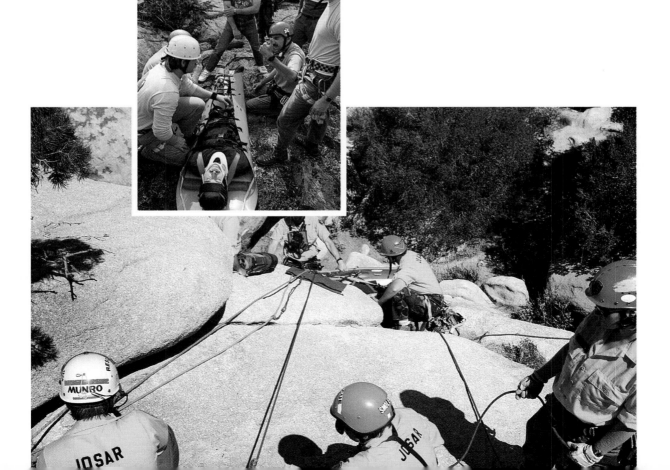

THE INCIDENT COMMAND SYSTEM: ORGANIZING AND MANAGING THE RESCUE EFFORT

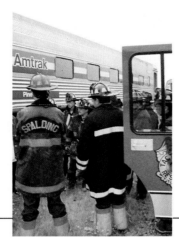

OVERVIEW

The primary key to a successful emergency rescue operation is a well-planned and carefully implemented incident management system. Rescue incidents require flexible and adaptable management structure to prevent deterioration of the situation.

This chapter describes the incident command system (ICS) commonly used to organize and manage emergencies. Included are discussions of preplanning, determining urgency, resource callout, and a resource tracking system. This chapter also outlines the organization of the ICS by functional areas with details of the incident command functions. It explains the incident action plan, and discusses incident communications.

In addition to describing the optimal incident command system, this chapter presents instructions for handling exceptional situations, such as a multi-jurisdictional/multi-agency incident, an expanding rescue incident, special rescue situations, an extended rescue operation, disasters, and a response system that lacks coordination and leadership. Finally, there are recommendations for coping with specific problems that may arise.

OBJECTIVES

The objectives of this chapter are to provide the rescuer with an understanding of the ICS. This will include defining and understanding:

- span of control
- the need for a rescue preplan
- the use of a callout sheet and a resource tracking system
- the requirement for an effective communications system
- how to minimize potential conflicts in multi-jurisdictional/multi-agency responses
- management techniques to deal with an expanding and/or extended rescue incident or a disaster.

Emergencies are stressful situations. However, there are some basic steps that enable rescuers and emergency managers to make correct decisions under stress and to reduce the possibility of events going wrong during a rescue.

The keys to a successful emergency operation are **resources, communications,** and **management** (Figure 1.1). To be successful, there must be the right resources in the right place at the right time. There must be good communications (radio, phone, face-to-face briefings) among those resources. There must be sufficient trained leadership to plan and manage the operation.

Rescue incidents often deteriorate because the management structure is unable to cope with the incident, is too rigid, or is unable to adapt to changing conditions. This chapter describes the incident command system (ICS), an incident management system commonly used in the United States to organize and manage a variety of emergency situations.

One of the most frequent errors of the person in charge in emergencies is attempting to supervise too many resources. The person in charge must maintain a manageable **span of control,** the optimum number of resources that can be effectively supervised by one person. The span of control for rescue operations is normally one person in charge for each three to seven subordinates or resources, with the optimum ratio being one to five. The type, nature, and location of the incident; resources; and safety factors determine the appropriate span of control for any incident.

PREPLANNING

In most emergencies, supervisors try to make critical decisions based on limited information gathered very quickly at the time of the incident. But the more information that can be gathered and analyzed before an incident, the quicker the rescuers can move from just reacting to the incident to managing the incident. The person in charge must make rapid decisions based on information collected and ana-

---

FIGURE 1.1

Keys to a Successful Emergency Operation
The keys to a successful emergency operation are resources, communication, and management.

RESOURCES ——————— Personnel/Equipment

COMMUNICATIONS——————— Radios/Telephone/Person-to-person

MANAGEMENT ——————— Trained leadership

lyzed by the staff. The more information included in the preplan, the better those decisions will be.

Based on predictable problems or situations, managers should make as many decisions as possible before a rescue incident occurs. In this way they can later concentrate on the unpredictable problems of the incident. Among the more critical decisions managers should preplan are incident command responsibilities, organization, management, and personnel requirements and qualifications.

Preplanning develops and maintains a plan for response to and management of a rescue. First of all, the preplan establishes who will be in charge and outlines the organization of the rescue. It also should include policies and procedures for responding to a rescue, including an analysis of the kinds of incidents in the local area that may require rescue operations.

The responsibility for managing a rescue is often set forth by law or regulation. In many jurisdictions, for example, the county sheriff is responsible for search and rescue management. In other areas, it may be the state police, the fire chief, or the park ranger. Sometimes the responsibility for rescue is determined by the kind of incident.

Like land areas, waterways may be under private, municipal, county, state, or federal control, each with a different management philosophy. For example, float planes are prohibited on most urban lakes, while mechanized equipment may be prohibited in wilderness or sensitive ecological areas. Preplans must contain options to resolve jurisdictional conflicts and accessibility problems.

In many areas, the fire chief is responsible for rescue from a burning building, while the rescue squad is responsible for extricating a patient from a wrecked motor vehicle. To avoid confusion or disagreement at the scene of a rescue, the preplan must specify who will be in charge of each type of rescue. Under the ICS, the individual in charge of the rescue operation is called the **incident commander**.

The preplan should also identify **resources,** both personnel and equipment. It should list resources by name, type, capability, and location with telephone numbers, radio or pager numbers, or other methods for contacting the resources. Because phone numbers, addresses, and personnel names will change, this listing should be contained in a separate resource **locator file** that can be easily updated without having to change the entire preplan. The resource list should be updated on a regular basis, at least yearly.

The preplan must include a **step-up plan** for expanding the rescue response if the size or complexity of the rescue grows. The step-up plan defines the responsibilities for determining the need for and requesting additional resources.

If the rescue becomes an extended operation, the preplan should guide the incident commander through the first shift or operational period (usually 8-12 hours) and help determine the resources needed for the second operational period.

Preplanning should also include:

1. An evaluation of the rescuers' area of responsibility, including terrain, hazards, attractions, potential incident base locations, staging areas, and helispots. These should be mapped with access routes noted.
2. A review and analysis of all previous rescues including types, locations, case histories, and preventive measures that can be taken to eliminate or reduce potential hazards to the rescue operation.
3. Identification of resources needed to respond to potential incidents. If needed resources are not currently available within the required response time, then additional personnel should be trained to meet the potential need.

In addition, part of preplanning for large operations should be to contact local chapters of community service agencies such as the Salvation Army to determine their capabilities and the conditions under which they will respond. These volunteer community agencies provide a wide range of services such as food, drink, and shelter. They can also care for residents displaced from the affected area. In addition, these service agencies can help evacuees establish contact with concerned relatives and friends.

Development of the preplan should be a joint effort of all organizations that may be involved in a rescue. These organizations should participate in joint training, exercises, and periodic review and evaluation of the preplan.

DETERMINING URGENCY

Every incident requires some form of immediate response, even if it is initially only an investigation and containment of the area. The first two to four hours are the most critical to the success of a rescue. A good preplan and early positive decisions often mean the difference between success or failure. It is usually not the number of resources initially called out that is important. Rather it is the callout of the right resources at the right time with the right assignments.

When the incident commander receives the first notice of a potential rescue, he determines the urgency and type of response that will be needed. The incident commander gathers critical information on the location of the incident, the subject's physical and mental condition, potential hazards, scene accessibility, and current and predicted weather conditions.

Often, the urgency of many rescues may not be immediately apparent. Because of the potential for severe injuries, a motor vehicle accident with unknown injuries might require a rapid response. But an uninjured person stranded on a ledge in good weather may be perfectly safe for the moment and only require assistance to get off the ledge. On the other hand, if the weather deteriorates, the person on the ledge becomes at risk and requires a prompt and active rescue. Thus, a careful, ongoing evaluation of the situation is necessary to ensure a response appropriate to the needs of the patient and the safety of the rescuers.

After establishing the urgency and determining the time available to accomplish the rescue, the incident commander must develop a plan for the rescue. The incident commander determines the **strategy,** a general outline of how the rescue will be conducted. An example of a strategy might be: "Evacuate the patient down the north side of the ridge to the road and meet an ambulance to transport him to the hospital." Another example might be to evacuate all the elderly above the fire floor in a high rise building to a safe zone below the fire.

Based upon the overall strategy, the incident commander or a subordinate develops **tactics,** the specific actions the rescuers will use to complete the rescue. Specific tactics developed for the above strategy might be: "Dispatch three teams. Team A will rappel to the ledge with a litter, stabilize the patient, package him in a litter, then do a high angle lowering to the base of the cliff. Team B will then do a steep slope lowering from the base of the cliff, down the boulder field to the meadow. Team C will carry the patient across the meadow to the road to the waiting ambulance for transport to the hospital."

Together, the strategy and tactics become the **incident action plan.** This plan establishes the priorities for action, guides the rescue efforts, and helps determine the number and kind of resources required. The incident commander must be skilled and experienced to determine the number and types of resources needed to carry out the rescue. Unlimited resources are rarely available. Thus, the incident commander must adjust the incident action plan to accomplish the rescue with available resources.

NOTIFICATION

Notification is the process of contacting needed rescue resources and providing these individuals with the information they need to get to the scene quickly, safely, and prepared for their assignment. This may be as simple as a dispatcher notifying firemen of a call or a complex callout requiring the identification, location, and activation of civilian or military resources not normally used in rescue operations. Before making the actual phone, pager, or radio call, the incident commander must evaluate the situation, determine the urgency for response, develop an initial incident action plan, and decide on the number and capabilities of the resources required for the rescue. Much of this should be outlined in the preplan.

Determining the size of a response requires judgment and the wise use of resources. While it is better to have too many resources than not enough, the incident commander should strive for the most efficient use of the resources in performing the rescue. For example, if the incident is expected to last more than one operational period, the incident commander would not call out the entire resource list but keep reserves for the second operational period. However, it is better to overreact to an incident than to underreact. There have been many cases in which rescuers found themselves overwhelmed because too few resources were called. This is particularly true when the exact nature and location of the incident are unknown, when there are multiple subjects, when the rescue is difficult or dangerous, or when it is complicated by weather conditions or unfavorable geographic features. It is always easier to cancel responding rescuers than to call them after the rescue effort gets in trouble.

When the required resources are identified, a **callout information sheet** is prepared. This sheet provides the dispatcher with the information necessary to brief the resources properly when they are requested to respond. The callout information sheet should include:

- Type of incident
- Location of the incident
- Anticipated assignment
- Special equipment, clothing, protection required
- Reporting location
- Reporting time
- Estimated length of time rescuers will be involved in the rescue
- Method of notifying rescuers if the reponse is cancelled while they are enroute

For extended enroute travel times, rescuers should be assigned a specific radio frequency to monitor or be given specific times to check in by telephone with the dispatcher. The dispatcher can then provide updated information if the rescuers' services are no longer required. The demobilization planning should begin during the initial callout so that once the incident is concluded, units can be returned to their home base as quickly and economically as possible.

A RESOURCE TRACKING SYSTEM

Once the resources are enroute to the rescue scene, the incident commander should maintain a method for **resource tracking** to monitor which resources are assigned to specific tasks, along with their leader's name, and their location. There are sophisticated and expensive systems for resource tracking, but a simple and inexpensive method is a **T-card locator file,** a plastic notebook with slots for the T-cards (Figure 1.2). The incident commander organizes resources in the file by function, assignment, capability, or location. Assignment changes are recorded by moving the T-card to the appropriate location on the locator file. Computer programs are also available to track resources but are expensive and require access to a computer and a trained person to operate them.

FIGURE 1.2

T-Card Locator for Use in Tracking Resources
The T-card locator file is a wall rack or portable file with slots for T-cards. It helps organize resources by function, assignment, capability, or location.

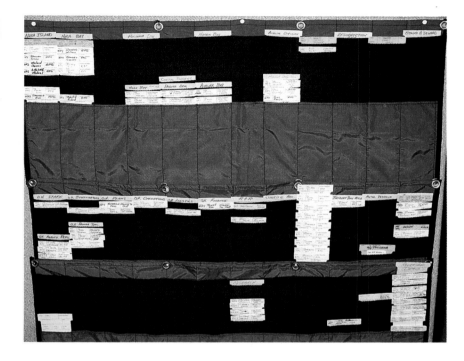

In the early stages of a rescue, the incident commander might keep track of resources with a simple list that includes the resource's name, identification, times of arrival, and assignments. But this information must be transferred to T-cards or another locator system so that he and others can easily track the resources. The resource locator file must be started at the beginning of the incident and kept current throughout the incident.

Using the resource locator system, each resource is assigned one of three current **status conditions.** *Assigned* means that a resource is actively performing a rescue-related task. *Available* means that a resource is available for assignment (that is, a resource in a staging area). *Out-of-service* means a resource is unavailable for assignment.

THE INCIDENT COMMAND SYSTEM

Why We Use the Incident Command System All incidents must be managed in a systematic way so that every rescuer knows what job he or she is to do, who is in charge, and where the resources are. If an organized system is not used, rescue efforts will become chaotic, ineffective, and possibly result in preventable death or injury to patients and rescuers. An emergency management system must be adaptable to different kinds of emergencies, different incident sizes, and different personnel. In addition, an emergency management system must be designed to allow the leader to *command the incident* and to prevent the incident from *commanding the leader*. The incident commander must be *proactive* to the incident and not *reactive* to it.

The **incident command system (ICS)** is a standardized emergency management system developed to organize and manage all the functions required to deal with an emergency situation. The ICS has been adopted by agencies across North America to manage a variety of emergency situations including rescues, lost person searches, fires, law enforcement incidents, and disasters.

Rescue Functions Under ICS

All rescue operations involve similar duties or tasks called *functions*. The ICS is organized by functional areas, each with specifically defined responsibilities (Figure 1.3). The major functional areas are:

1. Incident command
2. Operations
3. Planning
4. Logistics
5. Finance

All of these functions, along with a number of subordinate ones, are performed on almost every rescue incident. During initial response or on a small incident, such as a single vehicle accident or arrival at the scene where a child has wandered from a camp, one person might fulfill several responsibilities or possibly all of the functions.

However, one of the most critical considerations in managing emergencies is assuring that the management structure may meet the demands of the incident and grow when the size or complexity of the incident increases.

There can be increased needs for more or specialized resources. For instance, the lost child situation can become more urgent because of bad weather, or a fire can spread to threaten people and property. When these events happen, some crucial management functions must

FIGURE 1.3

ICS Functions
The Incident Command System (ICS) is organized by functional areas, each with specifically defined responsibilities. All of these major functions are performed on most rescue incidents.

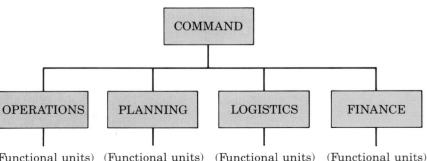

be delegated in order to maintain span-of-control (three to seven persons) and assure coverage. In such instances, the incident commander must appoint qualified individuals to lead the affected functions. When an incident expands or the situation dictates, the jurisdiction's responsible line officer may replace the incident commander with a more experienced or qualified individual.

Incident Command Functions

The following are the major functional areas of the ICS, along with their respective responsibilities. Remember, all of these responsibilities are carried out in almost every incident, whether by one person or by several people.

Incident Command   Incident command provides overall management of the incident. In the ICS, the command function includes the incident commander, the information officer, the liaison officer and the safety officer. In a small incident, all of these roles may be performed by a single person, the incident commander. But to preserve his or her span of control in a large operation, the incident commander may have to delegate the roles of safety officer, liaison officer, and information officer to other qualified staff members.

The incident commander:

- Ensures the incident is managed effectively
- Selects a strategy
- Determines incident objectives
- Approves the incident action plan
- Coordinates and approves requests for resources

The staff positions of **safety officer, liaison officer,** and **information officer** work closely with and under the direction of the incident commander.

The **safety officer:**

- Assesses and monitors actual and potential hazardous conditions or situations during the incident
- Develops measures or procedures to protect the rescuers and patient and makes certain these measures are used
- Monitors physical and mental stresses on rescuers during an extended operation and may recommend crew rotations

In a rescue involving an especially hazardous environment, such as a hazardous material spill, a collapsed structure, or a high angle rescue, the incident commander must appoint a safety officer. For other rescue situations, it is also a good idea to designate a safety officer to ensure that safe rescue tactics are used.

The **liaison officer** is the contact point for individuals or agencies directly or indirectly involved in the incident. In a politically sensitive incident, this person is a conduit for government officials. In larger incidents, the liaison officer coordinates interagency activities and resource utilization for the incident. When several different agencies respond to an incident, coordination becomes a difficult task, so the liaison officer becomes the primary contact among agencies at the scene. Good interagency communications and appropriate utilization of each agency's resources must be ensured. Each responding agency should designate a representative to coordinate with the liaison officer. Each agency representative then communicates through the liaison officer to the incident commander.

The **information officer:**

- Coordinates public information activities
- Provides the news media with timely, appropriate, and accurate information through live interviews or press releases
- Responds to special requests for information

Because the incident commander may not personally have time to deal with the media while managing the many demands of the response, the information officer becomes a key position in many incidents. A well-trained, experienced information officer provides the media, family members, and others with information on the current status of the incident. This leaves the incident commander free to concentrate on the response itself. If the media or other groups wish to talk with the incident commander directly, the information officer can set up a convenient time for a media conference.

Operations/Functions Rescues require skilled technicians to perform the tactical operations. In the ICS these tactical operations are grouped into one function. The operations section's function is to carry out the actual rescue tactics. The operations function may be the first one to be delegated as the situation grows in complexity.

The **operations section chief:**

- Assists the incident commander to develop the tactical portion of the incident action plan
- Directs the tactical portions of the incident action plan
- Supervises all air and ground operations

In a mass casualty incident, or when the patient requires medical care, the medical response function is under the operations section. If the medical response is in support of the rescue personnel, such as in a fire, the medical response function is under the logistics section.

In a small incident, the incident commander generally fulfills the additional role of operations section chief. But to maintain his span of control as the incident grows in size or complexity, the incident commander should delegate this function to a qualified rescuer.

To maintain span of control, the operations section chief may divide the rescuers into functional groups based upon the specific needs of the incident. For example, in a structural fire response, the operation may be divided into two groups: the rescue group to perform search and rescue and the suppression group to perform fire suppression. In a mass casualty incident, the operations section may be divided into five functional groups (Figure 1.4):

- Triage (casualty sorting) group
- Treatment group
- Transportation group
- Scene security group
- Traffic control group

Each of these groups would have a **group supervisor** responsible for managing its activities and coordinating efforts with the other group supervisors. It is generally more effective to assign all resources from one agency to a specific group, so they continue to work under their normal chain of command.

When the incident covers a very large area or when the area is divided by a barrier, the incident may be subdivided in terms of geography. For example, a multiple vehicle accident on a major interstate where the roadway divides the incident may require this type of subdivision. When the incident is broken down by geography in this manner, it is split into divisions. In the case of the freeway incident, the area might be split into a division north of the interstate and a division south of the interstate. Each division would have its own supervisor (Figure 1.5), who would report to a single operations chief (on a large incident) or to a single incident commander (on a smaller incident).

Planning The functions of the planning section are to collect, evaluate, and distribute all incident information. The **planning section chief**:

- Prepares and distributes the incident action plan (if it is written)
- Maintains incident maps
- Tracks and reports current and predicted events in the operation
- Tracks the current status of all incident resources (resource tracking)

FIGURE 1.4

Dividing Rescuers into Functional Unit Groups
In a mass casualty incident, the operations section may be divided into five functional groups.

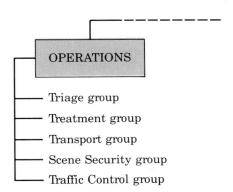

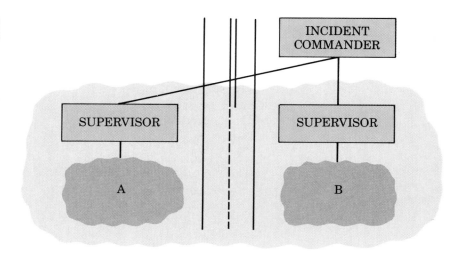

FIGURE 1.5

ICS Post Divisions
When an incident covers a large area or is physically divided by a barrier, the incident may be subdivided in terms of geography. In a multiple vehicle accident on an interstate, for example, the incident could be split into divisions on either side of the roadway.

- Conducts planning meetings
- Develops alternative plans to complete the rescue if the current incident action plan is not meeting objectives
- Documents all incident activities
- Prepares and distributes demobilization plans (in a large operation)

Technical resource personnel, such as hazardous materials specialists, structural engineers, physicians, or other individuals with specialized training, are assigned to the planning section though they may have operational or logistical duties as well. In the planning section, the specialists evaluate incident activities and assist in developing the incident action plan.

In a small incident the duties of the incident commander may also include the planning function. But if the incident involves a large number of resources from several agencies, or if the incident will last more than one operational period, the incident commander should maintain span of control by delegating the planning function to a planning section chief.

Logistics The logistics section provides personnel, supplies, materials, and facilities to support the incident. The **logistics section chief:**

- Requests all personnel and equipment
- Identifies and maintains staging areas
- Receives, records, stores, and distributes all personnel, equipment, and supplies
- Provides facilities for rest, feeding, and maintenance
- Supplies fueling, transportation, and repair service
- Provides and maintains communications for the incident, including equipment and personnel

- Establishes, staffs, and supervises the incident communications center, if one is required
- Provides medical services for incident personnel

In most rescues the logistical requirements are limited to ordering resources and, perhaps, feeding them. Communications at most rescues do not require a separate communications center but are handled by the agency dispatch personnel. Although medical services for incident personnel are often handled by medically qualified logistics personnel, in a mass casualty situation or if the patient requires medical care, medical services are under the direction of the operations section.

Finance   The finance section is responsible for all incident finances. Since most rescues are of short duration and do not involve complex financial issues, this function may be performed by the normal agency financial personnel. Incident personnel keep track of time and costs and submit these records to the appropriate agency for payment. In a larger or more complex incident, the **finance section chief:**

- Maintains personnel hours for payroll
- Investigates and processes claims for damage or injury to incident personnel or resources
- Maintains cost records for leases and rental of equipment

The Incident Action Plan

In any incident, all rescue personnel must know what their assigned duties are, while the incident commander must know what directions to give those he is managing. Each incident requires an **incident action plan,** a general outline or strategy on how to conduct the rescue. This plan establishes priorities for action, guides the rescue efforts, and determines the number and types of resources required. For simple incidents involving only one operational period, the plan may be developed by the incident commander and communicated orally to the rescuers. However, an extended, large, or complex incident lasting several operational periods requires a written incident action plan so that everyone follows the same strategy and tactics. While there may be specific incident actions for each operational period, there must be *only one plan* for an incident, regardless of the number of agencies or jurisdictions involved.

As part of the plan, the incident commander initially establishes **incident objectives.** These are results that must be achieved to successfully complete the rescue. Each objective must clearly communicate what must be done in a simple and straightforward manner. Some examples of an incident objectives might be "search segment C, to achieve a 70% probability of detection by 1800 hours," or "Using available equipment, safely move the debris from the southwest corner of the collapsed building by 1200 hours to gain access to the trapped person."

Using the incident action plan, the incident commander or the operations section chief selects the tactics needed to accomplish the incident objectives. On larger or extended incidents, a written incident action plan includes the incident objectives, an organization chart, tactical assignments, a resource locator file, and a map. It may also contain a medical plan, transportation plan, air operations plan, and any other plans that the incident commander feels are needed.

Communications

Incident communications are managed by a common **communications plan.** If the incident requires it, a communications center can be established solely for the resources working on the incident. Because there are so many different kinds of communications codes—such as "10 codes"—all rescue communications should be in plain English. No codes should be used except in certain tactical operations or to report fatalities if communication channels are not secure. All radio traffic should be restricted to essential messages. If radio traffic on certain channels becomes congested, **radio networks** should be established for various functions such as command, operations, logistics, or air operations.

In a rescue where several agencies work together, all personnel must communicate using commonly understood terms. The ICS uses standard terms to ensure that all personnel involved in an operation completely understand all communications (Table 1.1).

In the incident command system, incident posts have standard names. The **incident command post** is the location where the incident is managed. Depending on the incident, it may be the hood of a vehicle, or it may be an elaborate, mobile command center. The **incident base** is the location from which all logistical support is provided. **Staging areas** are locations where people and equipment are temporarily held until assigned. For instance, in a mass casualty incident an ambulance staging area holds available ambulances ready to move quickly to load patients in areas that need them. Thus, they are not wasted on areas that do not need them and they do not block traffic flow.

Multi-Jurisdictional/ Multi-Agency Incident Management

One of the most common problems in emergency response occurs when more than one jurisdiction or agency is involved in an incident. In multi-jurisdictional/multi-agency responses, there may be conflicts over who is in charge, differences over strategy and tactics, and inefficient allocation of personnel and equipment. Under the incident command system these conflicts are resolved in the same way the World War II allies won the battle for Europe: the unified command. In a unified command, each agency having jurisdiction over the incident appoints its representative for the incident. These representatives meet at the incident command post and jointly determine incident objectives and strategies for resolving the incident and approve a tactical plan. Together they select an operations section chief, usually an experienced person from one of their agencies, to carry out the tactical plan.

TABLE 1.1   List of ICS Terms

Branch	The organizational level having functional/geographic responsibility for major segments of incident operations. The Branch level is organizationally between section and division/group.
Camp	A geographical site, within the general incident area, separate from the base, equipped and staffed to provide food, water, rest, and sanitary services to incident personnel.
Clear text	The use of plain English in radio communication transmissions. No ten-codes or agency specific code are used when using clear text.
Command	The act of directing, ordering, and/or controlling resources by virtue of explicit legal, agency, or delegated authority.
Command staff	The command staff consists of all personnel within command function who report directly to the incident commander, such as the safety officer, the liaison officer and the information officer.
Committed resource	A resource checked-in and assigned work tasks on an incident.
Communications unit	A vehicle, trailer, or self-propelled unit used to provide the major part of an incident communication center.
Coordination	The process of systematically analyzing a situation, developing relevant information, and informing appropriated command authority (for its decision) of viable alternatives for selection of the most effective combination of available resources to meet specific objectives. The coordination process (which can be either intra-agency or inter-agency) does not in and of itself involve command dispatch actions. However, personnel responsible for coordination may perform command or dispatch functions within limits as established by specific agency delegations, procedures, legal authority, and so forth.
Dispatch	The implementation of a command decision to move a resource or resources from one place to another.
Dispatch center	A facility from which resources are directly assigned to an incident.
Division	That organization level having responsibility for total operations within a defined geographical area.
Element	Any identified part of the incident command system organization structure.
Equipment transport	Any ground vehicle capable of transporting a bulldozer or other heavy equipment.
Food services	Any resource capable of dispensing food to incident personnel.

General staff	The top incident management personnel consisting of:
	
	     incident commander (IC)
	     logistics chief (LC)
	     operations chief (OC)
	     finance chief (FC)
	     planning chief (PC)

Group	A division with functional responsibilities only for certain field operations such as air support, rescue, law enforcement, and so forth. Often not constrained by geographical areas on an incident (see also division).
Helibase	A location within the general incident area for parking, fueling, maintaining, and loading of helicopters.

Continued

TABLE 1.1 *Continued*

Helitack crew	A crew of two or more individuals who may be assigned to incident operations or to support helicopter operations.
Helispot	A location where a helicopter can safely take off and land.
Incident	Any situation man-made or natural, regardless of size or complexity, that requires action to protect life and property.
Incident action plan	The action plan, which is initially prepared at the first planning meeting, which contains general objectives reflecting overall incident strategy, and specific rescue, fire suppression, or law enforcement actions for the next operational period. When complete the incident action plan will have a number of attachments.
Incident commander	The individual responsible for the management of all IC activities at a specific incident.
Incident command post	The location from which the command functions are executed, usually co-located with the incident base.
Jurisdictional	The agency having jurisdiction and agency responsibility for a specific geographical area.
Operational period	The period of time scheduled for execution of a given set of actions as specified in the incident action plan.
Out of service	Resources assigned to an incident, but unable to respond for mechanical, rest, personnel, or other reasons.
Overhead personnel	Personnel who are assigned to supervisory positions. Includes incident commander, command staff, general staff and unit leaders.
Personnel pool	Unassigned personnel who may have reported to the incident without an assignment. They do not belong to a company, a strike team, or a task force.
Planning meeting	A meeting, held periodically during an incident, to select specific strategies and tactics for incident control operations and for service and support planning.
Rescue	Systematic removal of person(s) from a hazardous situation.
Resources	All personnel and major items or equipment available, or potentially available, for assignment to incident tasks and on which status is kept.
Section	The organization level having responsibility for an entire incident specialty function, such as operation, planning, logistics, and finance.
Staging area	A location near an incident where available incident resources are grouped together waiting for specific assignments.
Task force	Specified combinations of resources consisting of like units with a leader, personnel, and a common communications.
Strike team	A group of unlike resources with a leader, personnel, and common communications assembled for a specific mission.
Technical specialist	Personnel with special skills who are activated only when needed. Technical specialists may be needed in the areas of fire behavior, water resources, environmental concern, resource use, or training.
Unit	The organization element having functional responsibility for a specific incident or activity with the larger functions or planning, logistics or finance.

Under the unified command, the remainder of the ICS management system remains the same. There are staging areas for the unified operations section (not separate ones for each agency), a unified communications unit, (not separate ones for each agency), one unified logistics section (not separate ones for each agency), and so on. In this way, the incident is managed most effectively with the most efficient use of resources and with the minimal amount of conflict. Preplanning multi-jurisdictional/multi-agency incident management situations can significantly speed the operational response to an incident.

Managing an Expanding Rescue Incident

One common problem for an incident commander or his subordinates is losing control of the situation when the incident suddenly expands, such as when a large number of rescuers show up at the site or when the nature of the incident becomes more complex. The incident commander cannot control the incident with his original organization structure because the number of people involved will greatly exceed his span of control. The incident begins to command the incident commander.

To maintain span of control, the ICS provides for a controlled **step-up** or expansion of the organization by adding or subtracting modules to the command structure to keep the core management structure intact whatever the size of the incident. On an organization chart, these modules appear like a child's blocks that can be snapped together or pulled apart as needed (Figure 1.6).

Note that in the final form of the rescue organization, the incident commander may be managing an incident that involves 50 or 500 people. But there is still a manageable span of control, for he is *directly managing only three to seven people* (those people in charge of information, safety, liaison, operations, planning, logistics, and finance). In turn, all of these people are operating within their own span of control. None of them is supervising more than seven people.

The incident command system is the standard emergency incident management system. It is a flexible management tool for handling emergencies. Because of its modular nature, it can be adapted to the size and complexity of a particular incident. However, to maintain regional and national understanding by all personnel and agencies, the common terminology and principles of ICS must be adhered to by personnel utilizing the system.

Special Rescue Situations

Different rescue environments may present particular problems in organizing and managing a rescue operation. However, there are some common recurring problems in rescue situations.

Patient Evacuation The stabilization and evacuation of the patient should be planned and established before the patient is located. These plans should include having medical and rescue resources

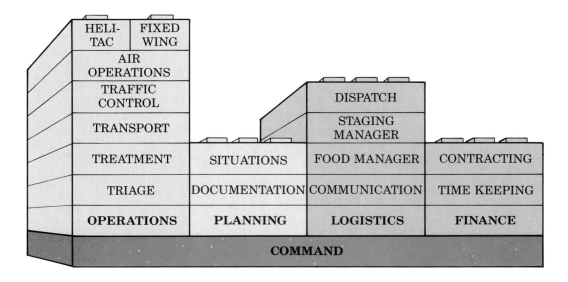

FIGURE 1.6   ICS Step-Up Plan
To maintain span of control, the ICS provides for a controlled step-up of the
organization but keeps the core management structure intact whatever the
size of the incident.

ready, notifying receiving hospitals, and preparing for all possible
medical contingencies for the patient and rescuers during the rescue.
There should be plans for the possibility of a rope rescue, bad weather,
or a rescue starting at the end of shift when everyone is fatigued.

Using Specialists Untrained in Rescue   Rescues often require
specialists such as physicians, paramedics, hazardous materials specialists, or structural engineers. These resources may not be trained
to handle the particular rescue environment of the incident. Nevertheless, rescue leaders can still safely and effectively use these
resources.

In some cases, the specialists may be used as advisors at the command post or base hospital where they communicate with the field
teams by radio. In this way, the specialists are not exposed to the
hazards of the rescue environment. However in these cases, their
decisions are based on information received secondhand, and some
incidents require them to be on scene.

Another method assigns trained rescue personnel to escort the
specialists in the rescue environment. The escort must closely supervise and assist the specialists to handle the rescue environment
safely by properly equipping and instructing them about the hazards
they may encounter. However, this method removes trained rescue
personnel from activities directly involved in rescuing the patient.

The advantages and disadvantages of both methods must be carefully weighed before a decision is made on using untrained specialists in the rescue environment.

Special Considerations for an Extended Rescue Operation

Most rescues are completed within a few hours or, at most, within one day. However, a small percentage of rescues last more than a day. These extended efforts challenge the rescuers' ability to organize and manage the incident. Rescuers cannot work effectively for long periods without food, water, and rest. The incident commander must ensure that there is advance planning for logistical support and for replacements of exhausted personnel. Logistical support includes food, shelter, sanitary facilities, transportation, and special equipment. It takes time to order these resources and transport them to the scene. Additional personnel are needed to provide these logistical requirements. Thus, the extended incident will require a larger and more experienced management team than would be needed for a smaller or shorter duration incident. In the initial stages of an incident, the incident commander must anticipate and plan for the additional requirements of an incident that is expected to last more than one operational period.

Obstacles to Overall Coordination and Leadership

Areas of emergency response that continue to cause problems in organizing and managing on-scene activities include:

- Lack of well-defined authority
- Lack of adequate communications (especially between different agencies)
- Lack of a staging area to assemble and control the flow of equipment and personnel
- Inappropriate use of specialized resources
- Poor media relationships
- Inability to identify and track responders at the scene
- Responders not completing their assigned tasks

For effective rescue operations, the incident commander must set up an on-scene organization to provide the coordination and leadership to manage these problems.

The incident commander should address each of the following elements on every search and rescue incident:

- Someone must be in charge of the overall scene and of each task.
- Leadership must be easily identifiable to the responders.
- An incident command post must be established in a safe, accessible, and visible location.
- A staging area must be established in an accessible and controlled location that does not impede incident traffic flow.
- Functions must be delegated to maintain the manageable span of control.
- Organizational staffing must be stepped-up early to stay ahead of incident requirements.

- The information flow on the incident must be coordinated and adequately disseminated to the media.
- Responders must know what they are expected to do and where and to whom to report.
- Responders must be provided with adequate communications.
- Decisions must be made carefully, based upon the best information currently available, and then reevaluated as more information is developed or as the situation changes.
- The incident action plan must be updated and revised as necessary.
- To delay a decision is to decide to continue the status quo. Critical decisions must not be delayed in the hope that more information will make the decisions easier or that the problems will solve themselves.

Decisive leadership, a well-organized response, and proper delegation of responsibility all improve the incident commander's ability to manage effectively when things go wrong. When problems arise, the incident commander must not lose sight of the incident objectives. The incident commander must only deal with the problems that directly affect the overall success of the incident. The incident commander must not get bogged down in unimportant details but should delegate them. Problems should be solved and actions taken at the lowest appropriate organizational level. If a unit or team leader can solve the problem, the incident commander should delegate it to that person.

The incident commander must evaluate problems when they occur and determine the best response based upon the specific situation. Preplanning for commonly encountered problems and possible solutions eases the stresses on the incident command staff.

Loss of Communications

Modern emergency response has developed a critical dependency on electronic communications. When these communications are lost, the rescue effort may be crippled, so preplanning should identify backup communication methods. If the rescue site covers a small area, runners might be used to relay information in case of communications failure. This requires a large commitment of personnel and is very slow, but it is a reliable method of communication. When using runners, all information must be written so that it is accurately relayed.

If radio communications are limited by "blind spots" caused by terrain features, radio relays can be established on high points of the terrain. These relays communicate messages between the incident and the communication center.

Communications are commonly disrupted in emergencies, particularly in disasters. The telephone lines may be destroyed by the disaster itself or the telephone links overloaded by civilian use. Even some base station radios will be lost because they are linked to transmitter towers by land lines.

Provisions for replacing these communications must be made in the emergency preplan. Possible substitutes for loss of land lines include the use of amateur radio operators (hams) or cellular phones with satellite linkage.

Breakdown in the Information Flow

The breakdown of the information flow inside a rescue organization will hinder the operation and endanger both patients and rescuers.
    The critical areas where information flow may break down are:

- Not reporting changes in the situation from field teams to incident headquarters
- Inaccurate reporting of conditions from field teams to incident headquarters
- Not reporting changing objectives or tactics from incident command to field teams
- Untimely and inaccurate recording of events in the log
- Inaccurate briefing of significant events by shift personnel to their replacements
- Breakdown in the flow of information inside the rescue organization, such as between planning and operations sections
- Interference in the chain of communication such as radio personnel who fail to pass along portions of messages or who add their own interpretation to messages
- Untimely and accurate reporting of information by the incident command staff to elected officials and the media

Communications between headquarters and the field teams can be improved by operational period briefings, briefing upon assignment, debriefing when every assignment is completed, and regular check-in reports from field teams. Communications inside the organization are improved by briefings at the beginning and end of each operational period. The incident commander must insist that all responders know and adhere to reporting requirements and procedures. Furthermore, the incident commander must ensure that all personnel document all messages.

If the incident commander suspects he is receiving inaccurate or inadequate information, field observers should be appointed to gather firsthand information and report back directly. The incident commander should ensure that all personnel write out all critical information and then route it to the appropriate people.

The liaison officer must keep elected officials and all affected jurisdictions in the information loop.

Disruption in Logistical Support

If critical resources are not available when needed, the best organized rescue operation will quickly deteriorate. For example, if shelter or food for exhausted rescuers is not available, rescuers' morale and efficiency decrease dramatically. When there is a disruption in logistical support, the incident commander must quickly identify the source of the problem. Adequate lead time is important for good logistical support of any operation. The incident commander must stress this to the staff.

The major reasons for logistical support disruption are:

- Required resources are not currently available or cannot be acquired
- The logistics section chief or staff cannot do the job effectively or are overwhelmed by the magnitude of the logistics requirements

If the problem is a lack of available resources, the incident commander must develop and carry out an alternate plan that does not require those particular resources. For example, if the expected evacuation helicopter does not arrive, alternate evacuation methods must be provided immediately. Incident commanders must possess the ability to improvise with available resources.

If inadequate staffing causes unsatisfactory performance by logistics personnel, the incident commander should add trained people to supplement the logistics staff. Sometimes, too, key personnel in the logistics section must be replaced to solve the problem.

Inadequate Leadership

If leadership deteriorates during an incident, the responsible individual must be replaced or assigned an assistant capable of providing the necessary leadership. If the incident commander is not effectively managing the incident, the agency head or other unified commanders must deal with the problem of leadership. If leadership failure occurs at or below the section chief level, the responsible supervisor for the failing individual must handle the problem. A rescuer working for an individual lacking adequate leadership should tactfully provide assistance. If the lack of leadership interferes with group performance, the rescuer should inform a higher level supervisor.

Preplanning must identify specific leadership needs for the organization and determine how appropriate leadership will be provided. Rescuers should have or obtain training and experience to assume command and provide effective leadership.

Loss of Span of Control

For rescue operations, the acceptable span of control is one supervisor for every three to seven subordinates. The optimum span of control is one supervisor for every five subordinates. There is only one way to deal with a loss of the span of control—delegate to trained individuals. Supervisors must constantly evaluate the efficiency and productivity of their units. When the number of subordinates assigned to a supervisor exceeds the supervisor's ability to manage the assigned task, the supervisor should appoint subordinate supervisors and provide them the necessary authority to accomplish the task.

Equipment Failure

Equipment failure can be minimized by:

- Using the right tool for the right purpose
- Maintaining and properly caring for the equipment
- Promptly repairing and returning to service
- Having backup equipment available to replace the broken equipment
- Improvising with available equipment or materials
- Discarding damaged or unrepairable equipment

The logistics section is responsible for obtaining, storing, issuing, and maintaining equipment. The logistics section chief should appoint someone to make certain equipment is ready for rescue activities. That person must ensure that adequate supplies are always available; that they are in good working order; and that backups, especially for specialized equipment, are available.

One problem that rescuers encounter is a dependence on specialized equipment that fails at a critical time. Rescue teams should undergo regular training using improvised equipment for common rescue tasks. In addition, rescue managers should always have backup plans ready. They must always remember that *what can go wrong, probably will,* and generally at the most inopportune time (Murphy's Law). They must be ready for that to happen.

When Initial Strategy and Tactics Do Not Achieve the Objective

One critical challenge for rescue managers is knowing *when* their chosen strategy and tactics are not working. This problem may occur because of the very human tendency to cling to apparently well-developed strategies. This problem often arises because the command center is physically away from the incident. For this reason, it is critical that information flow be kept flowing both ways. Briefings and debriefings must include honest appraisals by key personnel on success or failure of strategy and tactics.

The incident commander must continually reevaluate the progress of the rescue in terms of successfully meeting the incident objectives. The incident commander should also always have an alternate plan for completing the rescue. The incident action plan can then be adjusted or modified to meet changing needs.

Change in the Nature of the Incident

At times, the initial plan may fail because the nature or scope of the incident changes dramatically. One example would be when the weather suddenly changes to endanger patient and rescuers and ground all air support. Or while extricating the patients from one vehicle, another vehicle accident occurs at the scene. In such a situation, the operations chief should change the execution of the plan to fit the new developments and inform the planning section of his or her actions.

Jurisdictional Conflicts

Jurisdictional conflicts are common in emergency situations. The ICS helps reduce these conflicts by providing a unified command system in which each agency actively participates in incident management. Preplanning should establish the areas of responsibilities for each agency and the procedures to be followed at the incident scene. Despite this, however, jurisdictional conflicts may still occur. The incident commander must know the jurisdictions involved and responsibility of each responding agency. Knowing the rescuers in the neighboring jurisdictions and training with them on a regular basis before the incident occurs helps reduce and resolve jurisdictional conflicts.

When jurisdictional conflicts arise, responders must immediately locate the person in charge and attempt to develop procedures that meet the needs of the patient and all jurisdictions. If a unified command cannot be set up, the overall objective of the incident is always to provide care for the patients. Jurisdictional conflicts must not get in the way of providing adequate patient care. Rescuers must be willing to compromise to accomplish the rescue. As soon as the rescue is completed, the key people from the involved agencies should meet to resolve the problem to prevent a recurrence.

Disasters and Mass Casualties

An incident need not involve widespread destruction or hundreds of casualties to be a disaster. A disaster is any event exceeding the capacity of local resources to respond effectively in an appropriate time frame. In some areas, a complex vehicle accident can be a disaster.

Radiation leaks, chemical releases, and major transportation system accidents are man-caused disasters, while floods, hurricanes, tornados, volcanic eruptions, and earthquakes constitute natural disasters. Each disaster may cause different, specific problems, but the overall effect on rescue personnel is similar. Manpower and equipment resources are inadequate, transportation systems are congested, medical facilities are overwhelmed, and communication systems are overloaded or damaged by the disaster itself. Finally, rescuers, patients, and survivors in the field often have to fend for themselves for extended periods of time.

One common problem during disasters is the uneven distribution of patients to medical facilities. This often occurs because a few hospitals, close to the incident, receive the majority of patients, while other hospitals farther away do not receive as many patients as they can treat. A primary goal for triage and transportation personnel in disasters is to avoid transferring the disaster from the incident to the hospital. Before beginning to transport multiple casualties from a disaster, consult with the disaster medical coordinator or with the hospitals in the area. Remember that in many local disasters the medical facilities closest to the incident will be overloaded with "walking wounded" and other patients who have arranged their own transport outside the EMS system.

It is important that medical facilities at a disaster be organized to deal with the emergency. Figure 9.1 illustrates a typical incident command organizational chart for a medical branch at a disaster or multi-casualty incident.

Personality Conflicts

Personality conflicts commonly occur in stressful situations and often keep rescuers from maximal performance of their jobs. Personality conflicts must be handled early. If two individuals have a conflict and cannot work out their own problems, tact and diplomacy are required to resolve such situations. The supervisor must quickly mediate. The supervisor must be candid with the individuals, especially when discussing the effect of their conflict on the rescue and the patient. The supervisor should stress the need to work as a team to rescue the patient and that no one individual is more important than the team. If mediation is unsuccessful, the individuals should be separated and assigned tasks in which they will not come into contact. If a personality conflict cannot be resolved and interferes with the rescue, the individuals should be removed from the rescue scene.

Lost, Injured, or Deceased Rescuer

Safety of the rescuers is a higher priority than the safety of the patient. An injured rescuer cannot assist in the rescue. They also add another incident that diverts resources from the original objectives. Therefore, safety must always be a primary concern of the incident commander.

If a rescuer is lost, injured, or killed during a rescue effort, the incident commander must review the incident objectives, reevaluate priorities and tactics, and develop alternate plans to meet the changing needs. The incident commander must react quickly, decisively, and appropriately. The incident commander must first ensure that no other rescuers will be injured. While the injured rescuer is treated, the cause of the injury must be identified and specific steps taken to eliminate the unsafe situation. If the rescuer is lost, it may be necessary to establish a separate group to focus on that search. Rather than diverting a large number of rescuers from the original incident, new rescuers should be requested and assigned to deal with the second incident. If the rescuer is deceased, the scene must be protected. An investigation will be necessary to determine the cause of the injury or death. Whenever there is injury or death to a rescuer, trained individuals should monitor the stress levels of the remaining rescuers and their abilities to function. These stress levels must be taken into account when making assignments.

Injury to Patient Caused by Rescuers

An additional injury to the patient caused by the rescuers is managed in the same way as an injured rescuer. The rescuer must first take action to prevent another occurrence and then treat the patient for the injuries. An investigator first determines the cause of the accident that caused additional injury. The investigator then documents the accident scene, the actions of the rescuers involved, and the equipment in use at the time of the accident and obtains statements from the rescuers and the patient.

When Resources Are Overwhelmed

When rescuers reach the rescue site and face the reality of performing emergency care and rescue, it is easy for them to be overwhelmed by the size or complexity of the tasks that must be performed. After evaluating the overall situation, the incident commander must establish objectives and priorities for resolving the incident. If more rescuers or specialized resources are required to manage the incident, they should be ordered immediately. Initial on-scene rescuers should be assigned the highest priority tasks, such as scene control, triage, and priority care of the patients. The incident commander should initiate plans to expand the management organization to accommodate the resources required to accomplish the rescue. As was mentioned in earlier sections, rescuers arriving on-scene later must be tracked, assigned, and supervised to effectively perform their assignments.

SUMMARY

A well-organized management plan is essential to carry out a successful rescue operation. The incident command system (ICS) is such a plan that is used throughout North America to manage a variety of emergency situations.

The first step in developing the incident command system is a preplan, which enables rescue managers to make as many decisions as possible before an actual rescue operation. A preplan should be a joint effort of all the organizations that may be involved in a rescue.

The incident command system uses an incident action plan, a general strategy on how to conduct the rescue. As part of the plan, the incident commander develops incident objectives, results that must be achieved to complete the rescue successfully. Using the incident action plan, the incident commander selects the tactics necessary to accomplish the incident objectives. For larger or extended incidents, the incident commander may also develop medical, transportation, or air operations plans.

The ICS involves several functions, such as the incident command (which includes safety, liaison with other agencies, and public information), operations, planning, logistics, and finance. Incident command is responsible for the overall management of the rescue operation. The operations function is to carry out the actual rescue tactics. The planning function collects, evaluates, and distributes all incident information. The logistics function provides personnel, supplies, materials, and facilities to support the incident operation. And the finance function tracks all incident finances.

During a rescue operation, communications are extremely important and are managed by a communications plan. In a rescue involving several agencies working together, all personnel must communicate using commonly understood terms.

The ICS's incident facilities also have standard names. The incident command post is the location from which the incident is managed. The incident base is the area from which all logistical support is provided. Staging areas are sites where people and equipment are temporarily held until assigned.

The ICS minimizes jurisdictional conflicts by using the unified command concept. Each agency having jurisdiction identifies a representative to meet with the other representatives to prepare a joint operational plan. Preplanning the management of these situations is vital to avoid conflicts and problems.

To prevent loss of control when an incident expands, the incident commander must maintain the span of control by providing a controlled step-up of the organization, adding modules to the command structure to keep the core management structure intact whatever the size of the incident.

An extended rescue operation presents special considerations. There must be advance planning to ensure logistical support and to replace exhausted rescuers.

As a rescue gets underway, the incident commander must be certain that there is an on-scene organization to provide coordination and leadership to prevent or manage any problems. A well-organized response, strong leadership, and proper delegation of authority also help the incident commander manage effectively when things go wrong.

CLOTHING AND PROTECTION FOR THE RESCUER

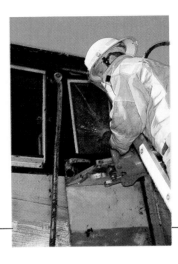

OVERVIEW

Protecting rescue personnel during a rescue situation is one of the primary goals of a successful operation. Thus, selecting appropriate protective clothing and gear for rescue personnel is vital to the successful outcome of the operation.

This chapter describes clothing options with recommendations for items to choose for each type of environment. The chapter also discusses personal gear that protects the rescuer from environmental elements.

OBJECTIVES

The objectives of this chapter are to enable rescuers to:

- choose appropriate protective clothing and gear for a rescue operation.
- determine the proper shelter and lighting for extended or remote operations.

- select methods of protecting themselves from personal hazards they encounter during a rescue operation.

Regardless of the environment, your first line of self-protection is clothing and gear appropriate to both the task and the environment. It is important that you become familiar with available clothing and gear and understand the specific features of each one. This knowledge will enable rescue workers to select the proper clothing and gear for the situation and adapt or change them as the situation and environment change.

Any personal protective equipment is only safe when it is in good condition. This is your responsibility when using the equipment at the emergency site. If you are unsure of the conditions of your protective equipment, consider it unsafe and unusable until you inspect it properly.

CLOTHING

For the greatest flexibility in protection from the cold, a layering system of clothing is much better than a single thick cover. By opening up layers of clothing or adding or removing layers, the wearer can control his or her body temperature. A cold weather system of layered clothing would consist of at least three layers. A thin, inner layer next to the skin, sometimes called the **transport layer** wicks moisture away from the skin to keep the wearer dry and warm. Materials such as underwear made from polypropylene or polyester work well for the transport layer except where flame is a possibility. Next comes a thermal layer of bulkier material that acts as insulation. Wool has been the traditional material for the thermal layer, but it is being replaced by other materials such as polyester pile. The outer layer is a shell of wind- and waterproof material to resist chilling winds and precipitation. The two outer layers should have front zippers to aid in venting body heat to prevent overheating. Some designs also have pit zips, zippers in the garment's armpits to dissipate additional heat.

Clothing Construction

The type of material used in clothing is very important in determining how well the clothing protects the wearer from the weather. Cotton is one material that should be avoided when chilling from wetness is a possibility. When it becomes saturated, cotton wicks heat away from the body, rather than insulating it. Cotton also tends to absorb moisture thoroughly. If a person wears cotton jeans, for example, and walks through wet grass, the cotton will wick the moisture from the cuffs up to the upper legs, chilling the wearer. Because it wicks moisture and heat away from the body, cotton is a good material for warm environments.

Down-filled clothing can be very warm as long as down retains its loft, which provides its insulative qualities. But if down gets wet, it loses its loft and its ability to keep the wearer warm.

For an outer layer, a plastic-coated nylon can provide waterproof protection. But it also may prevent the venting of body heat and perspiration that can make the wearer as wet inside as out. Newer permeable materials are designed to allow perspiration and some heat to escape while retaining their water resistance. Avoid flammable or meltable synthetic materials where there is a possibility of fire, such as in aircraft operations.

For Fire Fighting

Turnout or bunker gear is a fire service term for protective clothing/garments designed for use in structural fire fighting environments (Figure 2.1). Turnout gear includes clothing and equipment that protect the fire fighter from head to toe. Most current turnout gear utilizes different layers of fabric/material designed to provide protection from the heat of fire, to reduce trauma from impact or cuts, and to keep water away from the body. As with most protective clothing, fire fighting turnout gear adds weight and to some degree reduces the range of motion available to the wearer.

FIGURE 2.1

Bunker Gear
Turnout gear utilizes different layers of fabric/material to protect the firefighter from heat of fire, to reduce trauma from impact or cuts, and to keep water away from the body.

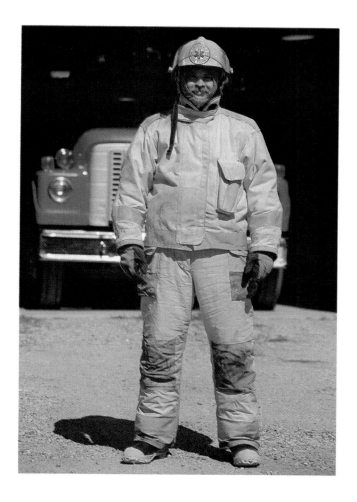

The exterior fabrics used in fire fighter turnout gear offer a barrier to high external temperatures while providing the fire fighter with increased protection from cuts and abrasions. The interior layers of fire fighter turnout gear do function as part of the external heat barrier protection, but these layers are also designed to keep out water. It is the interior layer that is designed to be replaced to meet changing weather conditions. For example, turnout gear worn in cold climates will likely have an insulated thermal inner layer of material that provides more retention of body heat than will the inner layer of turnout gear worn in hot climates.

For High Angle Rescue

Clothing worn for high angle rescue must be appropriate for the activity and the environment that will be encountered. The typical bunker gear worn in fire fighting, for example, is usually too encumbering. And the usual squad clothing may not offer adequate protection for exposure to the elements.

Clothing for high angle rescue must be loose fitting to allow the wearer to raise arms and legs to the fullest extent without restricting movement. Because most high angle rescues take place outdoors, the clothing must also provide protection against any weather that might occur, including both chill and wetness.

For Civil Disturbances

If the incident has a high potential of becoming violent, you should wear protective clothing. In civil disturbances, everything from dirt clods to bullets and tear gas may be hurled at you. Helmets with face shields, body armor (bulletproof vests), boots, and gas masks are a necessity.

There are several types of body armor that are currently being used by police agencies. These range from extremely light and flexible to heavy and bulky. Some types utilize steel chest and back plates. The lighter vests do not stop large caliber bullets but, because of their flexibility, are preferred by most law enforcement personnel. These vests are commonly worn under the uniform shirt or jacket, while the larger and heavier vests are worn on top of the shirt or jacket. You should be aware of the vests being worn by local law enforcement agencies and become familiar with how to remove these vests from patients. To access a patient, most vests can easily be removed by removing the Velcro™ strips or by cutting the shoulder and side straps (Figure 2.2).

FIGURE 2.2

How to Remove Body Armor
To access a patient wearing body armor, remove the vest by peeling the Velcro™ closures or by cutting the shoulder and side strap.

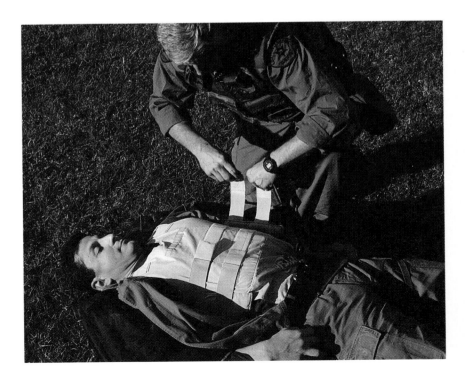

For Electrical Hazards

In situations where electrical hazards are present, you should use a helmet with chin strap and face shield. The shell of the helmet should be constructed of a certified electrical nonconductor. The chin strap should not stretch and should be securely fastened so that if you are knocked down or a power line hits your head, the helmet stays in place. The face shield must be lockable to protect your face and eyes from power lines and/or flying sparks.

A bunker jacket provides minimal electrical protection but may protect you from heat, fire, possible flashovers, and flying sparks. The bunker jacket opening must be properly secured with the front opening fastened and collar up and closed in front to protect the neck and upper chest. Proper fit is important to allow ease of movement.

For Cold Water

Emergency flotation and thermal protection can be provided for rescue personnel at water/ice rescue events by the use of full-body encapsulated flotation suits. These flotation/survival suits, originally developed for use by off-shore oil rig workers, were designed to provide emergency flotation and thermal protection for an individual that accidently fell into the ocean. These suits are NOT meant for use by rescue divers. The survival rescue suit has more recently found use by rescue personnel for emergency entry into water, for ice rescue, fast water rescue, and rescues during foul weather.

The emergency survival/rescue suit is generally constructed of a closed cell neoprene material. The suit encapsulates the body from the top of the head down to include the feet. The only exposed area of the body is a small area of the face including the eyes, nose, and mouth. There is no neck sealing ring to make the suit totally water tight. Therefore, immersion of the head area can result in water leaking down the neck into the suit. Nevertheless, even with some water inside the suit, you still have excellent flotation and thermal protection. It is important for rescue work that a harness be built into the suit or at least added to the suit. The harness provides for easy attachment of safety lines.

The survival/rescue suit can be put on over street clothes without the need for support personnel. Some suits have attached mittens (this gives less finger control) while others have attached gloves that allow for finger movement. The suit is so buoyant that you should use swim fins to provide direction and control when performing rescues in open water situations.

Headgear

In cold weather, a major portion of body heat can be lost through an unprotected head. Insulating hats are made from a variety of materials including the more traditional wool or the newer synthetics. For very cold weather, the hat should be a type that can be pulled down over the face and base of the skull to reduce heat loss.

Helmets Helmets should be worn by all rescue personnel but are mandatory for all personnel working in a fall zone. The helmet should offer both top and side impact protection and have a secure chin strap. Since objects frequently fall in a series, the first impact may knock off the helmet that has an inadequate chin strap, allowing the following objects to strike the unprotected head (Figure 2.3).

Most construction-type helmets are not adequate for the rescue environment. They offer minimal impact protection and have inadequate chin straps. Modern fire helmets offer impact protection, but those with a projecting rear brim may encumber the wearer in a rescue situation. Helmets that have passed certification by the UIAA (Union of International Alpine Associations) offer the kind of protection required for high angle work.

Patients in fall zones must also be provided with helmets unless they have injuries, such as to the cervical spine, which then require the patient to have other shielding. In addition to helmets, additional patient shielding may be needed. Other items used for shields include backboards and inverted litters. There are also commercially available plastic litter shields that protect the upper torso of the patient (Figure 2.4).

Footwear

Footwear should protect the feet from injury, cover the ankles to protect them and keep stones and snow out, be water resistant, fit well, and be supple so they are comfortable for walking. In colder weather, the footwear must also protect from the cold.

FIGURE 2.3

Headgear (helmet)
Rescuers working in a fall zone must wear helmets that offer both top and side impact protection and that have a secure chin strap.

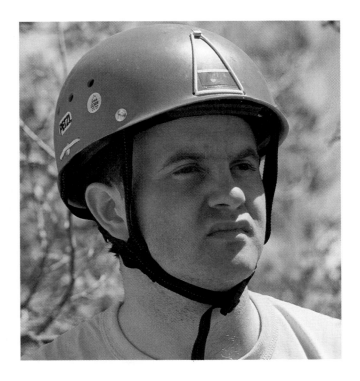

FIGURE 2.4

Patient in Litter Protected by Litter Shield
Litter shields can help protect the patient from falling objects.

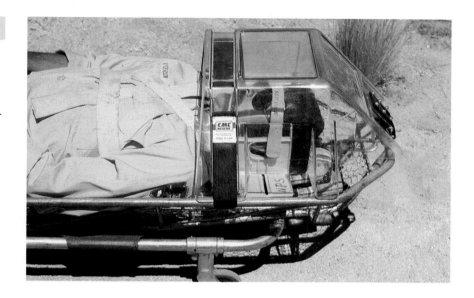

Traveling on foot in the backcountry requires footwear that provides thorough protection for the feet. You will become disabled if there is inadequate protection and your feet are injured by blisters, cuts, or bruises.

Leather still remains one of the best choices for footwear. However, footwear made at least partially of synthetics such as Goretex ™ is increasingly being used. Boots made completely of plastic are used in mountain climbing when the wearer is exposed to extreme cold. However, this type of boot does not flex as easily as other materials and may not be as comfortable for walking.

The soles of mountain boots must provide the adhesion needed for smooth rock and other slick terrain. For better traction, the lug-type soles are commonly used on mountain boots. They may grip well in some conditions, such as snow, but may become very slippery when caked with mud.

The fit of mountain boots is extremely important, since a minor annoyance can develop into a disabling injury. The feet must not move around in the boots, particularly when going downhill, or they will develop blisters and possibly cramped toes. There should be space enough to wiggle the toes. The boots should be fitted while wearing the socks that will be used with the boot.

Socks keep the feet warm and protect them from blows to the boots. In cold environments, two pairs of socks are generally preferable to one pair of thick socks. A thin inner sock next to the foot helps to wick perspiration away to a thicker outer sock.

For warm weather travel, a low **gaiter,** a leg covering reaching from the instep to the ankle, keeps small stones, forest debris, and mud from falling into the boot. For cold weather, a high gaiter keeps the feet and lower legs warm and snow and ice out of boots.

Protective footwear for structural fire fighting is designed to reduce adverse effects on the feet and ankles of fire fighters. Fire fighting boots may be purchased with varying levels of foot support and protection installed. There are three to four heights of fire fighting boots ranging from the ankle area up to the upper thigh. Many rescuers are now using short (ankle to lower calf area) fire fighting boots in combination with other protective turnout gear. This approach reduces the size and weight of the boot worn while providing good protection.

It is best to make sure that the fire fighting boots you wear have the maximum amount of puncture resistance, toe protection, and foot support that is available from the manufacturer (Figure 2.5). Many rescuers find it difficult to obtain a good fit on fire fighting boots. You may find it necessary to use shoe inserts or sock layering techniques to obtain a comfortable fit. The loose fit of some fire fighting boots may hinder you from working in mud or other materials that will tend to pull the boot off of the foot. You must also be sure to keep the top (throat) of the fire fighting boot "sealed off" (covered by pant legs or tight against the thigh) to keep rain, snow, glass, or other material from entering the boot.

Fire fighting boots often develop leaks from chemical or mechanical damage sustained during fire suppression activities. It is important that you frequently check these boots for deterioration of the exterior boot skin (checking, cracking, peeling, and flaking) and that any opening in the exterior barrier be sealed according to manufacturers recommendations.

FIGURE 2.5

Firefighting Boots and Mountain Boots
Firefighting and mountain boots offer different kinds of protection and are worn for different kinds of rescue operations.

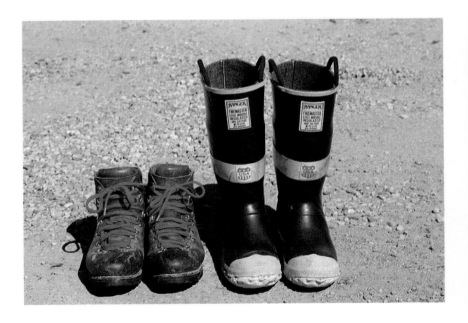

Gloves

All rescuers need protection for their hands and wrist. Select gloves that provide maximum protection for the working environment. Keep in mind that your gloves must provide the dexterity you need to use rescue tools and handle your rescue duties.

Structural fire fighting requires good hand and wrist protection for the fire fighter. The gloves designed for structural fire fighting minimize the effects of heat, cold, and cuts on the fire fighter's hand and wrist. These features are obtained at a cost of reduced manual dexterity.

During any incident in which you may be exposed to blood or other body fluids, you must wear rubber gloves and avoid direct skin to fluid contact.

GEAR

In high altitude areas, weather is unreliable, so you must provide for shelter. The most reliable form of shelter is the one that is carried by the team. This is usually a tent. A mountain tent must be lightweight, capable of easily being erected in darkness and severe weather, self-supporting, able to withstand the strongest winds, and capable of protecting against biting insects.

There are a great variety of designs and sizes of mountain tents. They range in size from accommodating one to four persons. While larger tents are heavier, they do allow more room to sit or stand and may help keep morale high if the rescue team must remain inside the tent for extended periods.

Most tents have waterproof floors and sidewalls to keep water out during rainstorms. A floor also helps insulate when the tent is pitched on snow. Tents that are completely enclosed should have some means of ventilation to allow for the escape of moisture. Otherwise, water vapor that is exhaled by sleeping occupants will condense on the tent walls and may soak sleeping bags and clothing.

Personal shelter can be provided though one-person **bivouac sacks;** temporary shelters which are lightweight but provide no extra room in which to stow gear.

Flotation

Personal preparedness affects the success of water rescue efforts. All personnel involved in a water rescue must wear a personal flotation device (PFD) when teams practice or respond to a water rescue (Figure 6.1). Type I or Type II PFDs are preferred for water rescue work, though Specialty Type III PFDs are suitable for some rescue situations. The problem with most Type IIIs is that they will not turn an unconscious person to a face-up position in the water. You should clean and inspect PFDs regularly as part of your equipment maintenance program. PFDs with torn covering or straps should be replaced.

Lighting

Many rescues occur at night where lighting or electricity isn't even present. You must frequently provide your own lighting sources. Each individual rescuer must have a light source for travel and for attending the patient. For extended operations, additional lighting for illuminating the base camp must be provided.

While flashlights may be reliable sources of light, they must be held in the hand, eliminating the use of that hand. Therefore, each rescuer should have a headlamp that either clips to a helmet or attaches to the head with a headband. You should always carry spare batteries and bulbs for each light source.

In the total darkness of confined space and underground environments, headlamps are an absolute necessity, for without light you are stranded. In the underground environment, you should carry three light sources plus spare batteries and bulbs.

Skin Protection

Sunburn is a threat in any outdoor environment. While it might be considered simply an annoyance, it is at least a first-degree thermal burn. Over the long term, excessive exposure of the skin to sun can result in premature aging of the skin and skin cancers. In remote areas, severe sunburn can be debilitating to rescuers.

In areas that are very reflective, such as sand, water, and snow, the risk of sunburn is magnified. In these places areas of the body that normally are not exposed, such as under the chin, inside the ears and nose, and around the eyes, may become sunburned. At higher altitudes, the solar radiation is much stronger than at sea level, and all rescue personnel must be particularly careful about sunburn, particularly on the lips and nose.

If you are going to be outdoors, particularly at high altitude or on a reflective surface, protect your skin by applying a sunblock with an appropriate rating from your personal kit. Since it is the ultraviolet (UV) rays that cause sunburn, skin can be burned even on a cloudy day. In addition to a sunblock, protective hats are also helpful.

Sun is not the only threat in an outdoor setting. It is wise to minimize the amount of skin exposed to potentially irritating environmental features, such as insects and poisonous plants.

For Eye Protection

You must protect your eyes and the patient's eyes against injury from foreign objects and the environment (e.g., plants, insects). Whenever tools are being used at an extrication scene, you must wear eye protection such as face shields or goggles. Whenever you are at risk for eye damage, then your patients are also, so the patient's eyes must be protected.

> YOU MUST ALSO WEAR EYE PROTECTION WHEN THERE IS A POSSIBILITY OF EXPOSURE TO BLOOD OR OTHER BODY FLUIDS.

Sun-induced eye injuries must be avoided. At higher altitudes persistent exposure to sunlight may cause serious damage. Sunlight reflecting on snow can result in snow blindness, a temporary but painful condition. To protect your eyes at higher altitudes and in snow or white sand, you must wear glasses or goggles that fully protect against UV exposure.

Goggles must be adaptable to the weather and physical demands of the rescue operation. Clear vision must be maintained regardless of temperature extremes and physical demands, and vision restrictions should be minimized. Goggles that perform well for one rescuer may be useless for another. Among the considerations are: Will they fit over prescription eyewear? How do they perform in varied light levels? (Figure 2.6)

For Ear Protection

If you routinely work around equipment with high noise levels, such as helicopters, hearing protection with higher noise reduction should be used. Soft foam industrial-type earplugs will usually meet the need.

FIGURE 2.6

Goggles
Eye protection, such as goggles, must be adaptable to the weather and physical demands of the rescue operation.

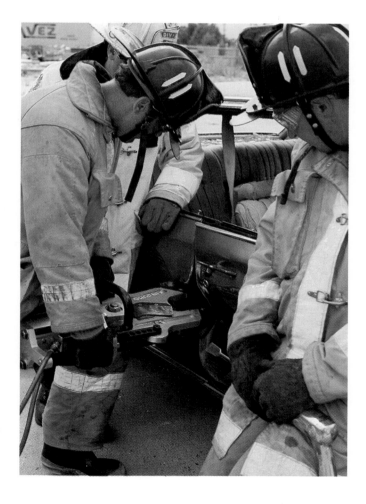

Along with noise levels, high winds can be extremely uncomfortable to patients and rescuers. This discomfort has direct effects on safety and morale. You should recognize the reduction or loss of hearing caused by plugs and adapt your personal communications as needed.

For Protection from Dust and Dirt Contamination

Contamination of the eyes, ears, and respiratory tract from dirt, dust, and wind can be devastating to the rescue operation. It is essential that eye protection, ear plugs, and some type of simple respiratory protection be incorporated into your packs and the patient packaging system. It is important to plan the kinds of equipment to be used for personal protection.

Even experienced backcountry personnel sometimes forget pieces of equipment during the rush of callout. For this reason, an equipment checklist is vital to ensure all the gear necessary for an extended incident rescue is available. "The 48-Hour Pack," is an example of a checklist for backcountry equipment. (Figure 2.7)

FIGURE 2.7

The 48-Hour Pack
An equipment checklist is necessary to ensure that all gear needed for a backcountry rescue is available when needed.

CLOTHING
Extra set of clothing
Cold weather clothing
Rain gear
Hat/Cap
Gaiters
Socks (2 pair)
Boots
Bandanna
Sunglasses/Goggles
Ear protectors
Mittens/Gloves

ACCESSORIES
Pocket knife (multipurpose)
Waterproof matches and case
Candles (two)/Firestarters
Compass (orienteering type)
Map
First-aid kit
Notebook and pencil
Whistle
Flashlight/Headlamp
Sunscreen/Lip balm
Insect repellent
Nylon twine (50 feet)
Flagging tape
Toilet paper
Leaf bag (heavy weight)
Quarters (for pay phone)

SHELTER
Tent/Tarp
Ground cloth
Sleeping pad
Sleeping bag
Bivouac bag

KITCHEN
Stove
Cooking/Eating gear
Water containers (2–1 liters)
Water purification tablets/Filters
Food
High energy snacks
Assorted small plastic bags

SPECIAL EQUIPMENT
Allergy kit
Extra eyeglasses
Binoculars
Camera/Film
Personal climbing equipment

SUMMARY

All rescue team members must be aware of the appropriate, protective clothing and gear to use for each type of rescue effort. Selecting clothing, including headgear and footwear, that will protect the body and help control body temperature is essential.

Rescuers often have to carry protective gear during all rescue operations. You may need to provide for shelter and/or some form of illumination.

In outdoor environments, sunburn is a threat. Therefore, rescuers should carry and apply a sunblock with an appropriate rating. Eyes and ears require protection from both the environment and from foreign objects. In addition, eyes, ears, and the respiratory tract must be protected from dust, dirt, and wind.

TOOLS AND TECHNIQUES OF RESCUE

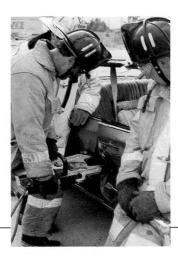

OVERVIEW

Familiarity with rescue equipment and its proper use is important to ensure a safe and effective rescue. Rescuers need to know how to select the most appropriate tools for each job and how to use each tool to accomplish the task.

This chapter examines the tools and techniques of high angle rescue and belay. It also discusses the equipment and techniques of extrication. The section on extrication includes detailed instructions about water and ice rescue and patient packaging and transport.

OBJECTIVES

The objectives of this chapter are for the rescuer to describe:

- the equipment used in a high angle rescue environment.
- the tools and techniques of belays.

- basic extrication tools and techniques.
- the tools and techniques of water and ice rescue.

There are different tools for a variety of rescue situations. Many tools conform to equipment standards established by various organizations. For example, certain U.S. and international organizations have set standards for equipment that is used in rescue activities. The National Fire Protection Association (NFPA) has set standards for rope and associated equipment when they are to be used on the fireground. The Union of International Alpine Associations (UIAA) has set standards for some high angle equipment used for recreational climbing. These standards may apply in some rescue situations but not in others. UIAA standards for rope, for instance, were developed specifically for dynamic rope that is used in recreational climbing and that has characteristics different from the static rope needed for rescue work. In another example, UIAA standards for helmets are appropriate for high angle rescue situations but would not be sufficient for helmets used on the fireground (See Chapter 2).

LITTERS

In many rescue environments, rescuers transport patients in litters. Litters used for extended transports must protect the patient from environmental factors, immobilize the patient, and be easily used in a variety of rescue situations and vehicles.

Stokes

Stokes litters are one of the most commonly used litters. They are manufactured with a variety of materials and types of construction. Older models include a woven wire basket (Figure 3.1) constructed with a frame and carrying rails of metal tubing. If the metal litter is subjected to high forces, such as occur in hauling, lowering, or attaching rescuers, the frame and rails should be constructed of steel. In addition, the wire basket Stokes is very uncomfortable for the patient unless the wire is padded. The unpadded woven wire has sharp ends that snag clothing, damage equipment such as air splints and pneumatic antishock garments (PASG), and may pierce the skin of the patient or rescuers. If the litter has a leg divider, the patient's groin must be protected with padding.

A particular disadvantage to the woven wire litter is that the chicken wire bottom is open, exposing the patient to cold and wet-

FIGURE 3.1

Stokes Litter
The woven wire basket is an older model of the Stokes litter. This type of litter must be padded for patient comfort and protection.

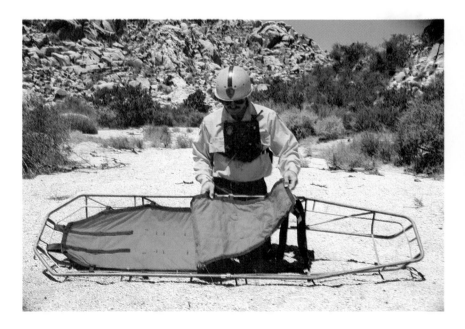

ness, as well as injury from stones or tree branches. If a wire basket litter is used, then you must protect the patient from these factors. If exposure to wetness is a possibility, both the bottom and top of the patient must be protected. Before the patient is placed in the litter, the bottom should be lined with a tough waterproof material. On top of this should be placed padding such as a closed cell foam pad.

If chilling is a possibility, the patient should be placed between blankets or in a sleeping bag that is accessible from all sides. After the patient has been placed in the litter, an additional waterproof layer should be placed on top and tucked in so that no water will run down onto the patient.

Since a full backboard will not fit most wire basket litters, you may have to use a conforming short board device for cervical and spinal immobilization. A body-shaped spine board (Figure 3.2) may also be used in litters with leg dividers. In some difficult rescue situations, such as confined space, vehicle, high angle, or high altitude, it may be easier to initially immobilize the patient with a conforming short board device. But as soon as possible, full body immobilization should be initiated with a long spine board.

In moving and maneuvering a litter, you should consider the structural weak points of a metal Stokes, namely, the butt welds where the frame and rails of the metal wire baskets join. You must avoid subjecting these butt welds to high stress. For example, when attaching a rope to the head or foot end of the metal Stokes (where

FIGURE 3.2

Body-Shaped Spine Board
A body-shaped spine board may be used for full body immobilization in litters that have leg dividers.

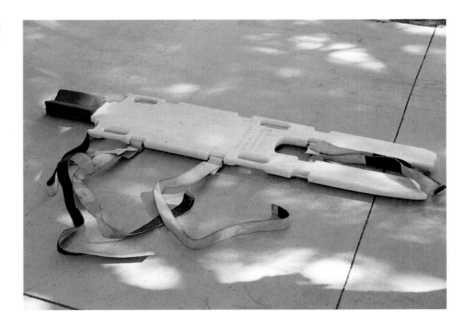

FIGURE 3.3

How to Attach a Rope to the Litter
When you attach a rope to pull a litter at one end, do not secure the rope at only one point. Spread the force of the pull over a wider area by wrapping the rope several times around the rail.

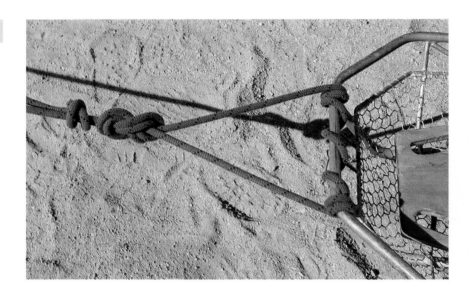

butt welds are usually found), the rope should not pull at one point but be spread across a wide area of the rail (Figure 3.3).

The plastic-type Stokes litter is a more recent design in which the main body is constructed of one piece of plastic riveted to a large diameter aluminum carrying rail. Early models were constructed of a plastic that cracked and deteriorated. However, more recent models have solved this problem with a slightly softer plastic and improved attachments to the rail. A plastic Stokes litter slides easily across snow and rock while protecting the patient (Figure 3.4). Current models of the plastic Stokes do not have a leg divider so they accommodate a full backboard.

All plastics, including those used in litters, deteriorate under prolonged exposure to sunlight. This deterioration should not be significant under normal rescue use. However, you should avoid exposing plastic litters to prolonged sunlight, such as storing them on tops of vehicles exposed to the sun.

If the patient is to be transported on wide trails or along forest roads, a detachable wheel may be used to help carry the load (Figure 3.5). However, the wheel is difficult to use over rugged terrain.

Both metal and plastic Stokes litters are available in two-piece versions that may be separated for easier carrying.

For over-the-snow transport, there are several litter designs including the Cascade toboggan (Figure 3.6) and the Akja,™ a European type. Both are available with detachable handles so they can be used as sleds.

Semi-Rigid

Semi-rigid litters have been designed for rescues in confined spaces but have also been adapted to other difficult rescue environments. One of the oldest designs is the Neill-Robertson litter, which was

FIGURE 3.4

Newer Stokes Litter
Newer models of the plastic Stokes litter will accommodate a full backboard. They also slide across snow and rocks easily.

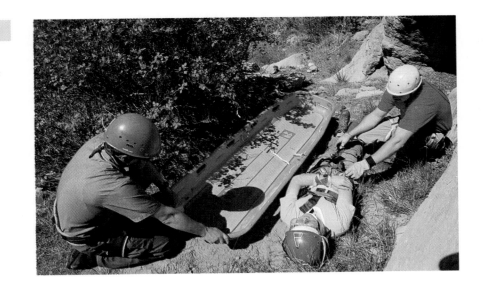

FIGURE 3.5

Detachable Support Wheel
A detachable support wheel can be used to help carry a patient over easy terrain.

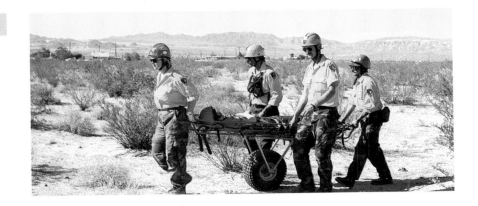

FIGURE 3.6

Over-the-Snow Transports
Several litter designs are available for transporting patients over snow.

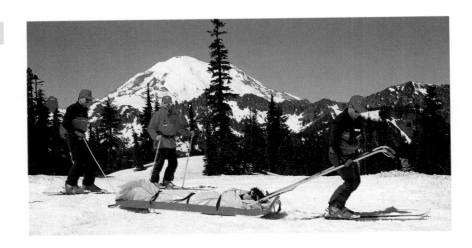

originally used for tight spaces aboard ships. In its basic design the Neill-Robertson has a narrow, rigid central spine board running from head to feet. Attached to this central spine board are fabric sheets containing wooden laths. The sheets are wrapped around the patient's body and are secured with buckles. A more recent version, known as the modified Neill-Robertson, provides more patient protection with stainless steel runners running lengthwise under the central spine-board and with an attached helmet. The Neill-Robertson can either be carried horizontally or hoisted vertically.

A recently developed semi-rigid conforming litter (SKED™) is con-structed of a large piece of flexible plastic that envelopes and protects most of the patient's body (Figure 3.7). There are attachment points and carrying handles along the litter, with lifting straps for using it in the high angle environment. When rolled into its cone shape, the

FIGURE 3.7

SKED™ Litter
When correctly formed into its cone shape, the semi-rigid conforming litter achieves a rigidity that allows it to contain a patient in a high angle environment.

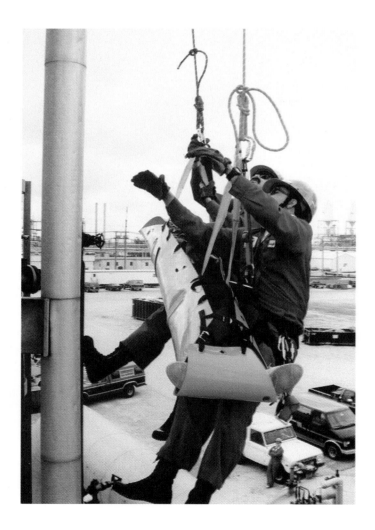

semi-rigid conforming litter becomes rigid allowing it to be carried or managed in a high angle environment. Because it does not add bulk to the patient, the semi-rigid conforming litter works well in a confined space. The material also slides easily over snow and rock. When used in snow, you should roll a blanket into a horse collar shape and put it in the stretcher around the patient's shoulders to prevent snow from collecting inside the stretcher.

ROPES, KNOTS, AND RELATED EQUIPMENT

The rope used in rescue should be of a **static** design, which means it has little stretch. This lack of stretch gives rescuers better control of the rope during most operations. The stretch of static rescue rope contrasts with the greater stretch of **dynamic** rope, which is often used in recreational climbing because it can absorb the shock of a falling climber.

Much of the static rope used for rescue is constructed with a tightly woven outer sheath that helps protect an inner core that supports most of the load on the rope. This kind of construction is known as **kernmantle.** It is derived from the German words, kern (core) and mantle (sheath). The outer sheath used on rescue rope should be denser and more tightly woven than that used on recreational ropes. This will help protect the rope from damaging cuts and abrasion.

Rescue rope is most commonly used in diameters of 7/16 inch (11.1 mm) or 1/2 inch (12.5 mm). Ropes with diameters larger than 1/2 inch will not fit many types of rescue hardware, are difficult to handle in the high angle environment, and are heavier to carry long distances. The specific rope diameter should be determined on the basis of local rescue needs while maintaining an acceptable safety factor.

Rope and other equipment used in rescue must have an adequate safety factor for the rescue work anticipated. A safety factor is the ratio of the highest likely load that might occur during a rescue to the strength of the equipment. A safety factor of 10:1, for example, means that if the highest expected load on a rope might be 1,000 pounds, then the rope should have a strength of 10,000 pounds. If the equipment has a safety factor of 15:1 and the maximum expected load is 1,000 pounds, the equipment would have a strength of 15,000 pounds.

In some high angle rescue environments, such as backcountry rescue, where the rope will not receive a great deal of abuse, where there is greater opportunity to inspect the rope for damage, and where weight may be a factor, rescue teams sometimes use a minimum safety factor of 10:1. In other environments, such as on the fireline, a safety factor of 15:1 is often used.

Rope breaking strength is expressed as **tensile test strength.** There are various ways of measuring this, but the standard now used by major rescue rope manufactures is Federal Test Standard 191A, Method 6016.

Rescue rope can be purchased in almost any length desired. The cut length for rescue ropes should be determined according to local needs and for convenience of carrying and storage. A convenient length for carrying is 200 feet. However, if rescues with vertical distances of more than 200 feet are common, then longer ropes should be carried.

As with all safety equipment, rescue rope must be inspected thoroughly and carefully after each use. Before rescue rope is returned to storage, every inch of it must be subjected to a *sight* and *feel* inspection. The rope should be carefully run through a bare hand and inspected. The inspector should look and feel for:

- Lumps, depressions, and changes in circumference that may indicate damage to the rope core.
- Broken sheath bundles; if rope core is exposed; or if over 50 percent of a sheath bundle is broken.
- Discolorations that may indicate damage from substances such as acids.
- Glossy marks indicating heat damage.

If any of the above conditions are found, the rope should be removed from rescue service. Alternatively, the bad section may be cut out leaving two shorter sections of good rope.

Rescue ropes are life safety equipment. They must be treated as such. They must be protected from damaging activities and substances. Abrasion is one of the most common destroyers of rescue ropes. Abrasion occurs when the rope is run over a rough surface, such as rock or a building surface. Abrasion is worse when the rope is loaded, putting weight on the rope. Use rope pads (Figure 3.8) or edge rollers (Figure 3.9) to protect from abrasion. Use great care to avoid walking on rescue lines. This grinds in grit and dirt that can damage the load-bearing fibers.

Heat fusion occurs from the heat of the friction of a moving rope running over a second rope *in one place*. This can happen when a lowering or hauling rope runs over an anchor rope. This sudden heat buildup can cut the rope.

Rope must be protected from damaging substances, such as acids, both during use and in storage. Acids from storage batteries is an obvious example, but wet concrete may also contain damaging acids. Other substances that can damage rope are soot and bleaches.

Rescue ropes must not be used for towing vehicles or lifting heavy equipment. If an organization has both rescue and utility ropes, precautions must be taken to make sure that rescue lines are not used as utility ropes. Rescue ropes should be a different color from utility ropes, be tagged for life support use only, and be stored separately from utility ropes.

FIGURE 3.8

Rope Pads
Rope pads help protect rope from damaging abrasion.

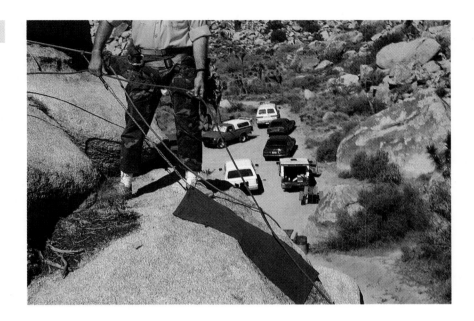

FIGURE 3.9

Edge Rollers
Edge rollers help a rope run more freely and protect it from abrasion.

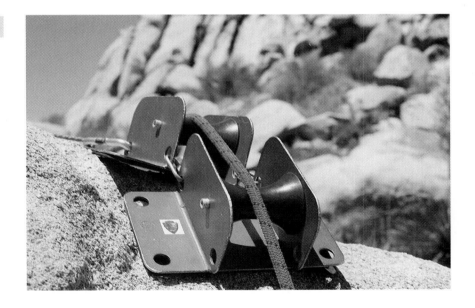

Rope should be stored in bags hanging in loose coils or in a protected place. To avoid damage from long-term overheating, store in a place that has temperatures comfortable for humans. Avoid long-term exposure to sunlight. To avoid mildew allow rope to dry completely before storage.

KNOTS

During rescue operations, a knot must remain tied despite flexing, manipulation, and being run through equipment or over rough edges. The knot must be easily remembered and easily tied, even when the rescuer is under stress or in adverse conditions such as rain, wind, and cold. The knot must not significantly diminish the strength of the rope.

It is not necessary for you to learn a large number of knots to be effective in tying rescue knots. A few general purpose knots, *well learned* are more effective than a great many knots *mostly forgotten.*

The following types of knots are commonly used and remembered by rescuers. With regular practice, you can easily remember them. The figure 8 family of knots will serve for most high angle rescue operations. The **simple figure 8** knot (Figure 3.10) can be used as a "stopper" knot. Tied in the bottom end of a rappel rope, it can help prevent a rescuer from rappeling off the end of the rope. Tied in the upper end of a rope, it can help prevent the rope from accidently running through equipment while it is being rigged. It is the "foundation" knot for other knots in the figure 8 family.

The **figure 8 overhand** knot (Figure 3.11) is usually tied in the end of a line as a "clip in" point to attach the rope to other things. You may use it to clip into a harness or a safety or lowering rope or as a tie-in while working as a litter tender. It can be clipped into a stretcher spider (see Chapter 17) for lowering or raising a patient or other rescue loads. Tied in the top of a rope, it can be used to attach the rope to the anchor.

FIGURE 3.10

Simple Figure 8 Knot
The simple figure 8 knot can be used as a "stopper" knot or as the "foundation" knot for other knots in the figure 8 family.

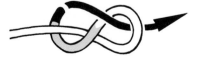 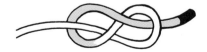 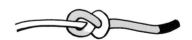

FIGURE 3.11

Figure 8 Overhand Knot
The figure 8 overhand knot is usually tied in the end of a line as a "clip in" point.

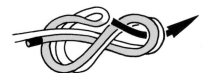 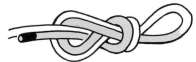 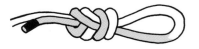

The **figure 8 follow-through** knot (Figure 3.12), like the figure 8 overhand, is usually used to form a loop at the end of a rope. But the figure 8 follow-through is used where a loop cannot be placed *over* an object but must be tied *around* it. Some examples would be a tree being used as an anchor that is too tall to drop a loop over or a structural beam closed in on both ends. In these cases the anchor rope can be tied around the object using a figure 8 follow-through. The knot is always begun by tying a simple figure 8 as a foundation knot. The running end of the rope is run around the object and then back through the first knot, following the contours of the simple figure 8 exactly.

A **bend** is a knot that ties two pieces of rope together. It can be used to tie two ropes together to make a longer line or to tie both ends of one rope together to make a continuous loop. The **figure 8 bend** (Figure 3.13) is one of the few bends that is secure enough to tie two ropes together for life support activities such as rescue.

The **water knot** (Figure 3.14) is used only for webbing. The water knot ties two pieces of webbing together to make a longer piece or ties two ends of one piece together to make a continuous loop. The flat shape of the webbing enables it to follow the contours of the knot while holding itself together.

For added security, you should tie a **safety knot** to back up the primary knot in rescue rope. Because most rescue ropes are stiff,

FIGURE 3.12

Figure 8 Follow-Through Knot
The figure 8 follow-through knot is used to form a loop in the end of a rope. This knot is used where the loop cannot be placed over the object, but must be tied around it.

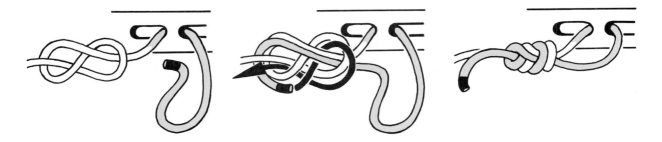

FIGURE 3.13

Figure 8 Bend
The figure 8 bend is used to tie two ends of rope together.

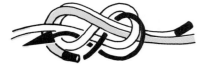 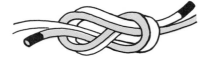 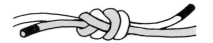

FIGURE 3.14

Water Knot
The water knot is used to tie two ends of webbing together.

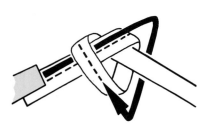
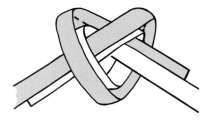
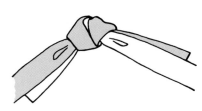

FIGURE 3.15

Barrel Knot
For added security, you should tie a safety knot to back up the primary knot in rescue rope. One knot that is often used as a safety knot is the barrel knot.

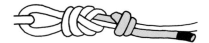
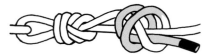
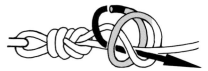

primary knots can become untied as they are flexed in the rescue system. One knot that is often used as a safety knot is the **barrel knot** (Figure 3.15). To use this as a safety knot, tie the primary knot so that there is about two feet of tail left in the rope after the primary knot is finished. Use this tail to tie the safety knot against the primary knot. To be effective, a safety knot must be snug against the primary knot.

Back-Up Knots and Webbing

Webbing is a woven fabric that replaces rope for certain specific indications. Because of its flat shape, webbing is more comfortable against the body than rope. Webbing is used for harnesses for rescuers or to secure patients in litters.

For anchor systems, presewn **runners** are more convenient. If the loops of webbing are well sewn, there is a greater assurance of safety, since they do not depend on someone properly tying a water knot in a continuous loop of webbing.

Webbing comes in two basic designs. **Flat webbing** is a single layer of material similar to automotive seat belt material. **Tubular webbing** is more commonly used in the high angle environment (Figure 3.16). It is a woven tube of material that is more supple and comfortable than flat webbing, especially when used in emergency harnesses. Webbing for the rescue environment is usually one inch wide. If very high loading is expected, wider sizes are available.

FIGURE 3.16

Tubular Webbing
Tubular webbing is commonly used in the high angle environment.

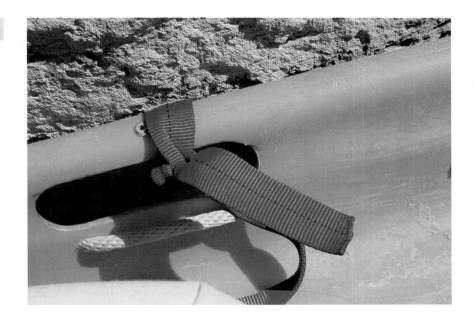

FIGURE 3.17

Seat Harness
A seat harness is the basic harness for rescue activities in the high angle environment.

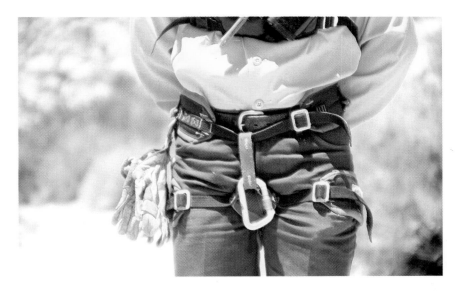

Harnesses

Everyone near or over the edge of a high angle rescue must wear a harness that is tied into either a main line or a safety line. There are three basic types of harnesses available for the rescue environment: seat harnesses, chest harnesses, and full body harnesses. The basic harness for rescue activities is the seat harness (Figure 3.17).

On occasion, chest harnesses may be used in combination with seat harnesses to hold a climber upright in case of a fall. However, *chest harnesses must never be used in the high angle environment without a seat harness, except in specific water rescue situations.*

Full body harnesses are very secure, but some persons find them too confining to wear for most high angle rescue work.

Safety and comfort are two main requirements for rescue harnesses used in the high angle environment. The webbing in the harnesses should be securely stitched to resist the stresses of shock loading. The stitching should be of a contrasting color so that you can determine when it is frayed. Hardware for attaching harnesses to the rope must be securely fastened, and attachment points should be reinforced to resist wearing.

In a rescue situation you may be hanging in the harness for extended periods of time. The harness should fit so it does not press on blood vessels and nerves. The webbing at critical support areas should be two or three inches wide, and the harness should have leg loops. In addition, rescue harnesses must be easy to put on in stressful situations.

Hardware

Carabiners are metal snap links that connect the individual elements of the high angle system. They may be used to connect a seat harness tie-in point to a rope or to attach a rope to an anchor system.

The basic parts of a carabiner are the spine, gate, hinge, and latch. The *spine* is the C-shaped main body that supports most of the load. So that the carabiner can be attached, the *gate* swings open on the *hinge*. A spring in the end of the gate at the hinge keeps the gate closed. At the end of the gate opposite the hinge, the *latch* helps keep the gate closed when the carabiner is loaded. The two main styles of latches are pin and hook and tooth latches (Figure 3.18).

FIGURE 3.18

Carabiner Latches
The two main designs of carabiner latches are pin (left) and hook and tooth (right) latches.

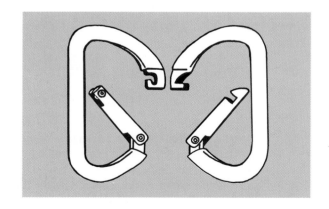

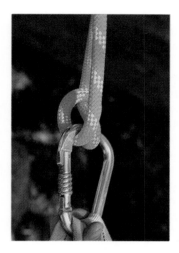

FIGURE 3.19

Correct Loading of Carabiners

The correct manner of function for a carabiner is lengthwise loading. Any other type of loading can damage the carabiner and possibly cause it to fail.

The weakest portion of any carabiner is the hinge/gate/latch assembly. Carabiner failures are usually failures of technique resulting from the individual not using this portion of the carabiner properly. Carabiners are designed to be used in a specific fashion or *manner of function.* It is critical that you use carabiners in their designed manner of function. Otherwise, the carabiner will fail, resulting in injury or death. The correct manner of function is to load a carabiner lengthwise (Figure 3.19). If a carabiner is loaded sideways, the gate assembly may fail.

You must make certain that carabiners are used in the correct manner of function when rigging a high angle system. You must constantly monitor the carabiners to ensure that they maintain the correct manner of function as the system is manipulated and equipment shifts.

Unsecured carabiner gates can be forced open by being pushed against rocks, ropes, webbing, or other objects. If this happens, material may slip out of the carabiner and cause system failure. Non-locking carabiners can be secured by arranging two of them together, *reversed and opposed* (Figure 3.20).

Locking carabiners are a more secure design. They have a locking sleeve that rotates up a threaded area on the gate to secure it closed. On most carabiners the sleeve locks the gate shut at the latch, although there are a few designs that lock the gate shut at the hinge. For most rescue situations, the added security of a locking carabiner is preferred. (Non-locking carabiners are usually preferred by recreational climbers.) However, locking carabiners are secure only *when their gates are locked.* Some carabiners have significantly less strength when their gates are not locked. As you rig a rope rescue system, you must develop techniques and habits to ensure you are locking your carabiners.

Locking carabiners may accidently become unlocked if the locking sleeve rolls open as it is rubbed against a rock or building face. The

FIGURE 3.20

Securing Non-Locking Carabiners

Non-locking carabiners can be made more secure by arranging them together in a position so that they are reversed and opposed to one another.

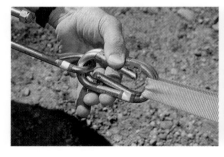
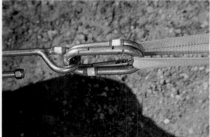

sleeve can also become unlocked through vibration. You must constantly be on alert to ensure that your carabiner gates remain locked.

Carabiners are made from either steel or aluminum alloys. Steel carabiners generally have higher tensile strength, but some aluminum carabiners have an adequate safety factor for rescue operations. However, the locking mechanism on steel carabiners will usually outlast the mechanism on aluminum carabiners, and steel locking carabiners usually withstand heavy shock loading better than aluminum carabiners. The sudden shock loading of a fallen climber, while frequent in recreational climbing, rarely occurs in rescue situations. When severe shock loading does occur in rescue situations, all involved rope and equipment should be retired from service. With the significant weight difference between steel and aluminum carabiners, rescuers who carry equipment for long distances may prefer aluminum carabiners.

Belays and High Angle Techniques

A patient should be belayed any time there is a danger of additional injury if there is a fall. The question of when to belay a rescuer depends on particular circumstances. Some experienced rescuers may find a belay encumbering in certain routine activities such as rappeling. The decision to belay depends on the judgment and experience of the individuals on the rope, the actual chances of falling, and elements such as rock or ice fall that could knock them off. Decisions on when to belay can be made by the safety officer on the scene or by policy in the preplan.

Because the loads and forces are greater in a rescue situation than they are in recreational climbing, you should use **direct belays.** These are belays directly attached to a **bombproof anchor** (Figure 3.21). A bombproof anchor is one that is stronger than any forces that will be placed on the system during the rescue operation.

FIGURE 3.21

Direct Belay
In rope rescue situations, you should use direct belays that are directly attached to a bombproof anchor.

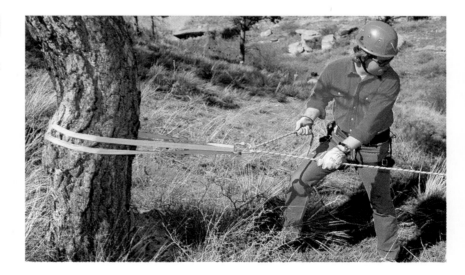

An **anchor** is a secure point to which the high angle rope system is attached. Since the high angle system will be only as strong as the anchors to which it is attached, a secure anchor system is a major concern in any high angle rescue system. The secure point might be a portion of a building, a strong tree, a large rock, or other objects that can withstand the stresses that will be placed on the system. If you use a single anchor point, it must be bombproof. If the single anchor is not bombproof, then the rescuers must establish a multiple anchor system with as many anchors as necessary to make the system bombproof (Figure 3.22). If the rescue load shifts or moves from side to side, it may cause uneven loading on the anchors in a multiple anchor system. This can overload the system and cause it to collapse. One solution is to create a **self-equalizing anchor system.** A self-equalizing system maintains equal loading on all anchors despite the angle of pull (Figure 3.23). A self-equalizing system is designed so if

FIGURE 3.22

Multiple Anchor System
If a single anchor is not reliable, then you should establish a multiple anchor system with as many anchors as necessary to make the anchor system bombproof.

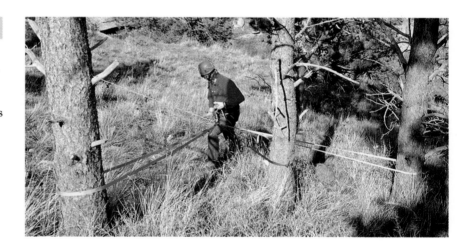

FIGURE 3.23

Self-Equalizing Anchor System
A self-equalizing system maintains equal loading on all anchors despite the direction of pull by the load. They should be designed so that if one anchor point fails, the system automatically equalizes the load on the remaining anchors.

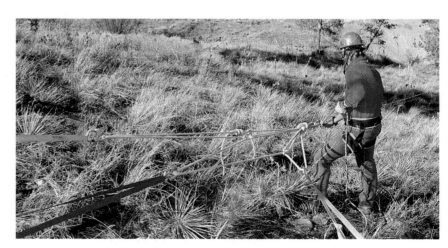

one anchor point fails, the system automatically equalizes the load on the remaining anchors.

For rescue work, direct belays are preferable to the body belays sometimes used in recreational climbing where the belayer creates friction on the rope by running it around his body. The large loads and greater forces present in a high angle rescue can injure or entrap the belayer so he or she is unable to assist the person who has fallen.

Among the various kinds of belay techniques used in rescue is the **Münter hitch**. The Münter hitch is a running knot in the belay rope tied around a carabiner attached to an anchor (Figure 3.24). The belayer allows the rope to slip around the carabiner in the Münter hitch while the person at the end is moving under control. But if the person starts to fall, the belayer pulls back on the Münter hitch to create a friction lock to slow or stop the fall.

The **belay plate** is used for belaying one person. Several different belay plate designs are available. Belay plates are usually designed for a specific diameter of rope, but they all work essentially the same way. The belayer pushes a bight (a slack part) of the belay rope through a slot in the belay plate, secures it on the opposite side with a carabiner, and attaches the carabiner to an anchor point. When the person attached to the belay rope falls, the belayer causes the plate and carabiner to come together to create friction to brake the fall.

FIGURE 3.24

Münter Hitch Tied to Anchor
The Münter hitch is a belay technique that uses a running knot in the belay rope tied around a carabiner.

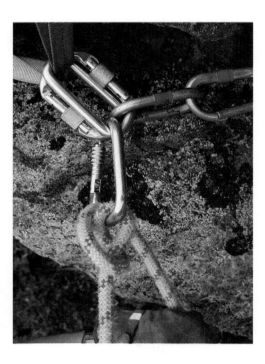

The advantage of the Münter hitch is that it requires only one action by the belayer, grasping the rope with the brake hand, to stop a fall. The brake plate requires two actions, grasping the rope and moving the plate against the carabiner. The advantage of the brake plate is the freer run of the rope that occurs when unloaded. This is particularly an advantage in recreational climbing.

Web Slings for Utility (Non-Life Support) Use

Synthetic fiber webbing for utility use can be configured into two general types of slings. One type is a single leg sling. This type has sewn eyes (loops) at either end. The eyes can have hooks or other hardware attached or can be set up as part of a bridle.

The second type of synthetic web sling is manufactured in a continuous (endless) loop with no end. One of the strongest continuous web slings is made with an outer jacket and a separate inner core. The core is made up of fiber bundles/strands that run somewhat parallel to each other. The inner core is made up of such fibers as nylon, polyester, or kevlar. The outer jacket, which carries only a small portion of the load, is manufactured of fiber similar to that of the inner core. The outer jacket primarily provides shape and barrier protection for the inner core.

There are three different hitches possible with the continuous sling. The vertical-horizontal hitch is used when the load is lifted straight up or the load pulls straight along a horizontal plane. In this case, the continuous sling is connected (using hardware such as a hook or a metal snap link called a carabiner) in a straight line between the load and the lifting device or anchor point. The cradle or basket hitch is the second hitch. The cradle/basket hitch loops around the load or the anchor. The ends of the continuous sling are brought together and joined with hardware such as a hook or carabiner. The basket configuration doubles the capacity of the continuous loop. The third hitch is the choker hitch (it is also called a girth hitch). The continuous sling is wrapped around the load or the anchor, and one end of the sling is passed through the other end. As the sling is loaded with weight, it tightens down on the load or anchor. The basket sling configuration reduces the load capacity of the sling by approximately 20 percent.

BASIC EXTRICATION TOOLS

The most common extrication problem facing rescuers is a patient trapped in a vehicle after an accident. The basic principles, skills, and tools used in the extrication of a patient from an automobile may be used in other rescue situations involving entrapped patients. A discussion of the common extrication tools follows (Figure 3.25).

FIGURE 3.25

Basic Extrication Tools
Common hand tools for
extrication can be used in
auto extrication and in other
rescue situations involving
entrapped patients.

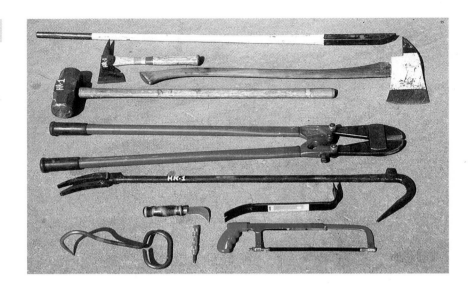

Cutting Tools

Air hammers/chisels may be used to cut sheet metal and supporting columns. The air hammer requires a compressed air source on the scene. A portable air compressor or a compressed air storage cylinder are two of the most common sources of compressed air used at extrication scenes.

Hydraulic shears permit fast cuts of supporting columns using the hydraulic power from pumps that may be manually activated or powered by a gasoline or electric motor. Extreme caution must be used to protect both the patient and rescuers from exposure to leaking hydraulic fluid, which is extremely corrosive. Use goggles or a full face shield to protect the eyes whenever hydraulic equipment is being used. Wear gloves to protect the skin, and cover the patient with a protective blanket.

The **electric** or **hydraulic saws-all** may be used to cut sheet metal and supporting columns. However, it requires an electric generator on the scene, and there is a risk of fire from sparking. **High-speed circular saws,** normally powered by a gasoline engine, are also capable of cutting sheet metal and heavier supporting columns. Again, the risk of fire and explosion from the sparks created must be a consideration.

Cutting torches, usually oxygen/acetylene, allow the rescuer to cut through heavy metal components, including vehicle frames. In addition to the considerable risk of fire and explosion, there is the potential for burning the patient from the heat generated during the cutting process. *Cutting torches should be used only when there is no other alternative.*

Spreading Tools

Hydraulic oil under pressure from a pump is used to power many spreading tools used in extrication. Small hydraulic spreading tools often require only a hand-operated pump to generate spreading forces in excess of 2,000 pounds. Larger hydraulic spreading tools utilize hydraulic pumps that are powered by gasoline, diesel, or electric motors. The larger power hydraulic tools generate spreading forces that are 6 to 10 times higher than those obtained from the smaller hand pump spreaders.

Air and hydraulic powered rams (tools with a piston that extends and pushes) are also frequently used to help extricate subjects. The pushing/spreading effect of the ram helps to stabilize or move objects. The portable rams frequently used in extrication generate pushing forces from 8,000 to 40,000 pounds.

Lifting Tools

A good choice for lifting objects during an extrication is the air bag. There are low-, medium-, and high-pressure types of air bags used in extrication. All air bags require a source of air pressure at the rescue scene. An air bag system should also include air pressure regulators, an air directional control valve (air into or out of the air bag), and a pressure relief valve.

Low-pressure air bags use less than 7 psi to obtain lifting capacities of 6,000 to 24,000 pounds. Medium-pressure air bags require less than 14 psi to lift from 6,000 to 34,000 pounds. High-pressure bags have lifting capacities from under 6,000 pounds to over 100,000 pounds. High-pressure air bags generally have a maximum working pressure of approximately 110 psi.

Pulling Tools

A **come-along** is a manually-powered tool with continuous pulling capability. It normally has a cable, a pulley, and a break-away handle. A come-along requires chains or other devices to anchor it to the vehicle. Most come-alongs can generate 4,000 pounds of pulling force.

Hydraulic-powered rams and spreaders may be used for pulling when anchored and attached with chains to a vehicle or other stable anchor point.

Vehicle Stabilization Tools

If there is a danger of a vehicle rolling, wooden cribbing or blocks should be placed to block the wheels. Wooden cribbing is also used to extend the base of support of the vehicle if it is unstable or is standing on uneven ground. In addition, cribbing may be used to build a force point against which a ram or spreader may apply its force.

Other stabilizing tools include ropes, cables, and chains, which restrict movement of the vehicle and broaden the base. Some rescue vehicles are equipped with special hooks to allow rapid attachment of these stabilizers.

WATER TOOLS AND WATER TECHNIQUES

Swimming rescues should be attempted only by trained and experienced rescuers with proper equipment. The water environment presents the challenges of complicated rescues and danger for rescuers. Rapidly changing weather conditions, for example, can add significant difficulties and risks to water rescue situations.

Waves, swift currents, runoff, and pollution may increase the water **turbidity** and decrease visibility. Low visibility may hide submerged objects, posing a hazard to swimmers, SCUBA divers, and rescue personnel. In addition, increasing numbers of rescue situations occur in bodies of water contaminated with infectious or toxic agents. Such situations require special techniques, equipment, and training to avoid injury or illness to the rescuer.

The **heaving line technique** uses a coiled buoyant line with a flotation weight on the end. Holding half of the coil in each hand, throw the weighted end underhand allowing the line to fall within reach over the victim's shoulder. The onshore/onboard end of the coil is paid out as the weighted end is thrown. The victim is then drawn to you (Figure 3.26).

A water **rescue throw bag** contains a line inside a floating stuff sack. Pull four to six feet slack line from the bag. Hold onto the slack end of the line but never attach it to your body. Throw the bag within reach over the victim's shoulder. Pull the victim to shore (Figure 3.27). Do not restuff the bag if you miss. The water in the retrieve bag adds weight for additional throws. The flotation in the bag is not sufficient to support a person.

A **ring buoy** with an attached line is grasped in the rescuer's hand like a big book. Holding onto the slack end of the line, throw the

FIGURE 3.26

Heaving Line Sequence
The heaving line technique uses a coiled buoyant line with a flotation weight on the end. While you hold half of the coil in each hand, throw the weighted end underhand to allow the line to fall within the victim's reach.

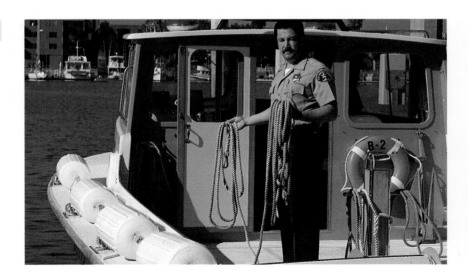

FIGURE 3.27

Throw Bag Sequence
The rescue throw bag contains a buoyant line inside a floating stuff sack. Pull four to six feet from the bag and hold onto the slack end of the line. Throw the bag within reach over the victim's shoulder.

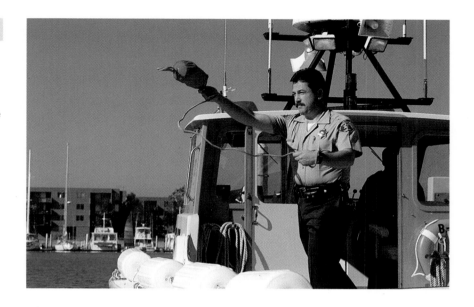

FIGURE 3.28

Ring Bouy
Holding onto the slack end of the line, throw the ring buoy underhand slightly beyond the victim, and pull it toward the victim.

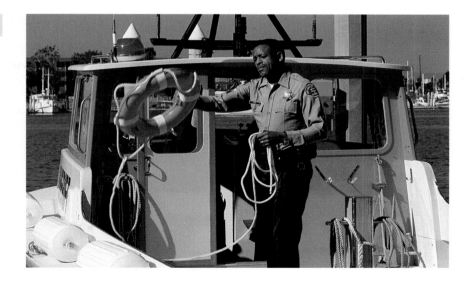

buoy underhand slightly beyond the victim, allowing for wind and current influences on the buoy. Pull the buoy toward the victim. When the victim grasps the buoy, draw the victim to shore (Figure 3.28).

These techniques assume the patient is responsive and within reach of these techniques.

You may employ **boat-assisted rescue** techniques if you cannot talk the patient into self-rescue or retrieve them by shore-based techniques. Operators of rescue boats require special training in navigation and boat handling in order to keep their boats away from hazardous areas such as strainers, eddies, jetties, docks, beaches, sandbars, boils, or dams. Although rescue boats may be effective in delivering lines, ring buoys, or throw bags to a victim, the churning propellers or possible collision present hazards to patients in the water. Furthermore, occupants of rescue boats risk capsizing or ejection in rough water.

Special Patient Treatment and Packaging Considerations

After reaching a patient in the water, you then follow standard spinal immobilization guidelines. A cervical collar or rigid neck splint is applied. Assistants submerge a backboard or semi-rigid immobilizing device under the patient and gently float it up beneath the patient. The immobilization device is centered in line with the patient's spine. The patient is then secured to the device and removed from the water. Check vital signs and neurological status regularly throughout the extrication process. The secondary patient assessment continues throughout the removal process.

There are several ways to assist a conscious, but fatigued patient onto a vessel. Before using either technique, place a personal flotation device (PFD) on the patient.

In the **stirrup technique,** loop a line or webbing over the side of the vessel to hang in the water. Secure both ends to a stable structure inside the vessel (Figure 3.29). Help the patient step into the loop, then swing the free leg up and into the vessel.

FIGURE 3.29

Assisting Patient Using Stirrup Method
The stirrup technique can be used to bring aboard a patient who is able to assist himself.

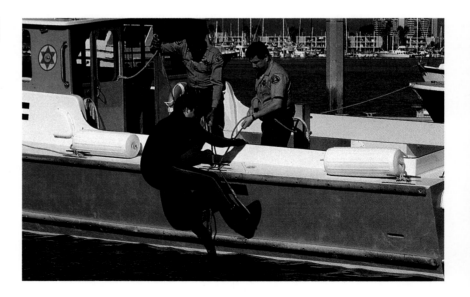

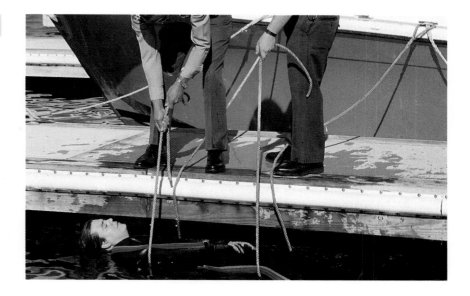

FIGURE 3.30

Assisting Patient with Roll Aboard Technique
The roll aboard technique can be used to bring aboard a patient who is conscious but unable to assist himself.

For the **roll aboard technique,** the patient is rolled over the side of the boat using a net or blanket (Figure 3.30). You must be certain that the top of the net or blanket is secured to a stable structure such as the gunwale edge or inside the boat. The patient is then placed in the net or blanket. Standing or kneeling in the craft, you slowly pull up on the free edge of the net or blanket to roll the patient into the boat.

If a net or blanket is not available, you can use a variation of this technique with lengths of rope or webbing. The lengths of rope or webbing are tied to stable structures inside the vessel, allowing loops to hang in the water. The loops are positioned under the patient's upper back, waist, hips, and calves, keeping the arms inside the loops. While maintaining a level position, you then pull on the loops to gently roll the patient aboard.

Ice Rescue Techniques

Basic ice rescue techniques focus on self-rescue. Team members face the same hazard as the patient. Responders develop a safe approach to the ice rescue incident by assessing ice conditions and available resources.

Emergency responders should initially try self-rescue and shore-based techniques in ice rescue. Try to direct the victim into self-rescue by having him grab a thrown rescue line. Do not use human chains that place additional stress on the irregular ice, resulting in further breakup. Human chains may result in multiple drownings. Public service organizations often place ring buoys and throw bags at popular ice recreation facilities. Rescue teams should emphasize shore-based techniques in public awareness programs.

Dry or **exposure suits** should be used for ice rescue (Figure 3.31). They are completely sealed to keep frigid water away from your body.

FIGURE 3.31

Dry Suit
Dry suits and exposure suits
are completely sealed and
insulated to keep frigid water
away from the body.

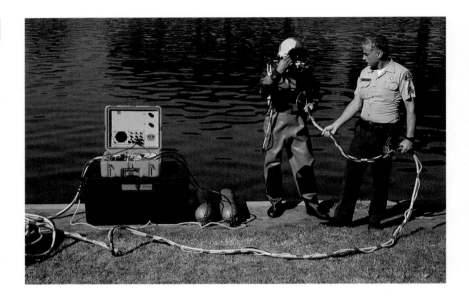

FIGURE 3.32

Ice Awls

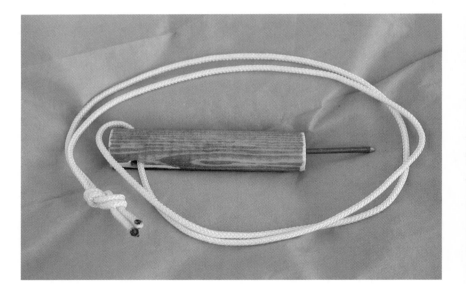

Ice awls, made of wooden dowels with a nail driven into the end,
must be carried around the neck for quick grasp in an emergency.
File the protruding end of the nail to a point. Upon breaking through
the ice, jab the ice awls into the ice surface, pull yourself out of the
hole and roll to safety (Figure 3.32).

The basic minimum equipment for an individual responding to an
ice rescue includes a dry suit, PFD, ice awls, ice staff, and an attached
safety line.

SUMMARY

Becoming knowledgeable about rescue equipment is an important priority for all rescue team members. The first step is to ensure that all equipment meets professional standards established by certain U.S. and international professional organizations.

Some of the pieces of equipment commonly used in a high angle rescue environment are litters, ropes, webbing, web slings, harnesses, and connecting hardware. Ropes and hitches are also used for belays.

Rescue rope and other equipment must have an adequate safety factor. A safety factor is the ratio of the strength of the equipment to the highest possible load factor that might occur during a rescue. For ropes, strength as well as diameter plays a part in maintaining the safety factor. All rescue equipment must be inspected thoroughly after every use for damage.

Equipment commonly used in extrication include cutting tools, spreading tools, lifting tools, pulling tools, and vehicle stabilization tools. Rescuers use air chisels, hydraulic shears, electric saws-all and cutting torches as cutting tools. Spreading tools range from simple pry bars and crowbars to hand-operated or power-assisted hydraulic spreaders and hydraulic rams. Low- and high-pressure air bags are the primary lifting tools. A come-along is a manual pulling tool, although hydraulic-powered rams and spreaders can also be used as tools for pulling. To stabilize a vehicle, use wooden cribbing, ropes, cables, and chains.

Basic tools used in water and ice rescue include personal flotation devices, safety lines, buoyant lines, rescue throw bags, ring buoys, ice awls, and ice staffs. Rescuers also use ropes, webbing, and nets to remove patients from the water.

PERSONAL SAFETY AND SURVIVAL

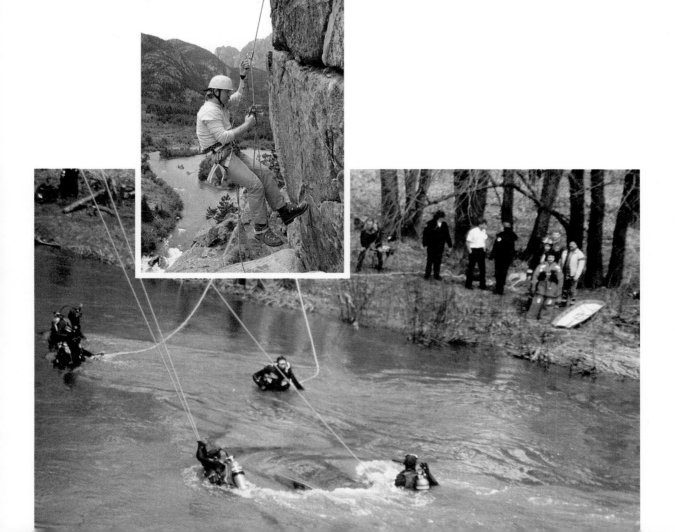

THREATS AND PREVENTION

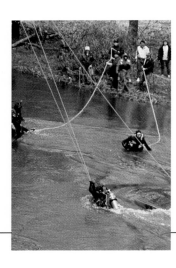

CHAPTER OUTLINE

OVERVIEW

Injuries or other hazards in emergency operations can jeopardize the successful outcome of a rescue. Therefore, the primary responsibility of members of the rescue team is to avoid injuring themselves or other rescuers while protecting the patient from injury or additional injury.

This chapter examines the various potential threats that rescuers may encounter in a rescue situation. Included are physical, medical, environmental, external, and psychological threats.

Avoiding and preventing these threats is the best means of reducing or eliminating injury or illness. This chapter offers recommendations about preventive techniques and procedures. In addition, each section outlines possible treatments and solutions for unavoidable injuries and problems.

OBJECTIVES

The objectives of this chapter are to enable the rescuer to:

- be physically prepared for rescue operations and to increase chances for survival.
- identify potential threats or hazards during a rescue operation.
- deal with unavoidable threats and problems in the rescue operation.

The primary responsibility of all members of the rescue team is to avoid injury to themselves or other rescuers while protecting the patient from additional injury. Injury, illness, stress, and the other hazards in rescues lessen the effectiveness and efficiency of rescuers in caring for their patient. Furthermore, these problems may jeopardize the rescue or result in injury or loss of life of the patient and among rescuers.

Prevention and avoidance are the best methods to reduce the risks of injury or illness during rescue operations. Knowledge and awareness of potential hazards are the tools rescue personnel use to reduce the threats inherent in rescue activities.

PHYSICAL THREATS AND SURVIVAL

Rescuers are exposed to many hazards that pose a physical threat to their survival. Different environments pose specific threats.

Obviously, one of the greatest physical threats is the contamination of the atmosphere leading to the inability to breathe in a safe atmosphere.

Another threat is a change in temperature. The human body functions efficiently within a narrow temperature range. When outside of buildings or vehicles, you must depend on clothing for protection from extremes of heat (sun and exertion) and cold (cold, wind, and precipitation). If you are on an extended operation, you should also carry a personal kit of essentials for survival in case of an emergency (See Chapter 2).

Hydration

Adequate fluid intake or **hydration** is important for proper functioning of the human body. In many environments dehydration is a common problem for both rescuers and patients. The environment does not have to be dry to cause this problem. Because the body is composed mostly of water, maintaining a high level of fluid intake is essential for efficiency and survival.

When persons leave their usual environment, they often fail to maintain an adequate fluid intake. This is a particular problem in cold environments, where drinking cold liquids is not appealing. Most active persons in high country or arid environments are dehydrated to begin with, and their efficiency is often diminished. Dehydration is a condition that will be present in all backcountry patients. Fluids are lost more rapidly with greater altitude and decreased humidity in the air.

The simplest way to replenish fluids is by drinking them. Any nonalcohol, noncaffeinated fluid is suitable. Water is the fluid most often available. It is absorbed faster by the body than any other fluid. Avoid fluids with high sugar and carbohydrate levels. They can actually slow the absorption rate and cause stomach discomfort and vomiting.

One convenient indicator of hydration is urination. Infrequent urination or urine that has a deep yellow color is an indication of dehydration. You should keep your fluid intake at a level that keeps your urine appearing clear or a light yellow color.

Nutrition

For its most efficient functioning the human body must have adequate nutrition. Food is the fuel on which the body runs. If you do not have a ready source of fuel, your performance will be impaired, which could endanger yourself, the patient, or your colleagues. The physical exertion and physical stress of rescue require a high energy output. You must have a ready supply of energy, otherwise you may weaken physically, lack coordination, and become irritable. You may also be more susceptible to such problems as hypothermia.

On the other hand, overeating may reduce physical and mental performance. After a large meal, blood required by the digestive process is unavailable for other body activities.

Simple carbohydrates such as the sugars found in candy and soft drinks are the foods most quickly absorbed by the body system and converted to fuel. But sugars also stimulate the body's production of insulin, which reduces blood sugar levels. For some people an abundance of sugar can actually result in lower energy levels. The body's need for sugar and the reaction to it varies depending on the individual.

Next in terms of energy production are complex carbohydrates. Some of these take hours to convert into usable fuel, but nutrition studies indicate that complex carbohydrates are among the safest, most reliable sources for long-term energy production during exertion. Some complex carbohydrates include rice, pasta, fruits, and vegetables.

After simple and complex carbohydrates, fats are the foods most easily converted to energy. Some fats are tasty and satisfying, particularly in cold environments, but the overuse of fats particularly by sedentary persons can lead to long-term health problems such as cardiac disease and obesity. Typical fats include butter, lard, chocolate, and sausages.

Proteins may satisfy the appetite but take several hours to convert to energy. Some proteins are meat, fish, chicken, beans, and cheese. Furthermore, at higher altitudes, the body has difficulty utilizing proteins and fats.

You should carry an individual supply of high energy food to help maintain energy levels. Several small meals throughout the day usually are more effective than a few large meals for keeping the body's energy resources at constant high levels.

Exercise

Every rescuer should participate in a regular program of exercise. Physical conditioning enables you to postpone dangerous exhaustion and enables the body to use body fuel efficiently to produce energy. The result is a well-conditioned rescuer who is better prepared to cope with the physical and mental stress encountered during a rescue.

MEDICAL THREATS AND SURVIVAL

Many medical threats encountered by rescuers are linked to pre-existing conditions. Whenever rescuers have a known medical problem, they should not participate in field activities where they could become a patient and an additional burden on other rescuers.

In addition to conditions that are already present, such as heart disease, diabetes, and so forth, rescuers face short-term medical threats that may develop during the rescue and become debilitating.

Many of these problems encountered by rescuers (headaches, mild stomach disorders, minor cuts, and scrapes) are annoyances rather than medical emergencies. To cope with these annoyances, you should carry a personal first aid kit. Pre-made kits are generally less versatile. The following is an example personal aid kit that can be packed into a plastic refrigerator box, sized approximately 12 × 12 × 3 inches (Figure 4.1).

Personal First Aid Kit

Case:
   Durable in temperature extremes
   Water- and dust-tight
   Sized to meet personal needs

Contents:
   Scissors
   Tweezers
   Hypothermia thermometer (reads down to 85° F)
   Over-the-counter pain medication
   Over-the-counter antihistamine
   Antacids
   Diarrhea medication
   Antibiotic ointment (such as mycin family or triple antibiotic)
   Sunburn cream
   Lip treatment
   Sunblock (SP15 or higher)
   Adhesive tape, one-inch cloth
   Roller gauze, two-inch
   Roller gauze, four-inch
   ABD Pad
   4 × 4s, sterile
   Non-adhering dressing
   Adhesive bandages
   Sewing kit (safety pins, needle, and thread)
   Soap
   Alcohol preps
   Acetone preps
   Cotton swabs
   Tongue blades
   Moleskin
   Disposable gloves
   Personal items (as needed)
   Prescription medications
   Eye care
   Allergy kit
   Water purification tablets or filter

FIGURE 4.1

Personal First Aid Kit
A personal first aid kit can
help rescuers cope with
minor medical annoyances.

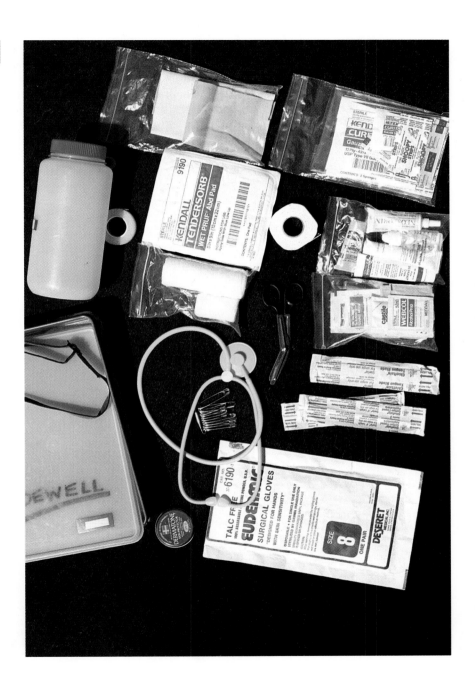

On some extended operations, some conditions require more than
simple first aid. Intestinal disorders may be the result of one of several
causes.

Acute gastroenteritis, also known by its common name, "stomach flu," is usually self-limiting. Though the person may be in discomfort while it runs its course, there are generally no long-term

effects. **Staphylococcal enteritis,** or "food poisoning" is the result of eating foods that typically require refrigeration, such as those made from mayonnaise, milk, and meat. It, too, is usually self-limiting.

Traveller's diarrhea is the result of fecal contamination of water or food. The culprit is one of the strains of *E. coli* bacteria. It is best prevented by careful sanitary practices, particularly when treating drinking water and preparing food. If prevention fails, an antibiotic may be required.

Giardia lamblia is a parasite that has increasingly infested water supplies, particularly mountain streams that appear pure. *Giardia* can be found in very cold, even ice-covered streams. Its mode of infection is through an extremely hardy cyst form that can live for months before activation through ingestion into the digestive tract. It may be two weeks or more before symptoms, which may be very debilitating, appear. It is usually characterized by sulfurous belching, foul-smelling flatulence, and severe diarrhea and cramping. It is usually treated by a prescription medicine such as metronidazole (Flagyl).

Waterborne contaminants, such as *Giardia* and *E. coli,* can be avoided by proper treatment of the water through one of three techniques:

- Boiling. Boiling water for 30 seconds at sea level is usually sufficient to kill bacterial and parasitic contaminants, even the hardy *Giardia* cysts. Since water boils at lower temperatures at higher altitudes, boil water for an additional 30 seconds for each additional 1,000 feet above sea level.
- Filtration. The filter openings must not be larger than 0.45 microns and must be used according to manufacturer's directions to safely filter the infectious *Giardia* cyst stage (Figure 4.2).

FIGURE 4.2

Water Filtration
Some waterborne contaminants can be avoided with proper use of a portable water filter.

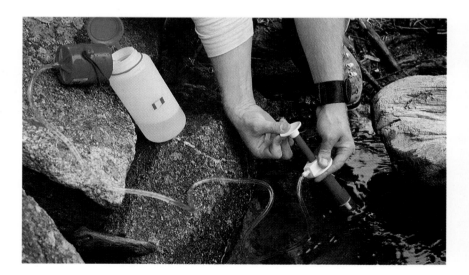

- Iodine. Iodine treatment will kill most contaminants when properly used in water. Iodine-treated water should be used only by healthy individuals who are known to have no reaction to iodine. It should not be given to pregnant or nursing mothers and should not be given to the rescuers' patients. One convenient form of iodine treatment is commercially available iodine tablets. Follow the manufacturer's instructions for the use of iodine tablets. The strength of solution and treatment time will vary depending on such factors as the temperature of the water and suspended solids.

ENVIRONMENTAL THREATS AND SURVIVAL

Weather is a prime concern for rescuers in any outdoor environment. Primary weather concerns will be exposure to cold, wet, and heat. However, temperature extremes may be a threat in any environment in which the temperature is not controlled. The human body works well only within a narrow temperature range, around 98.6° F (37.0° C). The difference of only a few degrees in the body core temperature causes body malfunction in terms of thinking, judgment, and coordination. Extremes in temperature cause brain dysfunction and reduce the likelihood of correct choices being made for necessary survival functions such as putting on or taking off clothing or seeking shelter. As the temperature continues to move away from the normal range, either up or down, there will be increasing dysfunction and possible unconsciousness. Unless this trend is interrupted, death may follow. Rescuers must continually monitor each other and their patients for dangerous temperature changes and to provide protection against temperature extremes.

Hyperthermia

Exposure to heat without proper protection that increases body temperatures above normal is known as **hyperthermia.** The human body can endure overheating even less than it can cooling. **Heat exhaustion** is the first indication that the body is being overheated. Heat exhaustion develops when the body loses excessive water and minerals called electrolytes through perspiration. The result is a mild **hypovolemic shock.** "Hypovolemic" refers to a reduction in blood volume caused by the loss of fluid from the body. To prevent heat exhaustion, shield yourself from the sun and other heat sources, maintain adequate fluid intake and reduce excessive perspiration. If you are in a hot environment or involved in a high exertion activity you should vent or remove some clothing *before* perspiration begins. You must also monitor your patients to ensure they do not become overheated by blankets and other protection.

If untreated, heat exhaustion may progress to **heat stroke,** a serious illness that results when the body is subjected to more heat than it can handle. Because the sweating mechanism has been overwhelmed, heat stroke victims do not perspire. They have hot, dry, flushed skin. Heat stroke is a life-threatening emergency. If untreated, it will result in death. To avoid tissue damage or death, cool the heat stroke patient immediately by any means available. Remove clothing and cool the patient by wet towels or sheets or immersion in water.

To avoid hyperthermia, you must wear proper clothing, vent heat away from your body, use shelter to protect yourself from heat sources such as the sun, and consume adequate fluids.

Hypothermia

Exposure to cold without proper protection may result in a potentially dangerous lowering of the body's core temperature known as **hypothermia.** It is particularly dangerous since the body's neurologic and psychologic systems do not function well at lower temperatures. Mental processes are affected, which endangers a person's ability to care for himself or herself. Because it may come on slowly in a very subtle way, you may not notice the onset of hypothermia in yourself.

Shivering occurs only during the initial stage of chilling. As body temperature drops further, the shivering ceases. The body is no longer able to create heat. The patient enters a dangerous stage of hypothermia. Lowering the temperature just a few degrees will result in loss of coordination and mental function. Below 95° F, the body enters a dangerous stage of hypothermia in which the individual may not be able to care for himself or herself. Below 90° F, the person usually lapses into unconsciousness (severe hypothermia). Unless the cooling process is reversed, the process usually ends in death. Protection from hypothermia includes adequate clothing, shelter, and nutrition.

Measuring body temperature in patients with hypothermia requires a special thermometer. The thermometers normally used for measuring body temperatures do not have reading points low enough to use in patients with severe hypothermia. To measure the temperature of hypothermic patients, you must use a *low reading* or *subnormal thermometers* that read down to at least 85° F.

See Chapter 16 for more information on hypothermia, hyperthermia, and heat exhaustion.

Frostbite

Frostbite is the freezing of body tissue. The most susceptible areas are the feet, particularly the toes, and the hands, particularly the fingers (Figure 4.3). Portions of the face, such as the ears and the nose, can also be frostbitten. Frostbite frequently develops because of exposure to chilling winds or water. It is often the result of inadequate foot- or handwear. Boots that may provide adequate protection may, if improperly fitted, also constrict circulation and lead to frostbite.

Another contributing factor is body temperature. As the body cools, circulation to the extremities is reduced to conserve warmth for the body core—the brain, heart, and lungs. But frostbite can also quickly develop by contact with cold metal on equipment or vehicles or by spilling cooled liquids such as gasoline. Anyone whose circulation has been compromised through a medical condition such as

FIGURE 4.3

Frostbitten Fingers
The toes and fingers are
among the areas of the body
most susceptible to frostbite.

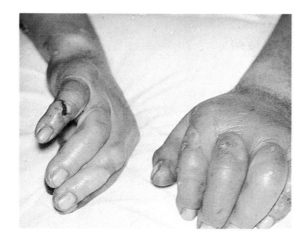

hypothermia or injury to an extremity is particularly susceptible to
frostbite.

Wind Chill

At lower temperatures, winds intensify chilling (Table 4.1). If there
is a combination of low temperatures and high winds, you must protect yourself and your patients from the danger of wind chill. You
should take particular precautions to protect exposed flesh from
frostbite.

TABLE 4.1   Wind Chill Chart

Temperature (F°)	Wind Speed (mph)							
	5	10	15	20	25	30	35	40
35	32	22	16	12	8	6	4	3
30	27	16	9	4	1	−2	−4	−5
25	22	10	2	−3	−7	−10	−12	−13
20	16	3	−5	−10	−15	−18	−20	−21
15	11	−3	−11	−17	−22	−25	−27	−29
10	6	−9	−18	−24	−29	−33	−35	−37
5	0	−15	−25	−31	−36	−41	−43	−45
0	−5	−22	−31	−39	−44	−49	−52	−53
−5	−10	−27	−38	−46	−51	−56	−58	−60
−10	−15	−34	−45	−53	−59	−64	−67	−69
−15	−21	−40	−51	−60	−66	−71	−74	−76
−20	−26	−46	−58	−67	−74	−79	−82	−84
−25	−31	−52	−65	−74	−81	−86	−89	−92
−30	−36	−58	−72	−81	−88	−93	−97	−100
−35	−42	−64	−78	−88	−96	−101	−105	−107
−40	−47	−71	−85	−95	−103	−109	−113	−115

Source: United States National Weather Service.

EXTERNAL THREATS AND SURVIVAL

Terrain

In many rescue environments, the location and terrain become a major obstacle to completing the mission. In some areas, the actual distances involved will be the concern. In some remote areas without roads, where foot travel is the only means of access, it may take several hours just to reach a rescue site. This means that you will have to carry everything you may need in with you. This may become a real test of endurance, particularly for those who are not in good physical condition.

Rugged terrain may complicate events further. In some areas, the difficulty of navigating the terrain will increase the difficulty and travel time. Such areas include boulder fields in mountainous areas, areas of fallen timber, and water hazards.

Potential of Falling

Where there is the potential for you or your patient to fall, preventive measures must be taken. **Exposure** refers to the danger of a fall that could result in injury or death. Wherever there is exposure, you and your patient must be protected.

If there is danger of falling, among your first actions at the scene should be to place a barrier line to prevent access to the edge. This should apply not only to onlookers but also to rescuers who have no reason for being at the edge. You should immediately establish **safety lines** and anchor them securely. Anyone who works at the edge must wear appropriate safety equipment.

When sufficient personnel are available, a designated safety officer oversees operations involving exposure to ensure that safety rules are followed. If there are not enough personnel available, then one of the rescue leaders must take on the additional duties of safety officer.

To **belay** a person is to attach a safety, or belay, rope and control the rope so that if the person starts to fall, the belay rope catches him or her. In most cases, the belay rope is controlled by a second person known as the belayer.

A belay is needed anytime you or a patient is at risk of falling. A patient in a litter must always be belayed where there is exposure during rescue operations such as litter lowering or raising. Your need for a belay may depend on the particular situation. But if you feel the need for a belay, ask for one. It should always be provided.

Unstable Surfaces

An unstable surface is any surface that must be negotiated where there is potential for a fall or loss of control.

The two distinct groups of unstable surfaces are natural and man-made. Natural unstable footing surfaces include creek beds, river rocks, cave surfaces, animal wastes, rotting vegetation, loose gravel, and ice. Some examples of man-made unstable surfaces include chemical spills, auto accidents, chemical reaction vessels, tank cars, large metal, plastic, or glass surfaces, animal processing factories, cooling systems, and coal slurry or grain storage facilities.

The best method of protecting yourself and your patients from the hazards of unstable footing is to be aware of the potential for mishap. The most common unstable surface mishap occurs when the rescuer slips and falls, sometimes creating an on-scene injury. The second common mishap occurs when the surface on which the rescuer is standing collapses under his or her body weight.

When planning for a stable access to the patient(s), remember that the overall safety of yourself and the patient is the prime consideration. First, develop an escape plan complete with standby gear (ladder trucks, ropes, boats, or whatever will be necessary). Have a backup crew dressed in the appropriate gear ready to take action. Whenever the possibility of a fall, collapse, or serious slide is present, have any rescuers and, when possible, patients that are on the unstable surface don a harness that is attached to a lifeline secured to a bombproof anchor.

Heavy, cleated hiking boots and structural fire fighting boots work well when you must walk over very rough and agitated surfaces. However, they can be extremely slippery when used on very smooth and wet or frozen surfaces, like the inside of glass or stainless steel tanks or reaction vessels. Consider using a good pair of heavy-duty *crampons,* spiked metal plates for the feet, on ice, mud, stainless steel chemical reaction vessels, tanks, mold-covered rock, or other hard surfaces that have a slippery covering. However, never use any steel-cleated shoes or crampons around flammable liquids that could be susceptible to a flash fire caused by sparks.

On some smooth surfaces, where an injury to the foot is not likely, the rescuer can increase the amount of friction by using smooth, soft rubber-soled shoes like tennis shoes. This works well on many wet, semi-smooth concrete surfaces.

The other method of increasing friction is to remove or alter the slippery surface as much possible. This may be as simple as washing down the surface to remove the mud, oil, fire-fighting foam, or other substance. Bulky substances can be shoveled or hauled away to help remove them from the area around a patient.

On occasions where a thin layer of ice has covered a hard surface, sodium chloride (table salt) or potassium chloride (road salt) can be sprinkled around the area. Most houses have at least a one pound container of salt that can melt a considerable amount of ice. However, when temperatures are below 10° F, chemical melting does not work well. Other items that work well on ice are poultry grit and sand.

There are chemical removing agents that can absorb a tremendous amount of moisture when sprinkled around a slippery area. These can be employed successfully when used by a person that has been trained in their application.

When the combination of the angle and the slipperiness of the surface to be traversed becomes too great for safe patient transport, a belay system must be employed.

The second common unstable surface does not have the strength necessary to support the weight of the rescuer or the combination of the rescuers, the equipment, the patients, and any associated debris. In this situation the pounds per square inch tolerance (psit) of the surface is less than the pounds per square inch (psi) of the weight of the rescuers.

Place or build a covering around the scene of the accident or evacuation site to lift the rescuers over the top of the unstable surface. On very loose materials like coal slurry or grain, place a large steel barrel over top of the patient (Figure 4.4). This protects the patient from further engulfment and helps to stabilize the surrounding area until the material can be removed sufficiently to gain access.

Grain storage facilities can also have unstable footing surfaces. Before entering the hazardous confines of a grain storage facility to search for a patient, consider passive removal of the grain. One method involves cutting large inverted Vs around the container. The inverted pattern will allow completion of the cut before the grain starts to pour out. When the cuts are completed, bend down the opening and allow the grain to pour out. Never use spark or flame-producing equipment to make cuts in grain storage facilities. Most pneumatic cutters will make short work of the cut.

When left standing for several months stored grain can develop a surface crust. This crust may remain in place above a void and a farmer or rescuer might mistake it for the top of a firm pile of grain, break through, and be engulfed by the grain.

Manure ponds and some chemical tanks may also have a crust that forms on top of the liquid surface. It is best to use a boat or similar

FIGURE 4.4

Large Steel Barrel Placed on Top of Patient
In very loose material, a large steel barrel placed over a patient can protect from further engulfment and stabilize the area for rescue.

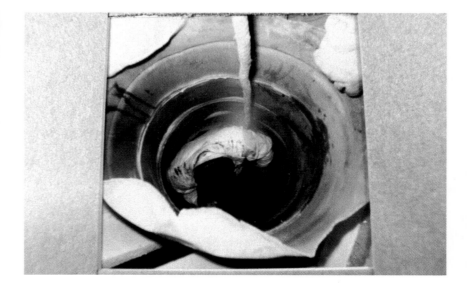

flotation device to gain patient access, regardless of how strong the crust appears.

Any questionable, untested surface must be assumed to be hazardous. Never stand alone and unsupported on top of any grain, coal, pea gravel, or similar type product. Always use a lifeline when involved in rescue on any unstable product substance. A lifeline may be also used to locate the person tied to it in the event of a secondary collapse of the substance. Always attach a lifeline to all rescuers and all patients as soon as possible. In a grain or coal slurry, a moving person will continue to sink, with movement, until supported from above. This support may be provided by placing plywood sheets on the product to distribute the patient's weight, supplemented by a rope in a haul and belay system secured from above.

Dilapidated structures of rotting wood or rusting steel may also provide a less than adequate surface on which to walk or work. If the stability of the structure appears too flimsy to walk on, use an alternate means of patient access, such as a fire department's aerial apparatus or a rope system. In circumstances where the structure is reasonably sound but the flooring unsafe, covering the old surface with plywood or ladders can spread out the weight of the rescuers enough to ensure a safe access.

In cold weather, or at higher altitudes, snow and ice can impede progress. In deeper snow, rescuers on foot may flounder unless they are traveling on skis or snowshoes. Traveling cross-country on skis requires skills and experience that cannot be gained the first time out. Snowshoes do not require the high degree of proficiency of skiing, but they do require some practice and a higher energy expenditure.

Steep slopes of hard-packed snow or ice require specialized climbing equipment and the skills and experience in using them.

Electrical Shock

Electrical shock can occur from two different sources: man-made or lightning. Both situations require evaluating the risks to the rescuers and to the patient. The level of skill of rescuers is the number one factor affecting the outcome in dealing with the victim of an electrical accident.

Man-Made Emergencies The severity of man-made electrical emergencies varies greatly and depends on the current involved. The local power company is the best available resource for in-service education on evaluating the risks and learning how to deal with electric lines once the risk has been identified. Rescue personnel should not attempt to deal with downed electric lines except to establish a danger zone around the downed wires.

Three common electrical measurements are voltage, resistance, and amperage. *Voltage* is a measure of the force of electricity as it travels along its path. The concept is similiar to the measurement of water pressure (pounds per square inch, or psi, in a pipe). A pathway's *resistance* to the flow of electricity is measured in ohms. A large overhead transmission line has little resistance to electricity, while a small wire has a lot. *Amperage* is a measure of the amount of electricity flowing along a path. The concept is similar to gallons per minute that flow through a pipe. Amperage, not voltage, causes damage to the human body.

Dealing with power lines is beyond the scope of most rescuers. The equipment that is necessary to deal adequately with electrical emergencies and provide personal protection requires in-depth training and specific storage and cleaning requirements. Simple deposits of dirt or other contaminants can render safety equipment, such as hot sticks, unusable and cause injury to the rescuers.

The moving of a downed power line has enormous potential danger. Energized power lines, particularly those carrying high voltage, behave in unpredictable ways. Lines carrying high wattage may arc and whip when attracted to a good conductor, like a rescuer or patient. Wires may also curl up unexpectedly.

Lightning Lightning is a complex natural phenomenon. When conditions are just right, a lightning strike will occur. Thus, it can be a fatal mistake to assume that "lightning will not strike in the same place twice." If a lightning strike has happened, the right conditions remain, and a repeat strike in the same area may occur.

If you are in the mountains and a thunderstorm approaches, move down from ridge lines and peaks as soon as possible. Make a safe camp, and suspend rescue action until after the storm has passed. There are warning signs that occur just before a strike. As the area of an impending strike becomes charged, you may feel a slight tingling sensation in your skin. Your hair may begin to stand on end. If this occurs, a potential strike is imminent. You must seek the lowest possible area. To avoid being hit by the initial strike, avoid projections such as lone trees. Avoid metal fences since they can transmit current from the initial strike for long distances. Drop all equipment, particularly metal items, that project above your body. The interior of vehicles are usually good protection from lightning. Continuing the rescue procedure in a charged environment may result in injury to the rescuers or further injury to the patient.

Lightning is a threat in two ways: a direct hit by the initial strike or by ground current. After the lightning bolt hits, the current drains along the earth, following the most conductive path. To avoid this ground current, stay away from drainage ditches, moist areas, small depressions, and wet ropes. The mouths of caves and overhangs may not offer ground current protection, since the charge may pass through a person's body as it crosses the opening.

Lightning will pass through the body along the path of least resistance. It may affect the body organs through which it passes. If the current passes from a hand to a foot, or from one hand to another, it might injure some of the most vital organs. A rescuer caught out in the open should present the smallest target both for the initial strike and the ground current. One of the least vulnerable positions is low crouch. This exposes only the feet to the current, while sitting on the ground would expose both feet and buttocks. To be in a low crouch on a nonconductive material such as a pack or sleeping bag would be even better.

Injury and illnesses resulting from electrical shock vary greatly and are a real test of a rescuer's medical knowledge. Burns may be the most obvious injury, though not always readily apparent. Other traumatic and internal injuries that may go unnoticed routinely accompany even minor electrical injuries. A thorough, in-depth patient examination is necessary to evaluate all existing injuries. How the injury occurred is of key importance in evaluating other potential injuries.

Falling Objects

In any high angle environment, there is danger to both patient and rescuers from falling objects, both tools or rocks. The **fall zone** is the area where rescuers are most likely to encounter falling objects. In backcountry, high angle or high altitude areas, fall zones include gullies, washes, and runs. In these areas, a person is at risk of being hit as falling rocks are funneled.

To reduce the risk of falling objects, you should immediately establish control of the area above the rescue site and forbid the entrance of any unauthorized persons. If it is necessary for you to travel up and down the slope or the face of a building, then you should establish a rappel/ascent line or safety line, depending on the angle of the slope to the side of the rescue site. Moving this line away from above the rescue site helps prevent rescuers traveling up and down from dislodging any material directly onto the patient or rescuers working below.

Running ropes may dislodge objects. Any rescue ropes should be rigged off to the side of the patient so they do not dislodge rocks or other objects. If there is the danger of falling objects, then the patient must be protected with a backboard or other hard shield.

During evacuations from the backcountry, high angle, or high altitude environment, the patient is often strapped down in a litter or stretcher. This means that he or she is unable to avoid falling objects, brush or tree limbs, rain, or building materials. Patients in litters must be protected with goggles, face shields, or litter shields.

In the high angle environment there is the risk of being hit not only by falling objects but also falling *people.* There is the possibility that a person above the rescue scene may slip and fall on those below. Therefore, when traveling up any incline, it is best not to travel one directly behind another.

Communications about falling objects must be quick and absolute. There must be no time lag in communicating the danger, nor any doubt about what is being said. In the high angle environment, a few standardized words are used to warn of falling objects. When anything hard (rock, hardware) falls, the warning word is *"rock!"* It must be shouted by whoever sees it first. It must be loud and distinct so that everyone hears the warning. If you are in the fall zone you should *not* look up, for you may well receive the object in the face. You should shield yourself and your patient as best as possible. Position yourself so that your helmet protects against the falling object and your body is as small a target as possible.

If the falling object is soft (rope, webbing, clothing), then the warning call is *"rope!"*

If the potential exists for falling objects to fall on the rescue site unseen, then a safety observer should be stationed to warn of any danger. If rescuers need to pass through an area that is prone to falling objects, scouts can "clean" the area with a deliberate dislodge before the rescue operation reaches the area.

Any time that you come into an area prone to falling rocks or other debris, you should immediately identify *escape routes* before tending to the patient. An escape route may not necessarily be completely out of the danger area, but it should be away from the fall zone.

Flying objects present a similar risk in operations using power extrication equipment, for example, metal fragments broken loose and thrown by a hydraulic spreader. You should take similar protective measures in such situations.

Avalanches

Thousands of avalanches take place in mountainous terrain each year. They can destroy a rescue party, but knowledge about the formation and behavior of avalanches can help you avoid being caught in an avalanche or save lives if caught.

Most avalanches occur during and shortly after storms because the weight of snow exceeds its adhesion to the surface of a slope. Many factors affect the creation and release of avalanches, including the incline of the slope, the direction the slope faces, the depth and type of snow, and the temperature.

The greatest avalanche danger is on slopes of 30 to 45 degrees, but they may also occur on slopes from 25 to 60 degrees. North-facing slopes are more likely to avalanche in midwinter, while south-facing slopes are more likely to slide on warm, spring days. Avalanches usually do not start where the snow is secured, such as in thick timber or boulder fields. However, slides may occur above these areas and overrun them.

Avalanches commonly follow natural chutes such as gullies. Broad, flat valleys are often safe zones, but large avalanches have been known to cross valleys and go up a distance on the opposite slope.

The science of snow conditions that lead to avalances is very complex, but some conditions typically lead to avalanches. Most avalanches occur during and shortly after heavy snowfall. They also tend to occur when the surface of old snow forms a poor bond with new snow.

Death in an avalanche is usually due to suffocation, so speed is essential in uncovering an avalanche victim (Figure 4.5). However, a person caught in an avalanche is likely to be swept some distance away, so it is difficult to know where or how deep a person is buried. The most commonly used device for locating an avalanche victim is

FIGURE 4.5

Avalanche
Death in an avalanche is usually due to suffocation, so speed is essential in uncovering an avalanche victim.

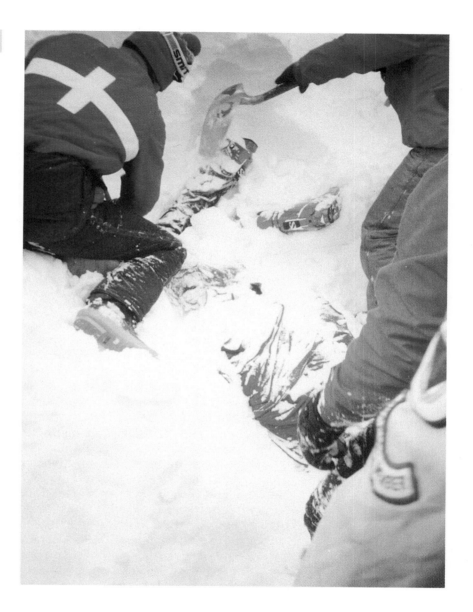

the **avalanche beacon** or **transceiver**. The avalanche beacon is a small battery-powered radio device that can transmit or receive a signal on 2275KHz.

Each person in avalanche country carries a transceiver that is switched to "transmit." If that person is buried by an avalanche, the rescuers switch their beacons to "receive" to home in on the patient. It is critical that users of avalanche beacons practice with each other to develop the skills necessary to use the device to find buried patients quickly.

In avalanche-prone areas, rescuers should cross danger slopes one at a time, trailing an avalanche cord or with their avalanche beacons switched to "transmit." If caught as an avalanche appears to be starting, do not try to outrun an avalanche but try for the nearest safe side. If caught in an avalanche, attempt to remain on the surface, moving as though swimming on your back.

Crevasse

A **crevasse** is in essence a large crack in a glacier. In glacier travel, crevasses are a great danger. You can easily fall into them, particularly since crevasses are often hidden by a snow bridge. Because the risk of falling into a crevasse is so great, all travel on glaciers should be done only by appropriately trained and equipped rescuers.

PSYCHOLOGICAL THREATS AND SURVIVAL

The psychological threats to rescuers include those common to emergency response personnel, such as stress. However, there are others that may relate to environment.

Fear of heights may occur in rescuers in the high angle or mountainous environment. This fear can only be moderated by experience in high places, for example, through group practice.

Claustrophobia, or fear of enclosed places, may appear not only in confined space rescue but also in other situations as well. You may, for example, also find it difficult to attend a patient in a vehicle, an aircraft, or in a tent during a storm for long periods. Claustrophobia is a common condition that many people suffer to varying degrees. In some cases, claustrophobia may not be moderated by experience in close environments but may require psychological counseling.

Stress

You have chosen a stressful career. Life and death crises occur almost daily. Sometimes there is little you can do to alter the effects of serious illness or injury. One of the most common problems in the emergency field is excessive emotional involvement with patients and their problems. It is natural and appropriate for you to care about the people you are helping, but excessive emotional involvement may hinder your ability to carry out emergency care effectively and objectively. At all times, you must strive to keep a balance between sympathetic concern and emotional involvement.

Another potential problem for you following a life and death crisis is that you may be criticized unfairly by a patient, the family, the community, or even by co-workers. It is very frustrating to hear criticism that is based on inaccurate information or sensationalism.

You are vulnerable to the stresses of rescue work; therefore, you must learn to recognize the symptoms of stress so that it does not interfere with your work or your life away from work, including family life. The signs and symptoms of chronic stress may not be obvious at first because they may be subtle and not present all of the time. The following may indicate the presence of excessive stress:

1. Irritability
2. Lack of enthusiasm (apathy)
3. Chronic fatigue
4. Feelings of not being appreciated
5. Difficulty sleeping
6. Excessive drinking
7. Drug usage
8. Change in social behavior
9. Change in appetite
10. Desire to quit work
11. Physical complaints (headache, gastrointestinal upset)
12. Rigid thinking (unwilling to adapt to new situations)
13. Sexual dysfunction

Any of these symptoms may indicate chronic stress. You should recognize them as such and take steps to relieve their cause. Concerns should be discussed with co-workers, many of whom will have had similar experiences. Such discussions may be enough to resolve the problem once you realize how common some of these symptoms are. Persistent and severe symptoms may require professional guidance from a counselor, a physician, or a member of the clergy. Early recognition of chronic stress problems is most important because a solution is much easier to achieve with early recognition. Persistent problems tend to increase in scope and complexity, making it much more difficult to reach resolution.

SUMMARY

Awareness of potential hazards and knowledge of preventive actions are essential to avoiding the threats inherent in any rescue operation. Rescuers must understand that their survival in the face of these threats may depend on their being informed and prepared.

Physical threats are common in rescue operations. Rescuers must maintain adequate fluid intake and appropriate nutrition standards to function in a safe, efficient manner.

Medical threats can include pre-existing conditions or short-term problems that develop during the rescue. A rescuer with a pre-existing medical condition, such as heart disease or diabetes, should not participate in a rescue in which the condition may cause him or her to become a patient. Short-term ailments, such as cuts or headaches, can often be managed by first aid techniques. Each rescuer should carry a personal first aid kit to treat these problems. Other medical threats, however, such as intestinal disorders caused by contaminated water, require more complex prevention or treatment.

Environmental threats often center around the weather, primarily exposure to cold, wet, and heat. Hyperthermia, above normal body temperatures, and hypothermia, below normal body temperatures, are equally dangerous and should be prevented. Frostbite, the freezing of body tissue, is also a concern in cold temperatures.

External threats can jeopardize many rescues. The location of the rescue operation and the terrain may become obstacles. Unstable surfaces, natural or man-made, can also cause falling or loss of balance. Other external threats include the dangers of electrical shock, falling objects, avalanches, and crevasses. In the event of any of these external threats, rescuers can take steps to avoid these situations and go on to a successful outcome.

Psychological threats encompass both stress, commonly encountered by all emergency medical service personnel, and emotional tensions that may relate to the environment. By far the most common psychological threat, however, is stress. Emergency service involves crises, and short-term stress is to be expected. Nevertheless, rescuers must learn the signs and symptoms of chronic stress. Early recognition of this long-term condition is important in order to treat and eliminate the problem.

FIRE HAZARDS

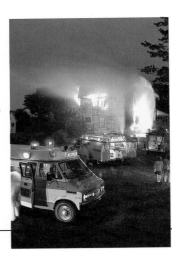

OVERVIEW

Emergency rescues involving fire present immense challenges to rescuers. Rescue situations involving fire will complicate your goals of avoiding injury to yourself, your patients, and other rescuers.

This chapter outlines what rescuers can expect and do when confronted with a fire rescue.

Beginning with background information about the phases of a fire, the chapter goes on to describe the hazards in a fire as well as the rescue hazards during fires. There are also sections discussing rescue and evacuation procedures in a wildland fire environment.

OBJECTIVES

The objectives of this chapter are for the rescuer to be able to describe:

- the phases of a fire.
- hazards inherent in any fire and hazards occurring in a fire rescue situation.

- ways to avoid injury and protect patients in rescue operations involving fire.
- rescue and evacuation procedures in the wildland fire envirnoment.

Fire is usually described by its physical characteristics. These physical characteristics include the heat that is felt and the smoke and flame that are usually seen. These physical characteristics that are seen and felt are the result of a chain reaction that involves oxygen, fuel, and heat. Two of the most common fire chain reactions seen are the smoldering fire and the free burning fire. A smoldering fire gives off smoke and heat, but has no visible flame present. A free burning fire has smoke, heat, and a visible flame present.

It is important to understand that fires are usually dynamic and unstable situations. The dynamic forces at work in a fire often place real time constraints on the rescue effort. There is usually only minutes to organize and implement a rescue. Rescue in a fire environment often occurs in building or structural types of fire situations. You should have a basic understanding of the phases and hazards associated with fire situations in order to be safe and effective in your rescue effort.

The fire triangle is a graphic representation of the three basic elements necessary for combustion: fuel, heat source, and an oxidizing agent (Figure 5.1). Combustion is the self-sustaining process of rapid oxidation of a fuel by an oxidizing agent, which produces heat and light. The initiation of combustion requires that the fuel be in a gaseous state. Liquids and solid fuels must be converted to a gas to have the potential for combustion. Thus, the need for a heat source.

PHASES OF A FIRE

The first phase of a fire is the **incipient phase.** In this phase the oxygen content of the surrounding air has not been significantly reduced. Water vapor, carbon dioxide, and a small amount of sulfur dioxide are being produced by the fire. Generally the room temperature does not rise significantly, but the fire may have a flame temperature of 1,000° F.

The second phase is the **free-burning phase.** The heat rising from the fire draws in air to support combustion. In a confined space the heat and smoke will rise to the ceiling and begin to spread out and down. The upper areas of the room can have temperatures near 1,300° F. As combustible items in the room are heated, they decompose and emit gases that add more fuel to the fire. This process continues until there is insufficient oxygen in the area to support combustion or there is no fuel left to burn.

The third phase is the **smoldering phase.** In this phase, as the oxygen is consumed, the open burning and flame may disappear altogether. The room fills with dense smoke and heat. Floor temperatures may reach 1,000° F. The oxygen content drops below 15 percent. New gases are added to the room by the continued heating and decomposition of the contents of the room (Figure 5.2).

FIGURE 5.1

Fire Triangle
The three elements necessary for combustion are fuel, heat source, and an oxidizing agent.

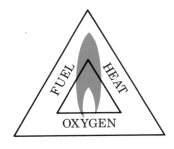

a.

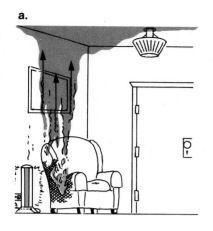

b.

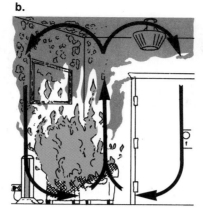

c.

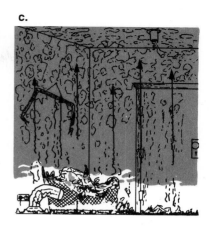

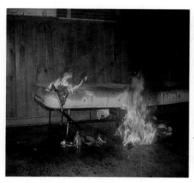

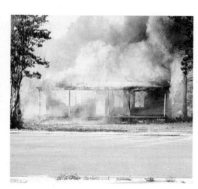

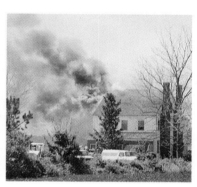

FIGURE 5.2

Phases of a Fire

a In the incipient phase, the oxygen content of the surrounding air has not been significantly reduced. Generally the room temperature does not rise significantly.

b In the free-burning phase, heat rising from the fire draws in air to support combustion. Heat and smoke rise to the ceiling and begin to spread out and down. Upper areas of the room can have temperatures near 1,300°F.

c In the smoldering phase, oxygen is consumed and open burning and flame may disappear altogether. The room fills with dense smoke and heat, and floor temperatures may reach 1,000°F.

HAZARDS IN A FIRE

There are four common hazards found in a fire environment: smoke, oxygen deficiency, high ambient temperatures, and toxic gases.

Smoke is made up of suspended particles of tar and carbon. Smoke particles irritate the respiratory system upon initial contact. This irritation often disappears after exposure, leaving the individual unaware of the continued presence of the irritant. Many of these particles are trapped in the upper respiratory system, but many smaller particles make their way into the lungs. Some of these smoke particles are not only irritants but may be lethal.

As the fire consumes the available oxygen in a room, anyone in the room will have increasing difficulty breathing. Table 5.1 demonstrates the effects of reduced oxygen in humans.

The high ambient temperatures in a fire can cause thermal burns and damage to the respiratory system. Breathing air heated above 120° F can damage tissue in the respiratory tract, causing reduced blood pressure and potentially fatal pulmonary edema or fluid in the lungs.

Toxic gases present in a structural fire situation include carbon monoxide, phosgene, nitrogen oxides, hydrogen cyanide, hydrogen chloride, and carbon dioxide. **Carbon monoxide** is a colorless and odorless gas that is present in every fire. This gas is responsible for more fire deaths each year than any other by-product of combustion. Carbon monoxide combines with hemoglobin in the blood cells about 200 times more rapidly than does oxygen. This blocks the ability of the hemoglobin to carry oxygen to the cells. Table 5.2 graphically displays the toxic effects and symptoms of carbon monoxide poisoning.

Phosgene is a colorless and tasteless gas with an odor of musty hay. In low concentrations it causes eye and throat irritation. When inhaled, it decomposes into hydrochloric acid, which chemically burns the lungs and causes pulmonary edema.

Hydrogen cyanide is a colorless gas with a noticeable almond odor. It blocks the exchange of oxygen and carbon dioxide in the lungs. Symptoms include gasping, muscle spasms, increased heart rate, and sudden collapse.

Carbon dioxide is a colorless and odorless gas that causes increased respirations, dizziness, and sweating. Breathing concentra-

TABLE 5.1   Effects of Reduced Oxygen on Humans

Percent of Oxygen in Air	Symptoms
21	None Normal Concentration
17	Increased respiratory rate/effort Some impaired muscular coordination (mild ataxia)
12	Headache Dizziness (severe ataxia) Fatigue
9	Unconsciousness
6	Respiratory/cardiac failure Death within minutes

Adapted with permission from the International Fire Service Training Association, Oklahoma State University, Stillwater, Oklahoma.

TABLE 5.2	Toxic Effects of Carbon Monoxide

Percent Carbon Monoxide in Air	Symptoms
.01	No symptoms—No apparent illness
.02	Mild Headache—Few other symptoms
.04	Headache following 1–2 hours
.08	Headache following 45 minutes, nausea/vomiting, unconscious following 2 hours
.16	Headache following 20 minutes, nausea/vomiting, unconscious following 45 minutes
.32	Headache following 5–10 minutes, nausea/vomiting, unconscious following 30 minutes
.64	Headache, ataxia following 1–2 minutes, unconscious following 10–15 minutes
1.28	Immediately unconscious, death following 1–3 minutes

0 1000 2000 3000 4000 5000 6000 7000 8000 9000 10000 11000 12000 13000

Carbon Monoxide parts per million (ppm)

Adapted with permission from the International Fire Service Training Association, Oklahoma State University, Stillwater, Oklahoma.

tions above 10 to 12 percent may cause death within a few minutes.

Hydrogen chloride is a colorless gas with a strong pungent odor. It may cause severe irritation to the respiratory tract and the eyes. It may also lead to an irregular heart rhythm. Inhalation may result in chemical burns and edema of the upper respiratory tract.

Nitrogen oxides decompose into **nitric oxide,** which converts to nitrogen dioxide in the presence of oxygen and moisture. This creates nitric acid that is reddish-brown in color and may cause pulmonary edema and death by suffocation.

RESCUE HAZARDS DURING FIRES

An uncontrolled fire is a very dynamic situation. Significant changes can occur rapidly. The four major hazards that you should consider when sizing up a fire are **flashover, backdraft, building collapse,** and **inadequate protective equipment.**

Temperatures in a free-burning fire can exceed 1,500° F. Most of the combustible material in a home will ignite at temperatures ranging from 400 to 1,400° F. These combustibles are preheated to their ignition temperature by the open fire situation. Flashover occurs when all of the combustible items within the fire zone ignite. This sudden ignition is a violent reaction similar to an explosion.

From the time an open flame appears, it takes just over *two minutes* for flashover to occur. Fire fighters who have survived a flashover describe it as like being in the middle of a blast furnace. Anyone exposed to a flashover without protective equipment will probably die. Rescuers with protective equipment in place during a flashover are still at risk of severe injury or death. Even the best protective fire fighting apparel is not designed to withstand periods of excessively high temperatures generated during a flashover.

In the smoldering phase of a fire, burning is incomplete because of the lack of oxygen. Adding air during the smoldering phase causes the stalled burning process to resume. It creates conditions ideal for a backdraft, an explosion of the gases of the incomplete combustion caused when the gases mix with additional air. Ominous signs of impending backdraft are

1. Little, if any, visible fire showing outside of the building
2. Hot exterior doors and windows
3. Puffing, grayish-yellow smoke coming from the building
4. Air or smoke forcefully reentering the structure
5. Audible sounds such as whistling or moaning emanating from the structure

An unsuspecting rescuer, lured by the desire to rescue, who opens a door or breaks a window supplies fresh oxygen and completes the cycle necessary for a backdraft to occur.

Vertical ventilation allows the heated gases to escape in a more controlled manner. Entering a building after ventilation requires extreme caution. Always stand to the side when opening doors and windows of a burning structure. Enter a building fire only when proper respiratory equipment, "envelope protection," and a backup water supply are in place and ready.

In structural fires there is the potential for collapse of floors and roofs. Warning signs of impending structural failure are frequently absent. Thus, hasty entry into burning structures may result in serious injury and possible death. Once inside the burning building, you are subject to an uncontrolled hostile environment. Fires are not selective about their victims.

RESCUE IN THE WILDLAND FIRE ENVIRONMENT

Wildland fire, including forest fires, brush fires, and range fires, are natural occurrences in many parts of the world. Wildfires are affected by three primary factors: fuels, weather, and topography. Together, the factors work to create *fire behavior*.

Fuels The rate of spread and intensity of a fire will be partially controlled by the types of vegetation and other fuels available to it. The moisture content, the amount (fuel loading), the vertical arrangement, size and shape, compactness, continuity, and chemistry of the fuels will all contribute to fire behavior. For example, a dense stand of dry, dead pines with branches reaching up from the ground will support a faster moving, more intense fire than scattered hardwood leaf litter.

Weather Weather conditions that affect a fire include the wind speed and direction, relative humidity, precipitation (or lack of), temperature, and atmospheric stability. For example, fires will be much more active during the heat of the day, driven by dry winds during periods of warm temperatures and low humidities. During periods of higher humidities and lower temperatures, fires typically will be less active.

Topography Fires burn upslope faster than downslope because the heat of the fire preheats the fuels, preparing them for rapid combustion. Other topographical factors include the position on the slope, elevation, and shape of the country. For example, a fire will be more active at midslope on the south aspect than at the bottom of a slope of the north aspect.

Fire Behavior Descriptions The following are generally considered to be low intensity fires:

- Ground fire: Fire that consumes the organic material beneath the surface litter (e.g., peat)
- Smoldering fire: Fire burning without flame and barely spreading
- Creeping fire: Fire burning with a low flame and spreading slowly

The following can be either a low intensity or high intensity fire:

- Surface fire: Fire that burns surface litter, debris, and small vegetation.

The following are generally considered to be dangerous, high intensity fire behaviors:

- Running fire: Fire that is spreading rapidly with a well defined head or flaming front
- Torching fire: Fire moving from surface fuels into the crowns of individual trees, but not necessarily from one crown to another
- Crown fire: Fire that advances from top to top of trees or shrubs more or less independently of the surface fire
- Spotting fire: Fire producing sparks or embers that are carried by the wind to start new fires beyond the main fire.

- Blowup fire: Sudden increase in fire intensity or rate of spread that defies control or forces a change in plans
- Firewhirl: A spinning, moving column of ascending air rising within a vortex and carrying aloft smoke, debris, and flames.

Low intensity fire activity will usually not pose a problem for you, although fire behavior can change significantly should one of the controlling factors change. If wind velocity suddenly increased, for example, a low intensity fire could become a high intensity problem. You should consult with fire management personnel regarding fire behavior occurring at a given incident. You should also be aware that one of the common factors preceding most fire fatalities is that the fire appeared to be inactive.

High intensity fires can actually control the environment and significantly modify weather elements near or adjacent to the fire. Fire can move with alarming speed, change direction, and pose a significant threat to your safety. Close coordination with fire management personnel is essential.

If the agency with fire management responsibilities is not on the scene, it should be notified and consulted prior to attempting rescue operations. You should assess the situation before beginning the operation. If you believe that the patient can be safely assessed, a plan, which includes the following precautions, should be developed:

- You should wear personal protective equipment, including flame retardant pants and shirt, leather gloves, a hardhat, goggles, and strong leather work boots, and carry an emergency fire shelter. The shelter can protect you should fire overrun your position. Proper and effective use requires prior training.
- Know what the fire is doing at all times. Post lookouts and keep in radio contact with observers if you cannot see the fire.
- Watch the weather closely. Be especially alert to thunderstorms, approaching cold fronts, and other such events that could change fire behavior.
- Plan escape routes that you and others can use if fire behavior changes.
- Avoid being in heavy cover with unburned fuel between you and the fire.
- Avoid routes where terrain or cover would make travel slow and difficult.
- Avoid entering areas where frequent spot fires are occurring.
- Avoid working at or near the head (i.e., the advancing flame front) of the fire.

If fire management personnel are available, or if the rescue situation allows for delay until such personnel arrive, you must coordinate activities with them. If you routinely work in a wildland environment, then wildfire preplans should be prepared, incorporating information from fire management agencies.

EVACUATION

If a fire occurs in an area where a large number of people may be exposed to fire hazards, the incident commander must consider evacuation of all individuals at risk. An evacuation should be a controlled movement of people from an area of danger to an area of relative safety. In many cases, the evacuation process has already been initiated by the building or area occupants because of their awareness of the immediate danger.

In most cases this spontaneous evacuation process helps to minimize the risk to the occupants. If there is no systematic process to the evacuation, it becomes difficult to account for all occupants and assess the need for an interior rescue. Quickly assigning people familiar with specific building areas or knowledgeable about specific groups of people to gather names and make head counts greatly improves the quality of the size-up.

Safe, controlled evacuations can require an extensive commitment of manpower. This is particularly true in high-rise buildings or buildings with special populations such as those found in jails, nursing homes, schools, or hospitals. Evacuation of such facilities must be conducted in an organized, methodical manner. Preplanning such evacuations is a real asset in these special situations.

The incident commander must have frequent updates on numbers of patients, location and status of the "disaster," and knowledge of reserve and special forces. Such incidents will have a high media profile. The incident commander should designate a public information officer to provide current information to the print and television media at the scene.

Evacuation of Special Populations

Evacuation procedures for special populations require much greater planning than does a general evacuation. It is necessary to have a designated plan that can safely provide the continuation of the same level of essential services with minimal disruption. This planning must be conducted before a fire occurs. A planned internal relocation may only take a few minutes whereas an external evacuation to a different location may take several hours.

An interior evacuation of building occupants to a safe zone through normal passageways or stairways is the safest method of evacuation and rescue. However, there are times when the interior evacuation is not possible because of unstable or uncontrolled incidents. In such life-threatening situations, an exterior evacuation can be performed using exterior fire escapes, ground ladders, aerial ladders, and/or elevated platforms.

If an external evacuation must take place, the best option is to locate facilities nearby that provide a similar environment. Moving a nursing home population of 80 people into other nursing homes is far better than moving this same group into a shelter designed only for the needs of the general population.

The following are some of the planning considerations associated with the evacuation of a medical facility.

- Total number of critical care, ambulatory, and nonambulatory patients
- Required patient life support equipment
- Amount of manpower and time required to move and monitor the population from one area to another
- Weather conditions that may cause significant medical stresses for the evacuees

Individual health records, medications, and personal belongings should be kept with each evacuee. It it helpful to tag each patient with name, age, diagnosis, and primary problems since some hospital and nursing home patients cannot or will not share this data in times of stress.

An uncontrolled exterior evacuation from a jail may present a more significant risk to inmates and rescuers than the incident itself. An unrestrained prisoner may attempt to escape by taking hostages or physically injuring rescuers.

A rescue in a fire situation is generally limited to a very brief "window" of time, usually between the appearance of an open flame and the moment when flashover potential exists. This is particularly true of rescue in the normal residence fire.

If an effective rescue is to occur, most of the tasks that must be carried out by a team need to occur simultaneously. These include the deployment of hose lines and ladders, ventilation, forced entry, and the rapid gathering of data from witnesses.

The solo, "heroic rescue" is usually ineffective and frequently results in greater risk to a rescuer than the situation requires. Effective rescue is the organized effort of a team of personnel trained and equipped to manage the situation.

Patients at the scene of a fire also require rapid evacuation. As soon as the patient is out of the fire site, rescuers must perform a rapid but thorough assessment and begin transport. The longer a patient waits for transport, the more serious respiratory distress and shock can become.

SUMMARY

Rescuers who confront a fire rescue situation must be prepared to manage the rescue without injury to themselves or their patients. Accordingly, understanding the physical characteristics and phases of fire is important for rescuers to be effective.

Rescuers must also be aware of hazards inherent in any fire. Even more importantly, rescuers must be familiar with rescue hazards that can occur during a fire. An uncontrolled fire is an extremely hazardous situation, and fires are not selective about their victims.

Fire fighting and fire rescue in an urban setting is different from that in a wildland setting. Rescuers who face wildfires must understand the factors, including fuels, weather, and topography, that create fire behavior in the wildland environment.

If a fire exposes a large number of people to danger, rescuers must be prepared to evacuate all individuals at risk. This requires a preplan for a safe, controlled evacuation. Even greater planning is necessary to develop evacuation procedures for special populations including those found in a high-rise or in public facilities such as hospitals, schools, nursing homes, or jails.

CHAPTER

6

WATER HAZARDS

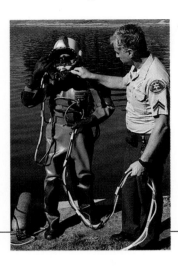

CHAPTER OUTLINE

Overview
Objectives
Personal Safety and Water
 Hazards
Summary

OVERVIEW

Water rescue requires specialized skills and concerns for personal safety. The chapter includes a discussion on water hazards and water rescue techniques.

OBJECTIVES

The objectives of this chapter are for the rescuer to:

- identify the types of water rescues based on the type of water environment.
- understand the forces that affect water flow.
- determine mechanisms of injury in a water rescue situation.
- select appropriate protective equipment.

Personal preparedness affects the success of water rescue efforts. All personnel involved in a water rescue must wear a personal flotation device (PFD) when teams practice or respond to a water rescue (Figure 6.1). Type I or Type II PFDs are preferred for water rescue work, though Specialty Type III PFDs are suitable for some rescue situations. The problem with most Type IIIs is that they will not turn an unconscious person to a face-up position in the water. You should clean and inspect your PFDs regularly as part of your equipment maintenance program. PFDs with torn covering or straps should be replaced.

PERSONAL SAFETY AND WATER

Occasionally, you will arrive alone at a water accident scene. You should not attempt a swimming rescue but use **shore-based rescue** techniques. Shore-based rescues are safer and more effective.

FIGURE 6.1

Personal Flotation Device
All personnel involved in a
water rescue must wear a
personal flotation device.

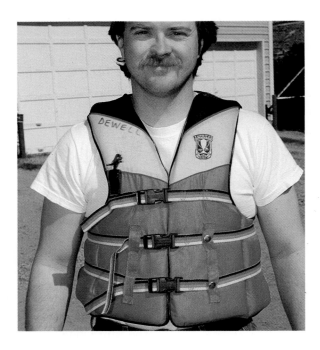

Solo water rescue attempts by an individual rescuer are unsafe. A
backup should be on hand to assist if the primary rescuer gets into
trouble. The backup may also assist in treatment or evacuation of
the patient.

Hazards

There are significant variations in the hazards you will face in each
of the wide variety of water environments you may encounter. As
part of preplanning, you must be aware of the types of water rescue
you can anticipate in your locale and the hazards inherent in those
situations. For example, river impoundments behind dams may contain submerged obstacles that become hazards as they are covered
by the rising water. Such hazards include terrain features such as
forests, buildings, bridges, and other man-made structures. These
may impede search and rescue activities by snagging or entangling
equipment or personnel.

You must also be aware that all water environments may contain
hazardous materials including bacteria, parasites, sewage, industrial
waste, and chemical spills. Appropriate precautions must be taken
and decontamination procedures done.

Eastern impoundments, western reclamation projects, and natu-
rally carved glacial lakes all have different bottom profiles. Well-
trained rescue units need a knowledge of local lake bottoms and currents and their effect on rescue operations.

In an ocean environment the offshore sandbars of the East Coast
barrier islands have currents that complicate rescues. The lush kelp

gardens immediately offshore in West Coast waters may hide swimmers and divers, impeding search or recovery operations.

Tidal influences are less pronounced in deep water than in shallower inshore waters. **Ebb** (falling) and **flood** (rising) **tides** may obstruct access to beaches near dunes and cliffs, or they may flood rescues occurring around marine structures and docks, especially near low tide marks. In coastal regions, rescue preplans must include local tide charts to provide responders with a necessary decision-making tool.

Undertows, or runoff, occur between the point of wave break onshore and wave reforming offshore. Swimmers caught in undertows fight the force of the current until they are too fatigued to make it to shore. They should relax and swim at an angle across the current to return to shore.

Water Flow Hazards   You can avoid problems by understanding the forces that affect water flow. Special training in river operations may enhance your competency and safety in moving water.

Water velocity increases in narrow-bore passages or where there is a rapid vertical drop. A tight bend in a river or stream diverts water away from the inner side of the bend, creating **eddies** (whirlpools) and **backwashes** (backward movement of water) with increasing turbulence on the opposite bank (Figure 6.2). A swirling upheaval called a boil indicates boulders or debris changing the speed and direction of water flow.

In rivers and streams, knee-deep flowing water may throw a wading person off balance into the river. Water flowing as slow as five miles per hour can pin patients under water. A person's abdominal and back muscles are no match for the force of water rushing over them.

Strainers are obstructions that allow current to flow through yet trap objects such as boats or people. The pressures generated by water

FIGURE 6.2

Eddies and Backwashes
A tight bend in a river or stream creates eddies and backwashes. Boulders or debris in the stream create boils.

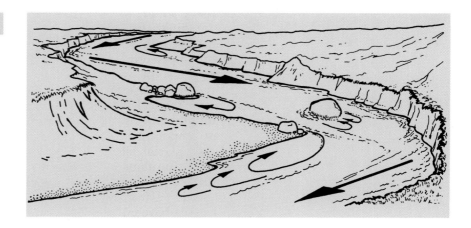

flowing around, over, or through a strainer, such as a partially or completely submerged tree branch (Figure 6.3), may cause major blunt trauma. The pressure of the flowing water may pin boats and bodies against the strainer. Untrained persons may attempt self-extrication but only further complicate their situations. Rescue teams must cautiously approach strainers to avoid their own entrapment.

Some alterations in water flow are man-made. Low head dams range in height from six inches to ten feet. They frequently show a boil line downstream from their dangerous hydraulics (Figure 6.4). The boil is the result of some of the spillway flow backwashing upstream toward the dam. The backwash of the hydraulic will push the victim back to the dam face, where water rushing over the spillway pushes them back underwater. The current moves them downstream along the river bottom back into the boil. There the backwash recaptures the surfacing victim and propels them through this cycle repeatedly. Those who are trapped often succumb to fatigue, hypothermia, or drowning. They also sustain traumatic injuries from impact with debris trapped in the water with them.

Water Temperature You will face additional problems depending on the temperature of the body of water. Hypothermia occurs rapidly in cold water; a person cannot maintain body heat in water below 92° F. In fact, water draws away body heat 25 times faster than exposure to air at the same temperature. For example, people in 35° F water for more than 15 minutes face a high probability of death

FIGURE 6.3

Strainer
Strainers are obstructions in a moving stream that allow current to flow through yet may trap boats or people.

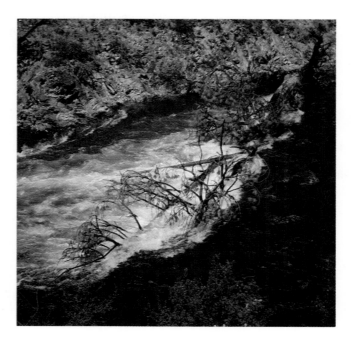

FIGURE 6.4

Hydraulic
Low head dams can create dangerous hydraulics which may trap people in a backwash. The trapped victims often succumb to fatigue, hypothermia, and drowning.

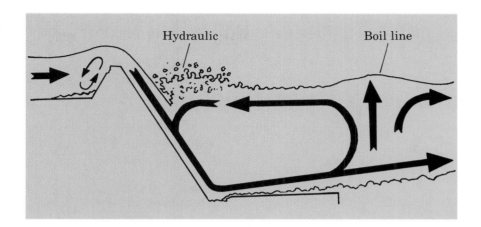

from **immersion hypothermia** (Table 6.1). As the core body temperature drops, muscle spasms develop. The body mass becomes denser, acquiring a "negative buoyancy" that can lead to submersion and drowning. You are at risk for developing hypothermia and must adequately protect yourself. To conserve heat, adopt the heat escape lessening posture, **HELP,** or **HUDDLE** together with other people (Figure 6.5).

Total immersion in cold water may obstruct the airway by triggering **laryngospasms,** a reflex constriction in the throat that prevents the person from calling for help or breathing. The resulting oxygen deficiency may lead to unconsciousness and asphyxiation.

Warm water above 70°F increases fatigue and may prevent patients from rescuing themselves. Warmer water also contains marine predators, such as sharks and barracuda, who may interpret a person's swimming actions as injured prey behavior and suddenly attack. The bites of these marine animals cause lacerations and puncture wounds that may result in significant blood loss. There is also significant risk of bacterial contamination. In addition, stings from jellyfish and man-of-war may cause local or systemic reactions that may deteriorate into life-threatening anaphylaxis.

Thermoclines are layers of water of varying temperatures. You may feel the temperatures of the distinct layers as you pass through them on a dive. Thermoclines may prevent bodies from surfacing until seasonal temperature changes occur.

Overboard Power vessel ejections create immediate threats to life. The most dangerous situation is when the operator is ejected. A vessel without directional control and with power applied, especially at full throttle, will make ever tightening circles because of engine torque and water pressure on the rudder. During this out-of-control period, the boat and propeller slice through the water increasingly closer to the victim until a collision occurs. Because of the possibility of ejec-

TABLE 6.1   Cold Water Immersion Survivability Chart

Temperature (°F)	Estimated Survival Time in Hours and Minutes		
	No Thermal Protection	Full Clothing	1/4" Wet Suit
80	6:00 / *	8:00 / *	* / *
75	3:30 / *	4:15 / *	12:00 / *
70	2:30 / 12:00	3:00 / *	6:00 / *
65	1:45 / 8:00	2:15 / 12:00	3:30 / *
60	1:00 / 4:30	1:20 / 5:45	2:30 / 8:00
55	:30 / 2:00	:45 / 2:30	1:30 / 5:00
50	:15 / 1:00	:25 / 1:30	1:00 / 3:00
45	:12 / :25	:20 / :40	:45 / 1:30
40	:10 / :15	:14 / :25	:35 / :50
35	:08 / :12	:10 / :15	:25 / :40
30	:05 / :10	:08 / :12	:20 / :30

Top number indicates time to unconscious state. Bottom number indicates time until death.

* Time over 12 hours.

Adapted with permission from Dacor Corporation, Northfield, Illinois.

FIGURE 6.5

HELP and HUDDLE
When floating in cold water, conserve body heat by using a body position that will reduce the escape of heat.

a If alone, use the HELP position.

b With other people, HUDDLE together.

a.
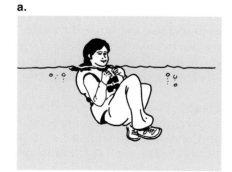

b.
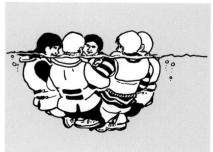

tion, rescue boats should be equipped with a tether between the rescue boat operator and the *engine kill switch* to stop the engine in case of an accident.

Rescue personnel face the hazard of being pinned against rocks, structures, and strainers when thrown overboard from capsized vessels. A river current approaching 10 miles per hour exerts several tons of force on objects in its path. All rescuers in the water must keep upstream of any vessels to avoid being pinned between the vessel and a rock or other obstruction.

All members of water rescue teams should be strong swimmers and trained in self-rescue techniques. Team members should learn and practice the survival swimming strokes, sidestroke, modified breaststroke, and elementary backstroke while wearing a PFD.

Diving Problems Water rescue teams using self-contained underwater breathing apparatus (SCUBA) divers should develop protocols to avoid the problems common to diving operations. When divers are in the water, a diver's flag must be displayed to warn surface vessels to stand clear. The flag also indicates a diver's location to attending surface crews. Attach the flag to an inflated inner tube or similar flotation device connected to an anchoring system that allows divers to move if it is necessary.

To avoid propeller injuries, all surface vessels, including rescue boats, should be kept away from a rescue incident when divers are in the water.

Diving with SCUBA has potentially a number of problems requiring the assistance of rescue personnel. The rescuer who treats SCUBA patients may recognize the characteristic cherry red lips and nailbeds associated with carbon monoxide poisoning. This condition occurs when gasoline-powered compressors fill SCUBA tanks with air contaminated with carbon monoxide from faulty exhaust venting or evaporation of the compressor's lubricating oil. An overabundance of carbon dioxide can also overcome a diver. All divers should obtain air tank refills from a reputable, inspected, and certified fill station.

Diving situations add another dimension to potential rescue problems. Pressure affects the solubility of gas in the blood, tissues, and organs of the body. Since air contains approximately 78 percent nitrogen, SCUBA divers inhale large amounts of nitrogen during a dive. At depth, the high partial pressure of the nitrogen causes it to enter into solution in the blood and tissues. Elevated nitrogen levels in the blood can lead to **nitrogen narcosis,** a reversible condition similar to alcohol intoxication that affects divers. Divers may exhibit impaired judgment, euphoria, or unconsciousness. The specific cause of nitrogen narcosis is not clear, and individual susceptibility to the effects of the nitrogen varies.

Decompression sickness, also known as "the bends," occurs when the nitrogen comes out of solution and forms bubbles in the blood and tissues during rapid ascents. The effect can be visualized as similar to the gas bubbles being released when opening a carbonated beverage. Nitrogen transfer from the tissues into the blood and from the blood into exhaled air takes a long time. When divers ascend too rapidly, the pressure on the body is reduced faster than the nitrogen can be exchanged and exhaled. As the partial pressure of the nitrogen within the tissue and blood exceeds the external pressure, bubbles may form, exerting pressure on nerves or depriving organs of blood. Pain, respiratory distress, and circulatory collapse can occur.

In a similar manner, breath holding during rapid ascents may result in overinflating the lungs. Alveoli, tiny air sacs in the lungs, may burst. Air enters the chest cavity, resulting in pressure on the outside of the lungs that may interfere with breathing.

Rupture of the alveoli may also result in an **air embolism,** an air bubble in the bloodstream that may lead to a blockage of circulation or a stroke. Air embolism patients may exhibit signs and symptoms similar to decompression sickness: skin blotches or petchiae; frothy, bloody sputum; pain; shortness of breath; nausea and vomiting; impaired vision; paralysis; or coma.

Units employing rescue divers must strictly adhere to dive tables that indicate accurate decompression information for the altitude from which the dive is made. This will help prevent air embolism and decompression sickness in rescue team members.

Because of potential problems from residual gas pressures in the blood and tissue, rescue team divers should wait 24 hours after a dive before an airplane or helicopter flight at altitude.

As in any rescue response, you must treat immediate life-threatening conditions. Personal safety is paramount. Therefore, secure the scene and protect the patient or remove him from hazardous situations.

SUMMARY

Water environments have their own unique hazards. Rescue personnel must be knowledgeable about the types of water rescue they can anticipate in their area and the hazards they will encounter.

Rescuers must understand the forces that affect water flow and the dangers of various water temperatures. All rescuers involved in water rescue must be strong swimmers, and they must understand their equipment. They must wear PFDs at all times, during water rescue operations. SCUBA divers, in particular, must become very familiar with the diving techniques and equipment to avoid problems. Rescuers who treat SCUBA diving patients must be able to recognize and treat conditions associated with SCUBA diving, including carbon monoxide poisoning and decompression sickness.

HAZARDOUS MATERIALS

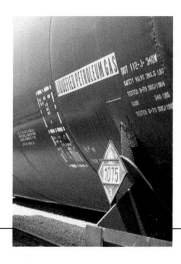

OVERVIEW

Potentially hazardous materials can be found anywhere. Rescuers must be prepared to recognize and manage hazardous materials at rescue sites.

This chapter outlines what rescuers can expect when they encounter a rescue operation that involves hazardous materials. The chapter explains how to identify and contain hazardous materials. There are also sections describing protection and decontamination of both rescuer and patient, and management of exposures.

OBJECTIVES

The objectives of this chapter are for the rescuer to describe:

- the initial assessment of an incident involving hazardous materials.
- hazardous materials warning signs, placards, or codes.
- the Hazmat Rule of Thumb to determine the size of a danger zone.
- ways to protect himself, other rescue team members, and patients from the dangers of exposure to hazardous materials.
- decontamination.
- management of exposures.

A **hazardous material** is a product or material that can cause damage or injury when released from its normal container or environment or when exposed to another agent or environment. Many everyday products may be considered hazardous materials, depending upon their volume, packaging, or use. Consumer products may not be classified as hazardous around the house, yet when found in larger quantities, or in specific circumstances, they can be hazardous. An example is the ammonia nitrate found in lawn and garden fertilizer as well as in blasting agents. When the fertilizer is mixed with petroleum products such as motor oil or transmission fluid and exposed to heat or flames, an explosion can occur.

Even though hazardous materials may be present at the site of an incident, there may be no immediate danger if they remain contained or controlled. The incident commander must determine the potential for a release or spill. The incident commander must continually monitor the potential spill and have plans to minimize damages or injuries should a release or spill occur.

IDENTIFICATION OF HAZARDOUS MATERIALS

Potentially hazardous materials are found everywhere. Rescue personnel must recognize the existence of potentially hazardous materials, but they may not be expected to stop spills or releases. Rescuers must have a solid, basic knowledge of the effects of hazardous materials in order to make rescue decisions. To avoid additional death or injury in dealing with potentially hazardous situations, you may need to delay entry until fully trained and equipped specialists such as a hazardous materials team are available to assess the danger and assist in the management of the situation. This can be a very difficult decision but one that is often required to avoid personal injury and additional injury to the patient.

The recognition of hazard potential begins with initial notification of the incident. Initial information should include the type of vehicle or building involved; whether smoke or fire is evident; location of the incident; topography of the location (mountains, river, etc.); description of the scene; and the presence of warning or identification signs, placards, or numbers. The preplan may contain a listing of hazardous materials stored at the location, as a result of legislation that requires such a listing be made public. If the presence of hazardous materials is suspected, approach the situation with caution. You should not enter a scene containing potentially hazardous material until the extent of the problem is known.

Upon arrival, perform a visual survey of the area from a safe distance upwind, preferably using binoculars. Maintain a safe distance until it is obvious that it is permissible to move forward to the scene or until properly equipped to do so. Before approaching the scene, look for evidence of a spill or release such as the presence of damaged ground cover, unresponsive people or animals in the area, chemical clouds or plumes, fire, or smoke.

If a truck or other commercial vehicle is involved, look for the presence of identification or warning placards (Figure 7.1). The U.S. Department of Transportation (DOT) requires vehicles transporting certain quantities of hazardous materials to have nine-inch, diamond-shaped placards on all four sides of the vehicle. These placards provide a limited assessment of the potential hazards of the contents based on an international agreement defining nine classes of hazardous materials.

FIGURE 7.1

Hazmat Placard on Vehicle
Vehicles transporting hazardous materials are required to have diamond-shaped placards on all four sides.

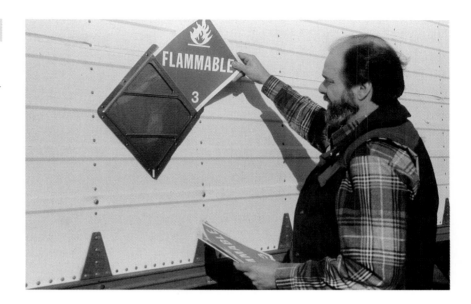

Though hazardous materials may fit into several areas of the classification system, they are identified by their primary hazard. Eight classes, identified by number at the bottom point of the vehicle placard are (Table 7.1)

Explosives	Oxidizers and organic peroxides
Gases	Poisons and etiological agents
Flammable liquids	Radioactive materials
Flammable solids	Corrosives

A ninth classification "other regulated materials," will often not be placarded. The placards for miscellaneous or other regulated materials may be color-coded (Table 7.2):

Red—flammables	Blue—water reactive materials
Yellow—reactives (oxidizers)	White on red—flammable solids
Green—non-flammable gases	Yellow on white—radioactive
Orange—explosives	materials
White—poisons	White on black—corrosives

Mixed loads will be placarded only for those categories that comprise over 1,000 pounds in the load. Loads less than 1,000 pounds in quantity do not require a definitive placard, except for radioactive materials. Vehicles with mixed loads will often have only a DANGEROUS placard with no indication as to the makeup of the load other than on the shipping papers. There are no miscellaneous designations; however, **other regulated materials (ORM)** will often carry a placard that indicates their primary danger.

The center of each placard contains a four-digit number to identify the material carried. For example, the number for gasoline is 1203.

TABLE 7.1   Nine Placard Classes

— Domestic label
— Domestic class number

Class Number	Nature of Materials
1	Explosives
2	Gases
3	Flammable liquids
4	Flammable solids
5	Oxidizers and organic peroxides
6	Poisons and etiological agents
7	Radioactive materials
8	Corrosives
9	Other regulated materials

Placards and labels may also use pictograms to describe the hazard involved (Figure 7.2). Thus, the placard provides an overview of the potential dangers that may exist with the materials.

For fixed facilities, such as storage or manufacturing locations, a similar placarding system has been devised by the National Fire Protection Association, the NFPA 704M System. Many communities require the use of this system in which a diamond-shaped placard is divided into four colored diamonds: blue—potential health hazard, red—fire hazard, yellow—reactivity, and white—specific hazards. Each diamond also contains a number to identify the degree of potential hazard (Figure 7.3). For example, in the blue or health diamond, 0 is normal while 4 is deadly. Fire hazard is also 0 (normal) to 4 (flash-

TABLE 7.2 Hazardous Materials Warning Placards	
	Red: Flammables
	Yellow: Reactives (oxidizers)
	Green: Non-flammable gases
	Orange: Explosives
	White: Poisons
	Blue: Water reactive materials
	White on Red: Flammable solids
	White on Black: Corrosives
	Yellow on White: Radioactive materials
	Red: Dangerous materials

FIGURE 7.2

Hazmat Pictograms
The center of each hazardous material placard contains a four-digit number to identify the material being carried. The number for gasoline, for example, is 1203. Placards and labels may also use pictograms to describe the hazard.

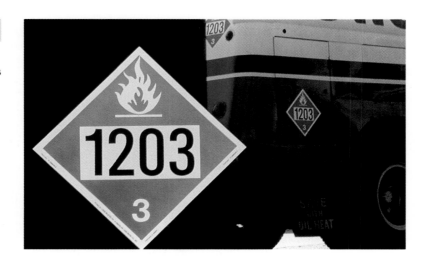

FIGURE 7.3

**NFPA 704M System
Placard**
The NFPA 704M System has
been devised for fixed facilities such as where hazardous
materials are stored or
manufactured.

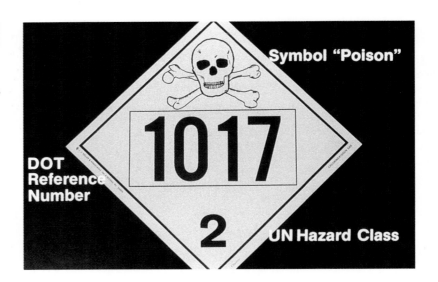

point below 73° F). Reactivity is identified as 0 being stable and 4
indicating a high probability of detonation. The white diamond uses
symbols to indicate special problems. Some jurisdictions use supplemental symbols in the white diamond to register corrosives, alkalis,
radiation, and other hazards.

Another immediate source of more information is Chemical Transportation Emergency Center (CHEMTREC), an organization coordinated by the Chemical Manufacturer's Association to provide information to field personnel needing to identify the problem.
CHEMTREC personnel can help identify the product and place you
in touch with the shipper who will assist in resolving the problem.
CHEMTREC can be reached at 1-800-424-9300, 24 hours a day (Figure 7.4).

All radioactive substances are kept in labeled and shielded containers when not in use. Radioactive materials shipped in interstate
commerce must be packaged with a label indicating the maximum
amount of external radiation. Vehicles used to transport radioactive
materials must be marked with a placard indicating a radioactive
shipment (Figure 7.5).

When hazardous materials are present, numerous clues usually
exist, for example, the presence of smoke. The color of smoke may
indicate the presence of a hazardous material, such as green or red
or yellowish vapors. Other clues you can look for include stained or
damaged vegetation in the area, people or animals lying down for an
unknown reason, unusual odors, and damaged pavement, particularly
asphalt. Anything out of the ordinary should be considered an indicator of the possible presence of hazardous materials.

Remember, you should maintain a safe distance, usually several
hundred yards upwind, while making the initial survey. Remember,

FIGURE 7.4

CHEMTREC Number
When a hazardous spill occurs, call CHEMTREC to help identify the hazardous material product and to contact the shipper who can assist in resolving the problem.

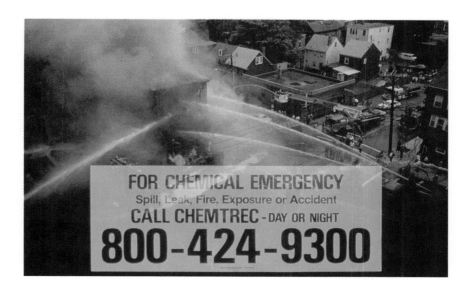

FIGURE 7.5

Radioactive Labeling
Vehicles transporting radioactive materials must be marked with special placards.

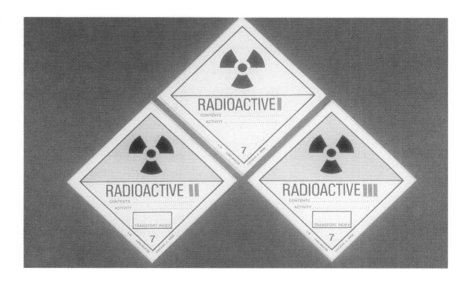

too, it does no good to approach the scene immediately if you will also be injured by the materials.

DANGER ZONE

The **Hazmat Rule of Thumb** is one way to determine the size of the danger zone. Using this method, hold your arm out straight with thumb pointing up. Then center your thumb over the hazardous area.

Your thumb should cover all the hazardous area from view. If the hazardous material can still be seen, you are too close. In addition, special precautions should be taken when toxic fumes are present. The safe area will be upwind from the site of the spill. But remember, wind direction can change quickly.

Once hazardous materials are suspected, the extent of the problem must be determined. Based on the information available, the incident commander must predict the possible behavior of the material, the area of potential danger, and the possible damage to people, environment, and property within the danger area. For example, if a tank or tanker containing a flammable liquid is involved with fire, a **boiling liquid, evaporating vapor explosion (BLEVE)** is possible. The fire will heat up the liquid in the tank, increasing its vapor pressure until the tank ruptures violently with a large release of energy.

BLEVEs will cause extensive damage for large distances around the area. Tanks have been blown as far as one-half mile. Explosive shock wave damage can extend even farther. Obviously, if a BLEVE threatens, distance and protection become important to you and others involved. Such a threat seriously affects the decision as to whether you should even enter the area.

Releases of materials without fire, such as the release of a vapor cloud of chlorine or ammonia, can also be extremely dangerous. Caustics may damage the container, roadway, or other structures introducing new hazards into the problem.

The incident commander must consider all of these issues in making the decision to enter the area and perform a rescue.

Based on the information available, the incident commander decides what has already been lost, predicts who or what is in danger but salvageable, and who or what is not in danger. There are occasions when the option of entering a danger area, even to save a life, is not an acceptable risk. If it is likely that one or more rescuers will be injured or killed, a rescue should not be attempted. There are numerous cases of rescuers requiring rescue because they entered a situation for which they were not prepared.

After evaluating the situation, the incident commander determines the goals and strategies based on available action options or tactics. These options may range from total resource commitment to immediate withdrawal. After evaluating the advantages and disadvantages of each option, the one with the greatest potential gain and the least risk is selected. Close monitoring of the situation is required to determine if modifications in strategies or tactics are required.

Initial decisions are critical to the outcome. Once resources and personnel are committed to a particular strategy, it is extremely difficult to change. If the incident commander cannot adequately assess the situation, the best option is to wait for qualified personnel, such as specialized hazardous materials teams. This is a difficult decision to make but avoids the risk of additional injury or death. Hazardous materials teams are organized and equipped to manage many of the incidents that occur or know how to access the right resources to accomplish the job with as little danger as possible.

DANGERS FROM HAZARDOUS MATERIALS

Though the dangers are present for both you and the patient, they must be evaluated differently. You must determine what hazards are present and the protective measures you must take. Do the hazards to the patients warrant rapid removal from the area of risk before initiating stabilization and treatment? Understanding the hazard potential is important in determining strategy and the level of protection required. Dangers from hazardous materials fall into six categories: thermal effects, mechanical effects, chemical effects, biological effects, radiation effects, and asphyxiation.

Thermal Effects

Thermal effects of hazards relate to temperature extremes. High temperature extremes are common at fire-related incidents. A fire fighter wears clothing specifically designed to provide some protection against high temperatures. Other rescue personnel may not have this protection available.

Hazardous materials injuries from extreme cold are often not considered. Many products, such as oxygen and other compressed gases, are stored or transported at extremely low temperatures and are called **cryogenics.** There is no placard for cryogenics. You must determine their presence by observing the tank, which is rounded on the ends and equipped with refrigeration equipment. Severe frostbite-type injuries can occur if you or the patient is directly exposed to these agents.

Protective clothing may be damaged by temperature extremes and thus fail to provide adequate protection. Equipment designed to protect against caustic materials or toxic gases cannot withstand temperature extremes. The suit will deteriorate rapidly, melt in heat or crack in cold, and place you in danger. It is important for you to understand the limitations of your protective equipment.

Mechanical Effects

Mechanical effects include explosions. There are three injury mechanisms from explosions. The initial pressure wave of the blast may cause internal injuries, frequently without external evidence. The pressure ruptures the small vessels and membranes in gas-containing organs such as the lungs and bowel. Central nervous system injury may also result from the initial blast. Secondary injuries result from the impact of material and debris being thrown by the explosion. The third type of injuries result from the impact of the victim who is thrown about by the force of the explosion.

Chemical Effects

Chemical effects are the result of chemical reactions on the object or body. Exposure to a corrosive, such as nitric acid, can cause severe burns to the skin or permanent eye damage. Other chemicals are hazardous when they are introduced into the body, for example, bone damage from hydrofluoric acid, internal burns from anhydrous ammonia, or nervous system collapse from parathion. When working in corrosive or chemical environments, specialized clothing is required, including a **self-contained breathing apparatus** (SCBA).

Biological Effects

Biological effects result from exposure to disease-causing microorganisms or their by-products. Tetanus, hepatitis, and HIV are examples of biologic agents. Biologic agents require special handling, specialized equipment, and decontamination of personnel and equipment.

Universal Precautions

Federal regulations require all health care workers, including rescue/ EMS personnel, to assume that *all patients* in all settings are potentially infected with HIV (AIDS) or other blood-borne agents. These regulations mandate the use of barriers and other protective equipment to prevent parenteral, mucous membrane, and skin exposure to the blood and certain body fluids of all patients. The Centers for Disease Control (CDC) **universal precautions** also emphasize infection control measures and urge caution when dealing with equipment subject to breakage or that might accidentally puncture the skin of the health care worker.

The primary assumption underlying the CDC's universal precaution recommendations is that protective barriers can be expected to reduce the health care worker's risk of exposure to blood, body fluids containing blood, and the other fluids to which universal precautions apply. The CDC notes that the type of barrier chosen depends on the clinical situation. In general, the selection of the type of protective barrier, protective equipment, or work practice should include consideration of (1) the probability of exposure to blood and body fluids; (2) the type of body fluid contacted; and (3) the amount of blood or body fluid likely to be encountered.

Because it is often not possible to know when a patient may be infected with HIV or other blood-borne agents, adoption of universal precautions represents one effective way to reduce the risk of transmission of HIV and other blood-borne agents in the health care setting. Thus, rescue and EMS personnel, regardless of HIV caseload, should adopt the use of universal precautions.

The CDC recommendations, amended in 1987, and in 1988, specifically provide that:

1. All health care workers should routinely use appropriate *barrier precautions* to prevent skin and mucous-membrane exposures when contact with blood or other body fluids of any patient is anticipated. *Gloves* should be worn for touching blood and body fluids, mucous membranes, or non-intact skin of all patients, for handling items or surfaces soiled with blood or body fluids, and for performing venipuncture and other vascular access procedures.

Gloves should be changed after contact with each patient. *Masks and protective eyewear or face shields* should be worn during procedures that are likely to generate droplets of blood or other body fluids to prevent exposure of mucous membranes of the mouth, nose, and eyes. *Gowns or aprons* should be worn during procedures that are likely to generate splashes of blood or other body fluids.

2. *Hands and other skin surfaces should be washed immediately* and thoroughly if contaminated with blood and other body fluids. Hands should be washed immediately after gloves are removed.

3. *All health care workers should take precautions to prevent injuries caused by needles, scalpels, and other sharp instruments or devices* during procedures; handling sharp instruments; during disposal of used needles; and when needles should not be recapped, purposely bent or broken by hand, removed from disposable syringes, or otherwise manipulated by hand. After they are used, *disposable syringes and needles,* scalpel blades, and other sharp items should be placed in puncture-resistant containers for disposal; the puncture-resistant containers should be located as close as practical to the use area. Large-bore reusable needles should be placed in a puncture-resistant container for transport to the reprocessing area.

4. Although saliva has not been implicated in HIV transmission, to minimize the need for emergency mouth-to-mouth resuscitation, mouthpieces, resuscitation bags or other ventilation devices should be available for use in areas in which the need for resuscitation is predictable.

Radiation Effects

Radiation effects result from the energy emitted by the radioactive source. The severity of the incident depends upon the intensity and the type of radiation—alpha, beta, or gamma. Protection required for rescue personnel will vary with the type of radiation source, container shielding, and duration and intensity of exposure. Alpha radiation requires minimal protection, since the alpha particle will not penetrate clothing or intact skin. Protection against inhalation and ingestion is very important, however, as alpha radiation can cause severe damage if taken internally.

Beta radiation will penetrate clothing and other common forms of hazardous materials protection. Therefore, the principles of time and distance become important protection against this type of radiation. Exposure can be decreased to one-fourth by doubling the distance from the source.

Gamma radiation will penetrate most forms of protection. They require very dense materials such as lead to provide protection (Figure 7.6). Again, time and distance become very important. The shorter the time and the greater the distance from the materials, the less exposed the individual is. Contamination with materials containing radiation emitting products can be a problem since this defeats the distance and time principles. Good contamination containment and control is important.

Types of Ionizing Radiation
The severity of radiation exposure depends on the intensity and type of radiation—alpha, beta, or gamma.

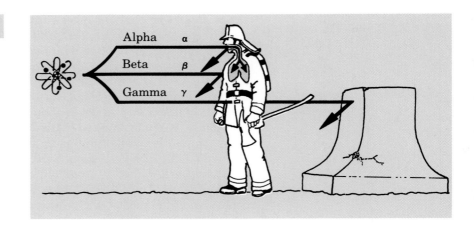

Asphyxiation

Asphyxiation can occur in two ways. Many materials such as nitrogen and carbon dioxide have the ability to displace oxygen when released in confined spaces. Asphyxiation can also occur when chemical reactions interfere with the respiratory process. For example, carbon monoxide reduces the oxygen-carrying capability of the red blood cells, and cyanide prevents oxygen from being absorbed into body tissue.

These types of injuries may be present in hazardous materials incidents. But rescue personnel must also consider the risks of contamination as well as the injury resulting from direct exposure.

PROTECTION

Protection must be provided to you and the patient to prevent further injury or contamination. You must consider all of the potential hazards and then develop a protective strategy to minimize the danger.

There are three main factors to consider when attempting to minimize the exposure: time, distance, and shielding.

Time The longer an individual is exposed to a hazard, the higher the probability an injury will occur. Extended exposure also contributes to the degree of injury, much like a sunburn. When managing a rescue, consider the time factor. Rotate rescue teams to reduce exposure to an acceptable level and keep the exposure time to a minimum.

Distance Radioactive materials provide a good example of exposure reduction as the distance increases. Doubling the distance from a radiation source decreases the exposure to one fourth. The distance principle applies to all hazardous material exposures, though the distance/intensity relationship will vary from product to product. The concentration decreases as you move away from the spill or release. Because a greater distance between you and a hazardous material means less exposure, all personnel not directly involved in the operation, including spectators, must be kept at a safe distance (Figure 7.7).

Shielding Though generally thought of only for radiation protection, shielding refers to all protective equipment used by the rescuer. It is an absolute requirement that you be familiar with the protective equipment and clothing you will use. What will happen when the shielding material is exposed to the agent? What is the amount of time required for the agent to break through the protective material? Are the materials compatible? You should not assume that your gear will protect you from the hazardous material. Your decisions must be based on fact.

Required protective garments and equipment vary according to the type of hazard and the degree of exposure. The U.S. Environmental Protection Agency (EPA) has a four-level classification for protective equipment to assist you in determining the level of protection required (Figure 7.8). The classification is based on the degree of protection provided to the skin and the respiratory tract. Level D provides minimal protection. It consists of the normal work uniform, including safety shoes, hard hat, gloves, and eye protection.

Level C adds chemical-resistant overalls, gloves, eye protection, and an appropriate respirator. This provides better skin protection as well as some respiratory protection.

Level B adds a SCBA for additional respiratory protection. Skin protection is still not the best; however, respiratory protection is excellent.

Level A is a totally encapsulated system with a SCBA . It provides the maximum level of protection to both skin and respiratory system.

Respirators should not be used unless the hazardous material is known, and its concentration is well below the Immediately Dan-

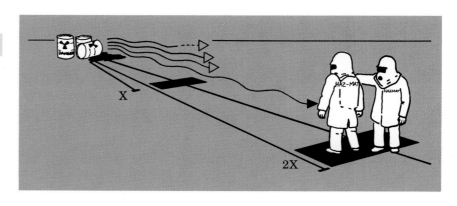

FIGURE 7.7

Exposure to Radiation
Doubling the distances from the radiation source decreases the exposure to one-fourth. All personnel not directly involved in the operation must be kept at a safe distance.

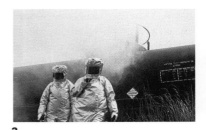
a.

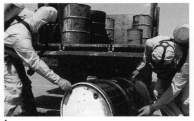
b.

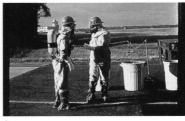
c.

FIGURE 7.8

Rescuer Wearing EPA Level Protective Equipment
The U.S. Environmental Protection Agency classifies its protective equipment based on the degree of protection provided to the skin and respiratory tract.

gerous to Life and Health (IDLH) level. Otherwise a SCBA must be used.

Levels A, B, and C require the use of specialized chemical-resistant clothing, gloves, eyewear, and so on. Most rescuers do not have this type of equipment immediately available. Those that do must make their selection based on the hazardous materials most likely route of entry into the body: absorption, inhalation, or ingestion (injection is not considered to be of significance). Most rescuers will use Level D or possibly Level B protection.

Accommodations to provide additional protection for very short periods of time can be made to Level D clothing. For example, if you are wearing fire service protective equipment, the use of a hood and turnout pants rather than three-quarter length boots and gloves with long gauntlets will help. Turnout gear, however, provides minimal hazardous materials protection because it is designed only for fire, heat, and water protection. The use of bands or duct tape around areas where openings occur, for example, wrists, ankles, waist, or zippers, will help reduce exposure. Chemical-resistant gloves, disposable booties, and SCBA enhance this level of protection. However, you must remember that protection is still limited and should be used only in the case of lifesaving emergency. Normal street clothing does not provide any significant protection.

A major problem with using substitute protection is that the hazardous material may enter and pass through the materials relatively easily, thereby reducing effective working time. In addition, substitute materials, especially natural fibers, may create absorption and contamination problems. Many materials are damaged by hazardous materials, both corrosive and noncorrosive. An example of damage by noncorrosive materials is Nomex™ material, used in fire protective clothing, that comes in contact with petroleum products. The petroleum product attaches to the Nomex,™ and, regardless of washing, will continue to adhere to the Nomex™. When heated, the petroleum product will vaporize, creating a hazardous, flammable condition that can endanger the wearer.

The degree of protection required is determined by the data collected in the early stages of the incident. If you know what the hazard(s) is, what task(s) must be performed, what protective equipment is accessible, and how much time is available to accomplish the task, you can make an informed decision about the advisability of entering the hazardous area to perform the required work.

DECONTAMINATION

Exposure to hazardous substances can be reduced by proper contamination control. **Decontamination** is the process of removing toxic and other harmful materials and properly disposing of them. It is an important part of all incidents involving hazardous materials, regardless of the materials involved or the size of the incident. Containment and decontamination must be included in the initial planning of all hazardous materials incidents.

There are four generally accepted methods of decontamination: dilution, absorption, chemical washes, and disposal and isolation. *Note that only the first three can be used on personnel.*

Dilution is the process of using copious amounts of water to flush hazardous residues from personnel and equipment (Figure 7.9). The runoff water must be contained and disposed of properly. The addition of soap or a mild detergent may speed the decontamination process.

Water is the most commonly used solution for dilutional decontamination. Other common decontamination solutions are

1. Sodium carbonate (washing soda)—5% to 10% aqueous solution, good water softening agent, effective for inorganic acids.

FIGURE 7.9

Flushing Hazardous Residues from Personnel
Dilution is the use of copious amounts of water to flush hazardous residues. It is one accepted method of decontaminating personnel and equipment after exposure to hazardous materials. Runoff must be contained and disposed of properly.

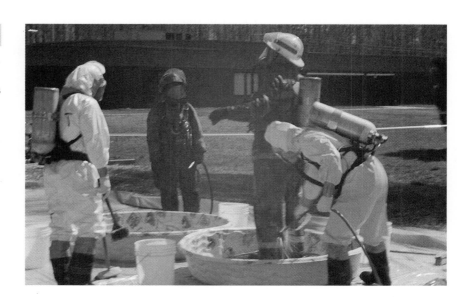

2. Sodium bicarbonate (baking soda)—5% to 10% aqueous solution, amphoteric (it can behave as either an acid or a base), effective with most acids and bases.
3. Trisodium phosphate (TSP, Oakite)—5% aqueous solution, good water softening agent and detergent, a general rinse solution.
4. Combination—an aqueous solution of 5% sodium carbonate and 5% trisodium phosphate.
5. Calcium hypochlorite (HTH)—10% aqueous solution, disinfectant, bleaching and oxidizing agent; care required in storage, mixing, and application; when heated above 212° F will explode; will react with water or steam to produce toxic and corrosive fumes; can react vigorously with reducing materials. This is the product used to purify water and treat swimming pools.

Absorption is the process used primarily for equipment but has limited application to personnel. Materials such as anhydrous fillers, soil, and other commercially available products are used to pick up the contaminant from the surface of equipment and personnel. Absorbents should be used only by trained personnel.

Chemical washes alter the hazardous material to a nonhazardous by-product. These can be used to wash down equipment, and some may be used on people.

Disposal and isolation is the process of discarding contaminated materials by prior packaging and shipment to an approved dump or incinerator. In some cases, there is no other option available except to dispose of contaminated equipment, no matter how expensive or irreplaceable it is.

Before you commit a piece of equipment to a hazardous material incident, you should consider the following:

1. Will the equipment withstand the required decontamination process?
2. After decontamination, can the equipment be sterilized, if required?
3. Can the equipment be tested for residual contamination?

If the answer is No to any of these questions, the equipment may require disposal after the incident. That can be an expensive proposition particularly if the equipment was not really needed for the rescue.

Decontamination should be done initially at the incident site. Selection of an appropriate location is determined by the following three questions:

1. Are required resources (for example, water) immediately available?
2. Can decontamination be conducted safely, considering personnel and the environment?
3. Can the equipment used during the process of decontamination be decontaminated?

Personnel decontamination should be done in a step-by-step process beginning with the removal of the outer layers of clothing without touching the contaminated portion. Gloves and respiratory protection should be worn throughout the process. During the decontamination process, assistants should wear protective clothing to at least the same level as those being decontaminated. Final decontamination may require a total body wash. Rescue personnel should shower again immediately after returning to their station.

MANAGEMENT OF EXPOSURES

Patients affected by hazardous materials may also have traumatic injuries or other illnesses because of the incident. You must avoid aggravating these injuries as you manage the hazard exposure.

The most frequent problem you face is determining whether the patient's medical condition or the chemical hazard requires management priority. Measures to control hemorrhage, shock, respiratory, or cardiovascular problems may be of equal or greater urgency than treatment for hazardous material exposure. All required assessment and treatment measures have to be performed in rapid sequence or by simultaneous team action. Patients sustaining an injury during a hazardous materials incident require a modified approach if a hazard exposure is known or suspected. If the patient is stable, decontamination prior to treatment must be instituted. The specific management of the injury remains essentially the same, that is, airway management, fracture immobilization using backboards and/or splints, and so forth. You must be protected at the appropriate level before providing treatment.

Rescuer Protection

To become proficient at providing medical care during a hazardous materials response, you should train while wearing protective equipment. At the same time, this will give you an understanding for what you cannot do. If the exposure is minimal and contamination can be contained, normal initial assessment steps should be taken for the patient. If you are not able to provide medical care (for example, you are wearing Level A protection), the patient must be moved as quickly, efficiently , and safely as possible to an uncontaminated area. Preparing the patient for movement may not be easy when you are wearing protective equipment. You must decide on acceptable risks both to the patient and the yourself.

Cardiopulmonary resuscitation (CPR) cannot be performed easily when you are wearing protective equipment. In addition, if the patient has been exposed to a toxic gas atmosphere, mouth-to-mouth resuscitation should not be done. You will then be exposed to the same toxic atmosphere even if you are not in the spill area. CPR should be performed in a contamination-free environment using respiratory assistance equipment, if possible. If you decide that the risk of working in the hazardous atmosphere is acceptable, all equipment and personnel should be protected as much as possible within the limits of the operation. You should expect to treat those individuals involved in the operation as possibly exposed and contaminated.

Managing Injured or Ill Patients

If patients with traumatic injuries or other medical illness are exposed to certain hazardous materials, such as radiologic, biologic, and certain chemicals, decontamination should be accomplished as soon as the situation permits. Lifesaving measures for a traumatic injury or some medical problems must be given priority over immediate decontamination despite the possible increase in chemical injury to the patient caused by the delay. The general principle is: *"Better blistered and living than decontaminated and dead."*

When a contaminated patient has other injuries or illnesses, the recommended order for emergency action is:

1. Control of respiratory failure with assisted ventilation
2. Control massive hemorrhage (bleeding) with pressure dressings
3. Administration of antidote, if available
4. Decontaminate the face
5. Remove contaminated clothing as soon as possible, and always before the patient is moved indoors or into the ambulance
6. Decontaminate the skin, where required
7. Provide additional emergency medical care and treatment for shock, wounds, and illness that are so severe that delay may endanger life (radiologic contamination is always secondary to other medical problems)
8. Manage and stabilize injuries
9. Transport to appropriate medical facility

Always alert the receiving facility as to the type of exposure, the extent of potential contamination, and the degree of decontamination accomplished on site. Then the hospital personnel may be adequately prepared and protected. *Remember to protect yourself and other rescuers during the decontamination process using the principles outlined earlier.*

Hazardous materials exposure may cause rapid changes in a patient's condition. Therefore, continuous monitoring is required. Medical personnel should be prepared for the potential changes caused by the patient's exposure and be able to recognize these changes. As with any other patient, basic airway support and monitoring of vital signs are essential. If advanced life support capability is available, it should be used as an extra measure of control for the patient. Appropriate shock management procedures should be followed.

Contamination Control During Transport

During transport, the patient should still be considered contaminated even though decontamination procedures were conducted at the site. Transport personnel should wear appropriate protective clothing. Contamination control procedures must continue during transport. Often the easiest method is to wrap the patient in an impermeable sheet to avoid further contamination, provided that this will not severely interfere with medical care.

Ambulances or other transport vehicles should be prepared before transporting a contaminated patient. The transport should be made in a vehicle with a partition between the driver and patient compartments to prevent the possibility of driver exposure. Drape the inside of the vehicle with plastic sheeting before loading the contaminated patient. Unnecessary items should be removed, and cabinet drawers and doors sealed with tape to prevent entry of contaminates. This will eliminate having to remove materials from the cabinets.

Equipment that must be used in the contaminated environment may be protected by covering it with plastic. However, a small part of the equipment must be exposed, such as the mask on a resuscitator. Proper protective measures significantly reduce decontamination problems after the incident and reduces equipment loss .

Remember to maintain contamination control at all times. Secondary contamination can sometimes become more devastating than the initial exposure. Proper cleaning and/or disposal of protective clothing and equipment used during the rescue will also ensure that adequate contamination control is maintained.

Secondary exposure of persons not actually involved in the incident have led to serious illness and, occasionally, to death. Many of these cases were the result of rescue personnel who did not use effective contamination control procedures properly. As a result, they carried the hazardous material into their homes.

If you recognize the possibility of hazardous materials being present and take appropriate action, you can minimize the risks.

SUMMARY

Incidents involving hazardous materials can be very dangerous to rescuers, but they can be managed. The rescuer must remember the principles to reduce exposure: decreased time, increased distance, and shielding. Often the only recourse for the rescuers arriving first is to wait for a hazardous materials team, which will be equipped and trained to cope with the situation. If you can recognize the possibility of hazardous materials being present and take appropriate action based on that knowledge, you can minimize your risks.

You must be prepared to make an initial asessment of a hazardous materials rescue site. Part of the training required to assess a site is knowledge of the classification system of hazardous materials with the identifying names, numbers, or codes. Another require-ment is the application of the Hazmat Rule of Thumb to determine the danger zone.

If the incident commander feels the rescue team can handle the situation without calling in specialists, three factors must be considered:

- Protection for both rescuer and patient from the hazardous materials.
- Decontamination control.
- Management of exposure and injuries.

Throughout the rescue operation, all rescue personnel must wear protective clothing, use the appropriate equipment, and participate in effective contamination control procedures to protect themselves and reduce personal risks.

CONFINED SPACES

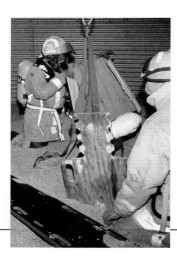

OVERVIEW

People trapped or disabled in confined spaces present rescuers with challenging situations. Confined spaces must be considered one of the most hazardous environments that face a rescuer.

This chapter defines and describes confined spaces and the hazards that can confront rescuers. These hazards include atmospheric, physical, and psychological hazards. In addition, the chapter explains how to manage potentially hazardous conditions in a confined space rescue.

This chapter also specifies the preplanning process. This section outlines a pre-incident plan to detail the hazards, map the area, and list qualified persons to help both the rescuer and the patient.

OBJECTIVES

The objectives of this chapter are for the rescuer to describe:

- a confined space.
- what determines whether a confined space is safe to enter to begin a rescue.
- a workable preplan.
- the atmospheric, physical, and psychological hazards in a confined space rescue operation.
- a safe ventilation system and when and how to use one.
- how to prevent physical injuries and hazards during a confined space rescue.
- how to avoid potential psychological anxieties by training and experience.
- how to make personal safety a top priority in a confined space rescue operation.

When people become disabled in very tight quarters, the rescuers are presented with a very difficult, unnatural, and dangerous situation. These locations are called **confined spaces.** They must be considered one of the most hazardous environments that confront the rescuer.

SPECIAL CONSIDERATIONS

A confined space is any space not intended for continuous occupancy, with limited or no ventilation and limited entrance/exit. Confined spaces include, but are not limited to, water and waste removal pipes and systems, wells, caves, grain storage facilities, reaction vessels, ventilation and/or other duct work systems, liquid storage tanks, tank cars, ship holds, and utility vaults. Confined spaces also include areas that are not small in size. The more important and potentially more hazardous factors are the limited entrance or exit and the limited ventilation. One example is a large grain elevator that must be considered a confined space even though many people could comfortably fit within its walls. It is not intended for continuous occupancy; it probably has little, if any, ventilation; and it is difficult to enter and exit. The contents also have the potential for engulfing the rescuer or the patient.

A major risk to the rescuer is that a confined space may look safe. Even experienced rescuers can develop tunnel vision, concentrating on the treatment of the patient. They may commit themselves to the dangers of the confined space, thus making themselves potential victims. The situation may be compounded when other rescuers attempt to save their team members and also become victims.

NEVER ENTER ANY CONFINED SPACE UNLESS IT HAS BEEN DETERMINED ABSOLUTELY SAFE FOR ENTRY.

Entry and patient stabilization must be attempted only with the proper equipment, after the appropriate training, and after the environment has been made as safe as possible.

PREPLANNING

Specific tactical decisions are based on the characteristics of the confined space. Confined space rescue involves extraordinary hazards. A pre-incident plan detailing the hazards, mapping the area, and listing qualified responsible persons can be a time- and a lifesaver for both the patient and the rescuer. The final incident plan should include the following steps:

- Gather as much information about the situation and the condition of the patient as possible. Locate responsible and knowledgeable people for advice. Most industrial concerns have strict entry requirements for their personnel. Locate the entry permits and double-check to make sure that safety requirements have been followed.
- Make certain an adequate number of additional personnel and a sufficient equipment have been called for. Examples include special rescue teams, air supply and lighting trucks, and special drilling, forcible entry, or hazardous materials units.

- Establish a clearly defined incident command network. Clear the entrance and exit areas of everyone except essential personnel. Stage all others to appropriate areas.
- Analyze the immediate environment of the confined space using gas detectors and information from knowledgeable people. Determine the exact oxygen content of the area. If there is a flammable product in the area, find out the limits of its flammable range.
- Reduce all hazardous conditions as much as possible. Begin a lockout procedure. The lockout procedure requires that all sources of power be identified. This lockout process may include electrical switches; hydraulic, steam, or pneumatic valves; and power take-off units from external machines. The term "lockout" means to shut off all power sources. Just as importantly, you must secure and control these power sources to prevent reactivation. The rescuer must lockout and prevent anyone from entering the area or gaining access to the controls of all power sources unless the individual is part of the rescue team and in direct contact with the rescue incident commander. When feasible, use employees of the facility to assist in securing all related electrical power, and post a guard. Cap or close all product transport devices and valves. Disable all electric or hydraulically-powered machinery within the confined space. Disconnect all steam or air operated equipment. If the atmosphere is immediately dangerous to life and health (IDLH), begin ventilation as soon as possible and eliminate any possible source of ignition.

DO NOT ENTER AN IDLH ENVIRONMENT

Rescuers who enter this environment without the proper training place themselves in great danger of becoming victims.

- Use a self-contained breathing apparatus (SCBA), preferably a supplied air system, if the air content is less than 19.5% oxygen. Use the buddy rescuer system, and place hose tenders at strategic positions. When there is no threat of fire or exposure to hazardous material, you may use less protective clothing, such as heavy coveralls, helmet, and gloves, if necessary to get into the confined space.
- Choose the best trained and most experienced personnel. Keep an identical backup team in reserve, ready to enter at a moment's notice.

Note: In caves and other confined spaces, conventional radio equipment may not work. You need to consider hard wire systems such as field phones. Because it is an arduous task to string and maintain a hard wire system in a cave, a special communications team should be assigned to this job. In a cave rescue, the telephone lines must be strung as soon as possible to prevent delays in the rescue. One recently developed alternative to the use of field phones underground is the so-called *Molephone*. The Molephone is a highly specialized unit that uses very low frequencies to penetrate the earth.

HAZARDS IN CONFINED SPACES

There are three groups of hazards in confined spaces. **Atmospheric hazards** are determined by the shape and configuration of the area, the degree of ventilation, and the presence of hazardous gases. The **physical hazards** include the presence of or potential for fire, the accumulation of hazardous materials, mechanical entrapment, electrical exposure, or product engulfment. **Psychological hazards** are those fears or anxieties that may profoundly effect your performance and the outcome of the rescue.

Atmospheric Hazards

Atmospheric conditions hazardous to the rescuer are those that present an unbreathable atmosphere. Air contains approximately 21% oxygen, 78% nitrogen, and 1% of other gases. Humans cannot function normally in an atmosphere much outside of these levels. Of primary concern is the oxygen content. Any confined space that falls under 19.5% oxygen content must be considered IDLH.

Anyone who enters an oxygen-poor atmosphere may not immediately notice the effects on his body, particularly when concentrating on a rescue. The effects of hypoxia (low oxygen) vary. But typically, the person becomes excited, agitated, or develops the symptoms of intoxication. The person may rush to escape the area, which only increases his oxygen demand. There are reported instances of people just sitting down and laughing. Disorientation, weakness, and lethargy are the factors that prevent self-rescue from the situation.

It is the lack of both adequate ventilation and inflow of sufficient fresh air that causes confined spaces to be so dangerous. In addition, oxygen can be consumed by many sources. In some settings, natural, rotting vegetation consumes oxygen. Rodents or other animals may consume additional oxygen. In most incidents, however, methane, hydrogen sulfide, or other gases produced by decaying matter displace the oxygen and can cause death by suffocation.

Oxygen can also be removed by certain chemical reactions. This can be particularly important around factories, chemical plants, and construction sites. Oxygen is consumed during rust formation on steel ladders, pumps, and other steel structures. Freshly poured concrete uses up a tremendous amount of oxygen. Special care should be taken when working around newly poured enclosed structures.

Toxic gases are also a threat in confined space. Hydrogen sulfide, for example, is an extremely toxic gas that is heavier than air. It can displace oxygen as it rests in the low spaces that may be present in confined spaces. Hydrogen sulfide can be fatal if even small amounts are inhaled. It must be avoided.

Grain bins, silos, and manufacturing vessels where the atmosphere is highly saturated with grain dust or similar materials must be treated in the same way as vessels with flammable vapors. The dust to air mixture can easily be in the explosive range. A single spark can have catastrophic results.

Combating Atmospheric Hazards   The solution to combating the atmospheric hazards encountered in confined spaces is twofold. First, the atmosphere must be tested with an acceptable testing device used by someone familiar with the equipment. The most important readings indicate a potential IDLH atmosphere: abnormal oxygen content and the presence of toxic and/or flammable gases and vapors. There are many different units available. Unfortunately, no two detectors operate in the same manner. More importantly, a gas detector that is being used by someone only marginally competent in its use can be a greater hazard than help. A rescue team could develop a false sense of security if the person using the detector makes an improper reading.

The single best source of information regarding the proper use of a particular gas detector is the manufacturer. Insist on training time with the manufacturer before purchasing a new gas detector.

The second tactic to reduce hazardous atmospheric conditions in confined spaces is to attempt thorough ventilation of the structure. This can often be done with the ventilation system built into the structure. However, you must first know the location and condition of the patient. You must also know any possible effect that ventilation may have on the patient's condition. You must be certain that the patient will not become injured by starting the ventilation system. One reliable and easy-to-use ventilation system is the smoke ejector that is located on most fire trucks. It will usually discharge between 5,000 and 10,000 cubic feet of air per minute (Figure 8.1). Always blow fresh air into the confined space. Never pull the air out of the confined space using just one fan. By pulling a suction, you pull the reserves of hazardous gases accumulated throughout the confined

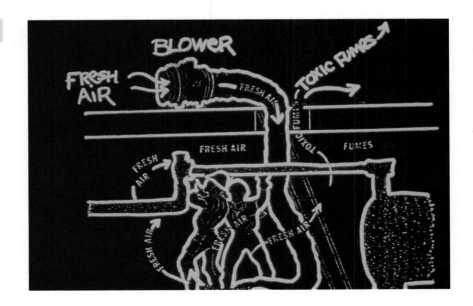

FIGURE 8.1

Ventilation Chart
A smoke ejector can be used to ventilate a confined space. The air should always be blown into the confined space, and never be drawn out of the space.

space across the victim, making the air supply worse instead of better. Always be certain that when blowing with forced air ventilation that the air source is not polluted by the exhaust of a truck or other source. Extension tubes on the fans can be used to help select air suction sites. Make certain that all fans and lights have explosion-proof motors and switches.

Another tactic is the use of positive pressure ventilation with the fans set up several feet from the entrance of the confined space. When it can be used, this technique increases ventilation because of the *venturi effect*, the increased volume of air created by the pressurized air stream. Also attempt to cross-ventilate the structure through doors or makeshift portals. Or use fans to blow good air in with the same number of fans on the opposite side to pull air out.

When making ventilation decisions, consider the content of flammable gases and liquids in a confined space. Flammable gases must have a specific mixture of gas and air to burn (flammable range). The **lower explosive limit (LEL)** is the point at which a gas mixes with just the proper amount of oxygen to burn (Table 8.1). This is similar to the concept of a carburetor mixing the proper amounts of gasoline and air. If the confined space has too much gas compared

TABLE 8.1   Lower Explosive Limit

	Percent by Volume in Air Lower Limit–Upper Limit
Liquids	
Kerosene	0.7– 5.0
Petroleum ether	0.1– 5.9
Benzene	1.3– 7.1
Gasoline	1.4– 7.6
Liquified Gases	
Butylene (Butene)	1.65– 9.95
Butane	1.86– 8.41
Propylene	2.0–11.1
Butadiene	2.0–11.5
Propane	2.12– 9.35
Gases	
Cyclopropane	2.4–10.4
Acetylene	2.5–81.0
Ethane	3.0–12.5
Methane (Natural Gas)	5.0–15.0
Hydrogen	4.0–74.2

The lower explosive limit (LEL) is the point at which a gas mixes with the proper amount of oxygen to burn.
Adapted from *Combustion Flame and Explosion of Gases*, B. Lewis and G. von Elbe, Academic Press (1951).

to the air (too rich), an explosion or fire cannot take place. But once ventilation is begun and the air/gas mixture falls and approaches the upper flammable range, an explosion is possible.

This could also happen in a confined space incident when air is inducted into a flammable liquid storage tank via a hose stream used to reduce sparks from a circular saw used in the extrication. The venturi effect created might allow the air/gas mixture to approach the flammable range and be ignited by the sparks from the saw. The safest alternative under these circumstances would be to breach the integrity of the tank wall by some other means, for example, a hydraulic spreader or cutter or heavy air chisel.

The only alternative to ventilating a too rich, flammable atmosphere is to enter the confined space with the proper breathing apparatus and protective clothing.

As stated before, entry into a confined space with dangerous atmospheric conditions is one of the most hazardous situations for rescue personnel. You must be properly equipped and have trained and practiced with competent instructors before considering such a tactic.

Because the air in many such incidents is unbreathable, the team must wear a SCBA. Because of the close quarters and the potential for entrapment in the confined space, the typical fire service, bottle-on-back SCBA is unacceptable for use in most confined space rescue situations. The most suitable equipment for the job is the supplied air or "in-line" breathing apparatus (Figure 8.2). This is a specially

FIGURE 8.2

In-Line SCBA
Supplied air or "in-line" breathing apparatus is used in confined spaces. During a confined space rescue, each rescuer should also have an escape bottle with at least five minutes of air in case the supplied air system fails.

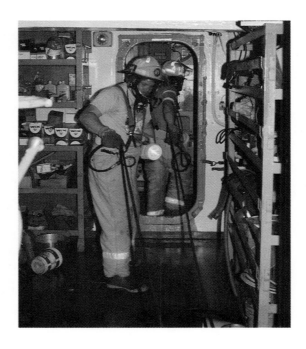

designed unit that is very lightweight. The wearer dons the face mask and straps a small escape bottle (a reserve air supply) to the waist. Air is supplied via hoses that are attached to breathing air regulators and compressed air cylinders or air compressors outside.

The advantage supplied air systems have over SCBAs is that they do not encumber the rescuer with heavy, bulky equipment. They also have a nearly unlimited supply of air, providing the compressor or compressed air cylinders are in good working order and are operated properly. However, a supplied air system is limited by the length of the air hoses. Using supplied air systems, you must be careful not to entangle or damage air lines. A hose tending team and buddy system inside the confined space can help reduce these problems. A minimum five-minute escape bottle is mandatory when using supplied air systems.

Physical Hazards

Among the numerous physical hazards of confined spaces are the potential for entrapment, electrocution, drowning, burns from steam, scalds from liquids, crush injuries, fall-related injuries, or impalement on sharp objects. You must locate and secure any mechanical, electrical, or product transfer device that could endanger you or the patient.

Combating Physical Hazards Locate the person responsible for the structure. In a factory this may be a maintenance supervisor or engineer. Establish direct communication with these individuals, and keep them at your side throughout the operation. They are an excellent resource.

Locate and secure all electrical and mechanized devices in the confined space. This may require locking electrical boxes and posting a guard to ensure that someone does not inadvertently turn on a switch. Remove or block off any product lines, including chemical, steam, and water lines. Secure other apparatus affecting the confined space.

Select the best trained and most experienced individuals for the initial access and patient assessment. A major consideration is the size of the rescuer. When all other factors are equal, the smaller the rescuer, the better.

Under extreme circumstances, such as a very hazardous environment with the potential for explosion or when hazardous material exposure is possible, the time the rescuer spends in the confined space should be short. The rescuer should take all the previously mentioned precautions and make a very rapid access to the patient. Once access is gained, a hasty connection can be made to the patient by the wristlet method (Figure 8.3), if the exit is no more than 200 feet away and the route not cluttered with obstructions. This method involves carrying a 10 to 15 foot loop of nylon webbing and attaching it to

FIGURE 8.3

Wristlet Method
One technique for quickly
removing a patient from a
confined space is the wristlet
method. Attach a 10 to 15
foot loop of tubular webbing
to the patient's wrists using
a girth hitch to haul the
patient from the area.

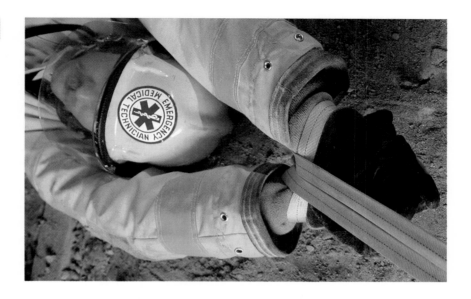

the patient's wrists using a girth hitch. This will enable a quick
retreat by the rescuer, while the patient is dragged out by rope.

Of all of the considerations required when making personnel decisions for confined space entry, the single most important factor is
the level of training and experience. To be a qualified rescuer, you
should have spent many hours training in confined locations so you
are familiar with the physical and psychological extremes present,
and to have the medical expertise necessary to assess and stabilize
the patient.

Psychological Hazards

Perhaps the most challenging aspect of confined space rescue involves
the psychological stress generated by the many potential hazards.
You may experience a high level of anxiety when entering a tight
enclosure under emergency conditions with limited escape options,
especially in the presence of electrical hazards, hazardous materials,
and little or no breathable air. However, training and experience can
prepare you to assist those that have been injured or disabled in
confined spaces.

Combating Psychological Hazards   Every person has some anxiety when entering a confined space. This anxiety is a normal and
natural part of the self-preservation instinct present in every person.
The way to control confined space anxiety is to train under realistic
conditions with a qualified instructor. As you train, you will become
more comfortable with the unusual surroundings and be able to concentrate more on the goals of access, patient care, and extrication.

The safety of the rescuer must always come first. You must answer YES to three questions before contemplating a confined space entry:

1. Am I absolutely sure that this area is safe?
2. If not, do I have access to specialized equipment to work in a confined space?
3. Am I trained in and do I feel comfortable with confined space entry and rescue?

If the answer to any of these questions is *no*, do not attempt the rescue until the situation improves and you can answer *yes* to all three questions.

A common confined space mishap parallels the following tragic incident. A utility contractor was installing supports for an underground waste pumping system. The worker was in a vessel constructed of steel and newly poured concrete, located 35 feet below grade. The only access to the pump location was a three-tiered steel ladder. Shortly after entering the structure, the worker became disoriented and called for help. From the top of the structure, a co-worker entered the vessel to assist the first worker up the ladder. He became too weak to make the ascent. After approximately 15 minutes, a foreman discovered the two dead workers. He also attempted entry, but fortunately realized the hazard when a short distance down the ladder. He managed to climb back up the ladder and escaped to call the fire department for assistance. The fire department ventilated the structure with a smoke ejector. Then rescue personnel with SCBAs were able to remove the bodies of the two workers.

The situation could have been much worse had the foreman not quickly realized the cause of the problem. In this case compassion helped to kill the second worker and almost disabled the foreman. Had any unprotected fire department personnel entered the structure, they also could have become victims. When this domino effect occurs, in which the rescuer becomes the patient and the next rescuer also becomes a patient, the situation becomes dangerously more complicated. With more victims and fewer rescuers, the odds of a successful rescue are drastically reduced.

SUMMARY

Confined spaces, one of the most hazardous environments facing rescuers, is any space not intended for continuous occupancy and with limited ventilation and limited entrance/exit. Confined spaces are not necessarily small in size. A large grain elevator is an example that fits the criteria of a confined space.

A major risk that a rescuer must address at the beginning of the rescue is the question of whether the confined space is safe. Rescue personnel should never enter a confined space that has not been declared safe for entry. Furthermore, entering and stabilizing a patient in a confined space must be attempted only with the proper equipment and only after the appropriate training.

A preplan is vital to a successful outcome of a confined space rescue. Because confined space rescues involve unusual dangers, the preplan details the hazards, maps the area, and lists persons who are trained to help both the rescuer and the patient. The preplan also determines the number and type of resources needed and establishes an incident command network.

At the beginning of the operation, you should clear the area of all but essential personnel. You must analyze the confined space for gas, oxygen, or any flammable product. If the atmosphere is immediately dangerous to life and health (IDLH), you should begin ventilation and eliminate any source of ignition. You should also wear protective clothing and gear, including self-contained breathing apparatuses (SCBAs), and use a buddy system.

Communications among rescuers is extremely important. Unfortunately, in confined space rescues, conventional communications equipment may not work. There are alternate devices that do function in confined spaces.

There are three types of hazards in confined space rescues: atmospheric, physical, and psychological. Atmospheric conditions are determined by the shape and size of the area, the degree of ventilation, and the presence of hazardous gases. To avoid atmospheric hazards you must first test the atmosphere to learn what, if any, threats exist. Second, ventilate the confined space if it does not endanger the patient or the rescuer and does not compound the hazards and dangers of the situation.

Physical hazards include fire or its potential, accumulation of hazardous materials, mechanical entrapment, electrical exposure, or product engulfment. Confined space rescues also have the potential for injuries, burns, or impalement on sharp objects.

Psychological hazards are fears or anxieties that can impair performance and the outcome of the rescue. Entering a confined space, especially when knowing its extraordinary hazards, can be very stressful. However, training under realistic conditions with a qualified instructor can prevent stress and help you focus on the goals of patient access, care, and extrication rather than on your anxieties and fears.

DISASTERS

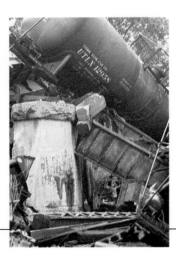

OVERVIEW

Many people assume that a disaster involves widespread destruction or hundreds of casualties. In some cases this is true, but any incident exceeding the capacity of local resources to respond adequately is also a disaster. It is, therefore, essential that you understand the nature of disasters.

This chapter describes the problems inherent in natural disasters such as floods, tornadoes, and earthquakes as well as technological disasters.

OBJECTIVES

The objectives of this chapter are for the rescuer to describe:

- rescue operations during a flood, tornado, or earthquake.
- tracking systems (National Oceanic and Atmospheric Administration and the National Weather Service) as a means of predicting disasters.
- how to perform triage at a disaster scene.
- how to recognize stress reactions, both immediate and delayed.

A disaster cannot be defined simply by the number of people injured. It is best defined as any incident that will overload the capabilities and resources of the local community. In some areas, a complex vehicle accident can be a disaster.

Disasters are often categorized into two types: natural or technological (man-made). Floods, tornadoes, and earthquakes are natural disasters while radiation leaks, chemical releases, and major transportation system accidents constitute technological or man-made disasters. Each disaster may cause different, specific problems, but the overall effect on rescue personnel is similar. Manpower and equipment resources are insufficient, transportation systems are tangled, medical facilities are overwhelmed, and communication systems are overloaded or damaged by the disaster itself. Finally, rescuers, patients, and survivors in the field often have to fend for themselves.

One common problem during disasters is the overload on medical facilities. This is often unnecessary because a few hospitals, close to the incident, are overburdened while other hospitals farther away have a light patient load. A primary goal for triage and transportation personnel in disasters is to avoid transferring the disaster from the incident site to the hospital. Before initiating transport of multiple casualties from a disaster, consult with the disaster medical coordinator or with the hospital. Remember that in many local disasters the medical facilities closest to the incident will be overloaded with "walking wounded" and other patients who have arranged their own tranport outside the EMS system.

It is very important that medical facilities at a disaster be organized to deal with the emergency. Figure 9.1 illustrates a typical incident command organizational chart for a medical branch at a disaster or multi-casualty incident.

FIGURE 9.1

Incident Command Organization Chart
A typical incident command organizational chart for a medical branch at a multi-casualty incident.

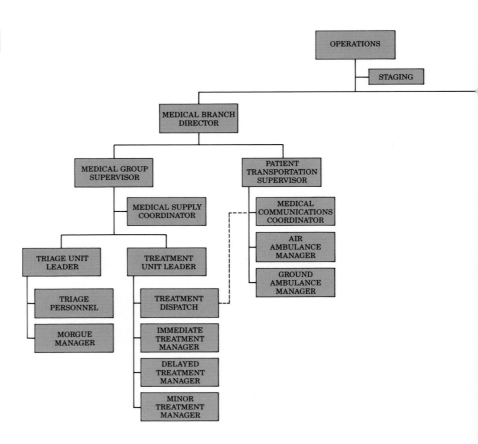

NATURAL DISASTERS

Floods

Floods have been a regular event in many regions. Because of the increasing population and economic development in many areas, people have been building homes and businesses in flood-prone areas at a risk to themselves and to their property.

For insurance purposes, the U.S. government uses historical records and hydrologic and hydraulic data to designate areas of waterways particularly at risk for flooding. Known as the *100-year flood level* or *base flood elevation,* this information is used by local government planners and zoning boards to define floodplains.

There are several types of flooding. **Riverine flooding** occurs in the inland watersheds of rivers and streams. The flooding usually results from a heavy or prolonged rain or a snow melt upstream. In most cases, there is adequate warning of the rising water to allow an orderly evacuation of persons living in the danger area.

During **flash floods,** the rise in the water level may occur so rapidly that individuals are caught without warning. Flash floods usually occur in steep-sided valleys as a result of sudden heavy downpours upstream. But they may also occur in flat terrain when there is a sudden release of water following a heavy rainfall, a dam failure, or the breakup of an ice jam. Flood damage is increased by high-velocity flows and by debris carried by the water (Figure 9.2).

Because of increasing land use in the southwestern United States, another type of flooding is becoming more frequent, **alluvial fan** flooding. This occurs in desert and semi-arid regions where sudden

FIGURE 9.2

Flood Damage
In riverine flooding, there is usually adequate warning for rescuers to perform an evacuation.

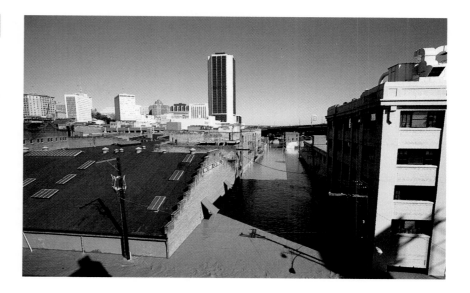

rainfalls flow down steep mountain drainages to empty suddenly onto flat valley floors. The name, alluvial fan, indicates the characteristic cone shape of the drainage. Alluvial fan floods are less predictable because they have no designated floodplain. At the upper parts of the fan these floods are extremely destructive because their high velocity flows carry large amounts of silt and heavy debris.

Coastal flooding results from storms in maritime areas. Heavy damage results from floodwaters driven ashore by heavy winds, such as occurs under hurricane conditions. The damage will be worse when the flooding coincides with high tides.

Flood Safety and Rescue Measures If a flood is predicted, monitor National Oceanic and Atmospheric Administration (NOAA) weather radio and other reliable weather sources. If you are in a floodplain, prepare to evacuate. If a flash flood warning is issued for your area, evacuate immediately, taking the shortest route to high ground. If you are driving, do not drive into any floodwaters unless you are certain of the water depth and the condition of the roadbed. If your vehicle is engulfed by floodwaters, abandon it immediately and move to higher ground.

Floodwaters often have a high velocity water flow. Do not enter floodwaters over your knees or where there is fast-moving debris. Do not go into any swiftly moving water unless you have the training and equipment for swift-water rescue. All rescue personnel involved in flooding incidents should wear a personal flotation device (PFD) at all times. Use a lifeline during any entry into flowing water.

Tornadoes

Tornadoes are extremely violent storms with wind speeds in their whirling center exceeding 200 miles an hour (Figure 9.3). Their destructive footprint may range up to a mile wide. Tornadoes do not generally last long, but can destroy buildings and cause many injuries and deaths in a matter of minutes. Although more common in the midwest and southern regions of the United States, tornadoes have been documented in all states. They usually occur in late spring and early summer, but have been recorded during all months of the year.

The National Weather Service (NWS) uses two terms to alert the public to severe weather conditions. The NWS issues a *watch* when conditions are right for the development of severe weather such as a tornado, but before severe weather has been spotted. Watches may be in effect for several hours to several days. A *warning* is issued when severe weather has actually developed and has been observed, such as when a tornado's echo has appeared on radar. A warning is usually in effect for periods from minutes to a few hours.

Tornado Safety and Rescue Measures There is little you can do during a tornado other than warn others and seek shelter. If time permits, secure outdoor objects such as furniture and garbage cans that could become windblown missiles. Seek shelter in the southeast

FIGURE 9.3

Tornado Damage
A tornado can cause extreme destruction, and result in many injuries and deaths along its path.

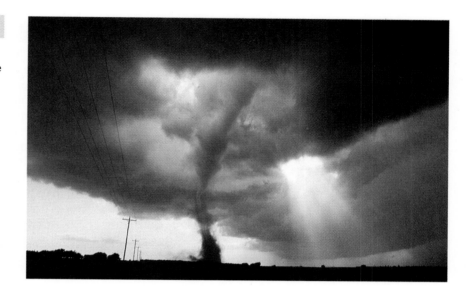

corner of a basement or in a closet or small inner room. Tornadoes can easily toss vehicles about, so if driving, leave the vehicle and seek shelter in a depression such as a ditch or culvert.

The rescue phase occurs after the tornado passes. It consists mainly of extricating victims from collapsed buildings or from under debris, attending to their medical needs, and evacuating them to the nearest undamaged medical facility.

Earthquakes

Earthquakes have the potential for causing widespread property destruction, loss of life, and serious injury. Although the most publicized North American earthquakes have occurred in California, destructive earthquakes have also happened throughout the United States and Canada.

Most earthquake-related injuries and deaths are caused by falling objects and collapsing buildings. Other damage, injury, and deaths are the result of secondary effects such as landslides, flooding from dam collapse, or earthquake-generated ocean waves known as **tsunamis.**

Earthquake Safety and Rescue Measures As a rescuer, your first responsibility is to protect yourself so that you can eventually help others. If you are indoors during an earthquake, avoid falling objects and structurally weak portions of the building. Stay away from bookshelves, mirrors, cabinets, and chimneys. Seek shelter by standing in the strong frame of a doorway, or crawl under a bed or strong desk or table. Do not go outside until the shaking has stopped and the building has settled. Do not use an elevator, but descend through a stairway.

If you are outdoors when the earthquake hits, stay away from power lines, poles, and walls. Seek open areas away from structures.

After the earthquake, immediately check utilities for damage. If there is damage to the electrical system, cut the electrical power at the main switch. If there are any suspected gas leaks, shut off the gas at the main valve. Extinguish any small fires, since fire equipment may not be able to reach the area immediately.

The greatest rescue demands will be in extricating victims from collapsed buildings and debris, attending to their medical needs, and transporting them to undamaged medical facilities. This may be an overwhelming challenge. The number of critical injuries may far surpass available resources. Streets may be blocked by debris. Hospitals may be destroyed. The best procedure for dealing with a widespread earthquake will be strong triage management and a well-developed, area-wide disaster preplan.

TECHNOLOGICAL OR MAN-MADE DISASTERS

An airplane crash, train derailment, hazardous materials leak or spill, building collapse or fire, are examples of technological or man-made disasters. Technological disasters tend to be localized and leave more of the infrastructure (communications systems, roads and bridges, hospitals, governmental systems and services, and so forth) intact, making it easier to manage the situation.

Triage Organization at a Disaster or Major Mass Casualty Incident

In a disaster or mass casualty incident, where medical resources are overwhelmed, **triage** is used to sort patients and allocate resources according to a system of priorities. This ensures the most efficient use of limited manpower, equipment, and facilities. At a major disaster, the triage process sorts patients into four categories:

- Deceased. This category is for patients who are obviously dead, mortally wounded, or unlikely to survive because of the extent of their injuries, age, and overall medical condition.
- Immediate care. This category is for patients with injuries threatening their airway, breathing, or circulation but who can be saved.
- Delayed. Patients who do not fit into the immediate or minor categories are classified as delayed.
- Minor. This category identifies patients who have only minor injuries. They are also known as "walking wounded."

At minor disasters where you can count on eventual assistance and where the medical facilities are not overwhelmed, you can do your triage using the modified **CRAMS scale:** circulation, respiratory, abdomen, motor, and speech (Figure 9.4).

However, at major disasters where resources will be limited for some time, where transportation resources are overloaded, or where hospitals have been destroyed or overwhelmed, you may wish to use **START**, the simple triage and rapid transport program (Figure 9.5).

FIGURE 9.4

CRAMS Scale
The CRAMS score for trauma patients is determined by adding the scores from the five body areas. A score of six or less indicates a critically injured patient.

Source: Clemmer, et al., *J. Trauma* 25(3): 188–91, Mar. 1285.

Circulation
2—Normal cap. refill and BP >100 mm Hg systolic
1—Delayed cap. refill or BP 85-99 mm Hg systolic
0—No cap. refill or BP <85 mm Hg systolic

Respiration
2—Normal
1—Abnormal (labored, shallow, or rate >35)
0—Absent

Abdomen
2—Abdomen and thorax not tender
1—Abdomen or thorax tender
0—Abdomen rigid, thorax flail, or deep penetrating injury to either chest or abdomen

Motor
2—Normal (obeys commands)
1—Responds only to pain—no posturing
0—Postures or no response

Speech
2—Normal (oriented)
1—Confused or inappropriate
0—No or unintelligible sounds

_____ Total CRAMS score (add the five areas)

START allows rescuers to triage patients in 60 seconds or less. It depends on only three physical assessments: ventilation, perfusion, and mental status.

After assessment, triage team members must attach a **triage tag** to all patients. (Figure 9.6). This allows rescuers who arrive later to stabilize the patients with the greatest need.

Stress Reactions

There are a number of psychological problems that can result from a disaster that affect both your patients and you. These are primarily stress reactions that may appear immediately or long after the event.

Some individuals may exhibit weeping, hysteria, panic, or loss of control. These individuals are a potential danger to themselves and others at the scene of a disaster. They may wander into dangerous areas, be combative, and spread their hysterical behavior.

If possible, these individuals should be transported to a hospital for psychiatric attention. If transport is not possible, they should be placed in the care of a responsible person and removed from the scene of the disaster. If another person is not available to care for hysterical patients, rescuers should attempt to calm them with firm and direct orders. Never slap or employ unnecessary force to subue a hysteric.

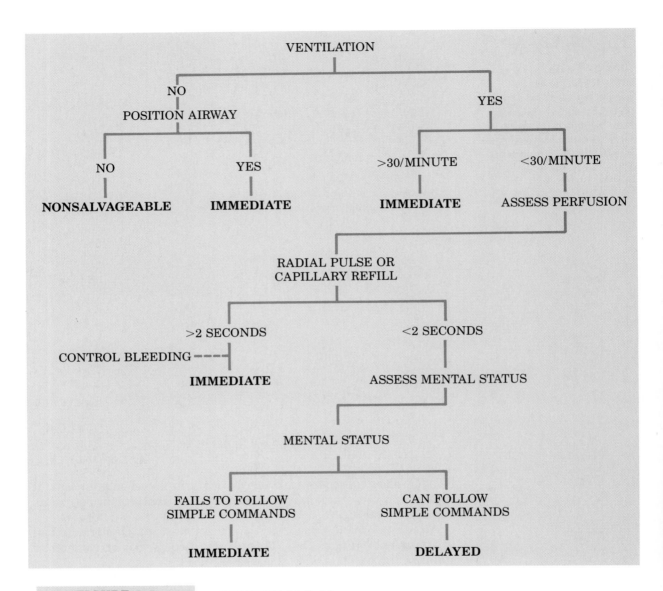

FIGURE 9.5   **START Field Guide**
START is a system of casualty rating using the simple triage and rapid transport program.

This may only aggravate the behavior. Rescuers must themselves appear calm and under control when dealing with such persons.

On the other hand, the depressed patient may appear subdued, yet be having serious emotional problems. The subject may only sit and stare or wander aimlessly. This person may be mentally confused and disoriented. If possible, remove the patient from the scene as soon

FIGURE 9.6

Triage Tag
As soon as they perform their quick assessment at a disaster scene, triage team members must attach a triage tag to all patients. This will allow rescuers who arrive later to attend to the patients with the most critical medical problems.

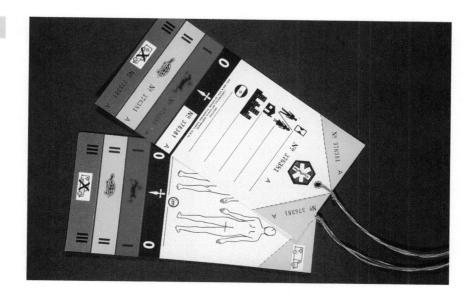

as possible. If transport is not possible, have the patient sit or lie down, and block the disaster scene from view. If possible, do not leave the patient alone. If a rescuer is not available, a calm bystander may be of assistance. Remember that confusion and disorientation may also be symptoms of a head injury or lack of oxygen.

You, too, may suffer a profound psychological impact immediately after dealing with a major incident or disaster. This is a very common and natural reaction to a major stressor. Post-incident debriefing and counseling should be provided to all rescue personnel involved in such situations.

Experiences encountered at disasters can also cause long-term emotional effects to both patients and rescuers called **delayed stress reactions**. Manifestations include sleep disturbances, loss of appetite, problems with alcohol, sexual dysfunction, feelings of guilt for having survived while others did not, and family problems. For your patients, the extent and depth of these emotional problems may depend on your initial response to the emergency.

Rescuers' long-term stress reactions from a disaster or multi-casualty incident may be the result of the degree of suffering or devastation at the incident or the horror of the carnage. Some rescue workers who normally receive great satisfaction from assisting living patients may be frustrated and dismayed having to deal only with dead and dying, especially if on a large scale. Following major incidents, agencies and organizations should obtain professional crisis intervention counseling for their personnel. You should feel free to discuss your feelings with others and to vent your emotions.

SUMMARY

A disaster can be one of two types: techno-logical or natural. Radiation leaks and chemical spills are examples of technological disasters while floods, tornadoes, and earth-quakes are natural disasters. Each disaster poses its own specific problems, but the over-all effect on rescue personnel is similar: insufficient resources and overwhelmed trans-portation, communication, and medical systems.

One serious problem common to all disas-ters is the overloading of emergency resources. Rescue teams must be careful during triage and transportation to avoid transferring the disaster from the incident site to the medical centers.

There are several types of flooding, includ-ing riverine flooding, flash flooding, alluvial fan flooding, and coastal flooding. Rescuers in any floodplain should prepare to evacuate if a flood is predicted. All rescuers involved in floods must wear a personal flotation device and use a lifeline when entering flow-ing water.

Tornadoes are extremely violent storms, usually of short duration. During a tornado, you can do little more than warn others and seek shelter. After a tornado has passed, the rescue operation begins. It usually involves extricating patients from debris, meeting their medical needs, and transporting them to a medical facility.

Earthquakes can cause widespread destruction and loss of life. Most injuries are the result of falling objects and collapsing buildings. As with tornadoes, rescue demands will be for extricating patients and attending to their medical needs. Strong triage manage-ment and a well-developed disaster preplan are your best tools for dealing with an earthquake.

Triage at a disaster sorts patients to ensure the most efficient use of limited facili-ties and resources. Depending on the extent of the disaster, you can use routine field triage scores or a rapid method that allows you to triage patients in less than 60 seconds.

No matter what type of disaster occurs, this type of incident places tremendous stress on both you and your patients. Individuals who are hysterical or out of control must be removed from the scene. Depressed persons may appear to be subdued but are really suffering serious emotional problems.

Rescue personnel, too, can suffer psycho-logical stress during and after a disaster. This is common, and you and your colleagues should be debriefed and counseled after the incident. In addition, you should be alert to the possibility of delayed stress reactions.

LOCATE

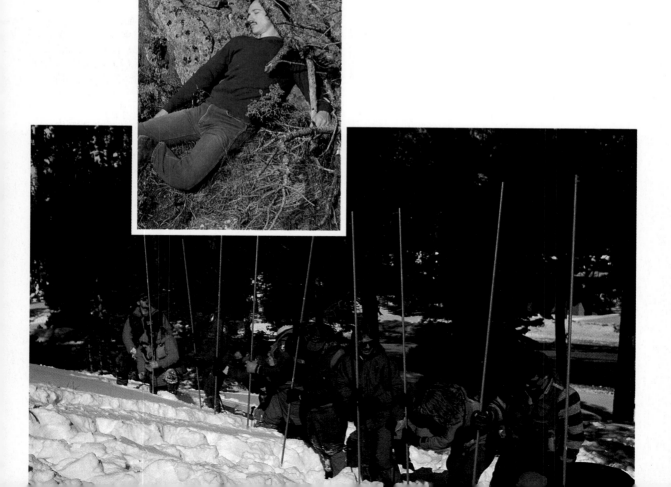

LOCATE

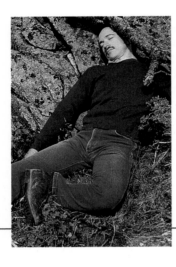

OVERVIEW

The search for and location of the subject is one of the first steps in a rescue mission. This chapter discusses the "locate" portion of a rescue. There are descriptions of initial response actions and types of searches. This chapter examines each type of search from the standpoints of initial actions, strategy and tactics, and effective resources. In addition, the chapter outlines the locate and access phases of a rescue at a structural collapse.

OBJECTIVES

The objectives of this chapter are for the rescuer to describe:

- the range and complexities of searches.
- the three primary search environments.
- how the environment influences the search and locate components of a rescue.
- the generic initial response actions for any rescue situation.
- the initial response actions for specific search environments.
- the strategy and tactics necessary for a successful outcome in each search environment.
- the most effective search resources to use in each search environment.
- the response considerations for structural collapse.

The techniques involved in searching for lost, overdue, or missing persons can vary greatly depending on the environment. In some cases, finding someone whose location is not known might be as simple as driving to an overlook and looking up to the side of a cliff with binoculars. You have then located that person. However, to access him and provide medical assessment, stabilization, and transport might be extremely difficult and time-consuming. In a different example, one or more subjects entrapped by the collapse of a building after an earthquake might present no problem because of the confined search. But accessing the patients might be extremely difficult and dangerous because of the need to move or cut through the debris. Another completely different search problem might involve finding someone who is several days overdue from a hike in a large, remote area. Finding this person might be extremely complex. Such a search will consume a great deal of time and resources. However, once you have found the missing hiker, you have probably accessed him. If your assessment shows he is not ill or injured, his stabilization and transportation might be as simple as escorting him to the trailhead.

The "locate" phase of a rescue mission involves solving problems related to the specific search environment. There are three primary environments where searches might be necessary:

- Natural areas, such as forests, deserts, and mountains
- Water, especially underwater
- Structural fires and collapsed structures

Although there are similarities in the response required for each of these environments, there are also significant differences.

The success of a search mission in any environment depends on:

- How long the subject has been missing before the response is initiated
- Information known about the circumstances of the lost person
- The resources used to find the missing person
- The strategy and tactics used to apply the resources to the search

GENERIC INITIAL RESPONSE ACTIONS

No matter what circumstances are involved when a person is missing, every search problem *must* initially be treated as urgent. In every situation, actions taken during the first six hours after a person "goes missing" are crucial to finding the person alive and well.

The first critical phase of a search occurs when the initial report comes in. At this point, the search team must gather as much information as possible. (A guideline for information gathering is provided below.) Some of this information may eventually prove to be unimportant. Not all of the requested information will be available in every case. But it is best to gather as much information as possible about the lost person and the circumstances. Later, you can determine its importance. It is easier to disregard unneeded information already obtained than to go back later and try to retrieve or reconstruct critical information.

In every search you must obtain information about each subject involved. The following checklist covers information most often needed to plan a search.

Subject Information This includes important indications about what the subject might do, where and how far he might go, how easily the subject might be spotted, how well he or she might survive. This information should include the clues that could help indicate the subject's whereabouts as well.

Activity You need to determine what the subject was doing (hiking, climbing, diving, or other activities), plus consider the following:

- Age
- Mental and physical condition of the subject
- Medical history
- Experience in the activity in which the subject is involved
- Equipment and belongings in the subject's possession
- Personality traits of the subject

Location Information Specific starting point(s) for the search, terrain or structure considerations for use by search resources, what actually happened, how far and what direction the subject might travel, and safety considerations for the searchers are some facts derived from this information. Also, searchers need to know the following:

- Specific last known position or point last seen
- Where was subject located, coming from, or going to
- Details about the surrounding location in terms of vegetation, water conditions, terrain, condition of the structure, and hazards

Weather Information What was the weather at the time the person was lost and since that time? How will the current and anticipated weather affect the subject, clues, and the searchers?

Other Information Who reported the incident and how can they be reached for more information? Who are the nearest relatives and others who might have information about the subject or who need to be notified?

To help guide rescuers teams in asking the right questions, search specialists have developed very detailed "lost person questionnaires." Some of these guidelines are very specific for search situations. They are available to rescue personnel for help in taking detailed information during the initial report. These questionnaires are very useful because they organize and structure the information-gathering process. This assures that you do not overlook a piece of information that could be critical to making important decisions early in the search.

THE ROLE OF "CLUES"

In most searches, especially land and water searches, clues are crucial to the success of the mission. The adage, "search for clues, not the subject," should always be kept in mind. In a search, there might only be *one* lost subject who is difficult to find. But most of the time, there are *many* clues because every person generates clues. These could be physical clues such as footprints, dropped clothing, broken vegetation, discarded candy wrappers. Clues may be a scent that could be detected by a search dog, or other indications that the person has been in the area. There are also clues in the information obtained about the subject. These clues might include the subject's personality type, his or her particular interests, outside influences on him or her, and other indications of how the subject might behave or where he or she might go when lost. Clues are extremely useful in determining search actions. As a rescuer, you should train yourself to be "clue-conscious" in any situation involving lost, overdue, or missing persons. All clues must be *protected* from any disturbance so that they can be properly cataloged and used by the incident commander and trained searchers.

NATURAL AREA SEARCHES

Natural area searches can occur in many different kinds of environments. They may occur in suburban, rural, and remote areas. However, natural area searches are not limited to those areas. Searches for a lost child who strays from his house or a patient who wanders away from a nursing home often occur in adjacent natural areas. But whatever the search environment, there are certain priorities in natural area search management that are always the same. The search team will employ essentially the same strategy and tactics for all searches. The exceptions to this approach will be when searching in water, structures, and debris.

We often read of searches that are conducted by hundreds of volunteer helpers who line up shoulder-to-shoulder and move through the woods trying to find the lost person. Years of experience by many different search groups has shown that this approach is about the least effective method of searching. This kind of effort is extremely inefficient and usually has poor results. A line search also destroys the clues left by the lost person. These clues are essential if the search team is to find the lost person quickly and efficiently.

Initial Actions

As soon as you receive a report of a lost or overdue person, you must immediately gather the extensive information described earlier in this chapter. In addition, it is extremely important to identify and protect the *last seen point* or *last known position* and the immediately surrounding area. This location can be very important to the identification of clues, such as the lost person's direction of travel, that are crucial to the early stages of planning the search effort.

Do whatever is possible to keep "unofficial helpers" from forming their own loose "search" organization and running about through the search area. Keep these people in a staging area, if possible, until the incident commander can initiate his or her own actions and before the outsiders inadvertently destroy important clues.

It is important that the incident commander *confine* the search area early in the rescue operation. During **scene confinement** the incident commander begins to confine the search area first by defining the "possible" search area. The "possible" search area is defined by determining within reason, how far the person *could have* traveled by considering how long the person has been lost, the physical and mental condition of the person, the nature of the terrain, and other conditions. To confine the search area, the incident commander must take all reasonable actions to keep the search area from getting bigger. Placing people at key locations or patrolling routes to try to intercept the missing person are actions that will help to confine the search area. A search in the area after a missing person has left is nonsense!

Another initial action may be a **hasty search**. This is an immediate search of those locations where the subject or clues are likely to be found. Such locations include places where the lost subject might be attracted. Typical "attractions" include water, scenic vistas, and hilltops. The hasty searchers should also check likely routes of travel along with hazardous areas where the person could have gotten in trouble. A hasty search is usually done by small teams of readily available, highly mobile persons who are skilled at finding clues left by the lost person.

If possible, locate and preserve a "scent article." A scent article is an object in which the lost person has left his or her own individual scent and is used to find a person. Body scent consists of skin cells that are constantly being shed by the body. This scent becomes affixed to articles we wear and carry. Scent is left along routes that we travel, and scent is picked up by air currents and potentially transported long distances.

As will be discussed, dogs often rely on a scent article. The best scent articles are unlaundered items of clothing worn close to the body (such as underwear) or unlaundered bedding. To prevent contamination with other smells, scent articles should not be directly touched by anyone. They should be stored in such a way that they are not contaminated by other scents, such as garbage bags with manufacturer's perfume in the plastic, grocery bags that have held food items, or day packs that have contained your gloves or clothes. If an uncontaminated container is unavailable, it may be best just to hang the article somewhere in the open until the dog handler can arrive.

Another important initial action in a lost person search is for the team to perform what has become known as the *bastard search*. The bastard search gets its name from what you would like to call the subject when, after hours of searching, you find he or she is not actually lost but in a safe and comfortable location. Some examples would be the hunter you find is not lost but in a warm bar, or the "lost" teenager who has been discovered holed up someplace with his girlfriend.

The bastard search includes identifying and searching locations that normally might not be considered part of the search area. Many "lost" children have later been found hiding under their bed or asleep in a closet. Also in this category of search are those occasional "staged incidents," in which a person may leave an area to make it appear as if he or she is lost to divert attention from financial problems or a criminal incident. Or a person may commit an act of foul play and make it appear that the victim is lost. Although these types of incidents are unusual, all searches should include a detailed investigation to help determine whether any of these possibilities could be involved.

Strategy and Tactics

After a logical search area has been identified and confined, the incident commander should *segment* the search area into smaller more manageable search units. The search management team determines the size of each unit according to how big an area can be easily searched by a team in one operational period (usually about ten hours). The boundaries of each unit can be determined by features such as rivers, ridges, fence lines, and power lines. The management team then assigns each segmented area a "probability." This probability is the percentage that represents the "odds" that the lost person is in that particular segment compared to all other search areas.

To establish these **probabilities of area,** the search management team relies on a combination of information such as statistical data of lost persons, history of searches in the area, terrain barriers, logical routes of travel, lost subject profile information, deductive reasoning from clues, and the experience of search team members.

When the areas have been segmented and assigned probabilities, the incident commander then assigns resources such as hasty teams, search dogs, or helicopters to search areas. These search resources should have a known high **probability of detection**, a high chance of locating the subject or a clue, given that either are in the assigned area. The probability of detection for each resource is determined through its past experience in search, its proven competence, its obvious ability, and other factors. The resources with the highest probability of detection are assigned to the area(s) with the highest probability that clues or the person, are present.

As additional clues become available and as segments are searched without results, the probabilities of area are updated. These updates provide the incident commander with alternatives for shifting resources during subsequent operational periods.

Effective Resources

Search Dogs Search dogs are able to locate lost humans in three general ways. **Tracking dogs** scent by following ground disturbances cause by a person's footsteps. This disturbance is commonly crushed vegetation and bacterial action in disturbed soil, though some tracking dogs may detect human scent in the tracks. Tracking dogs tend to follow close to the person's footprints regardless of the wind conditions. **Trailing dogs** are trained to follow human scent which has fallen from the lost person to the ground or on surrounding vegetation along the person's route of travel. A trailing dog may work some distance from the actual footsteps of the missing person, depending in part on the wind in the area. **Air scenting dogs** are trained to orient to a human scent carried by air currents. The dog will search for any human scent in the area. An air scenting dog may detect scent articles that the person has dropped or the person himself, whether living or dead. Air scenting dogs may also be able to locate humans even if covered by water, snow, or rubble.

Some dogs have the breeding, ability, and training for **scent discrimination.** They are able to distinguish scents distinctive to individual humans. These dogs are first allowed to smell an uncontaminated scent article belonging to that person. Then they try to locate the person through tracking, trailing, or air scenting. A dog that is truly scent discriminating would be an advantage, since it would be able to work in areas of human activity such as parks or urban areas.

Air scenting dogs are trained to pick up airborne human scent and follow it to its source. Unless they are scent discriminating, air scenting dogs often do not differentiate a specific human's scent and will locate any human (or source of human scent) in an area. As a result, air scenting dogs that are not scent discriminating usually work most effectively in segments of the search area that are not contaminated by the scent of other humans, such as other searchers. Air scenting dogs usually work "off leash." They are trained to range through an area ahead of their handlers until they find an air current with human scent in it. They then "alert," a behavior specific to that dog that has the appropriate meaning to the handler. They follow the scent to its source, or until they lose it, and then return to guide the handler to the source (Figure 10.1).

Trailing and tracking dogs are most effective in areas that have not been contaminated after the subject passed through or when the scent has not been destroyed by time or bad weather. The effectiveness of air scenting dogs is not so dependent on time, since as long as the source exists they can detect it. Even if the person is dead, the body may still be emitting scent.

Dogs that are well-bred and well-trained can be highly efficient search resources. When combined with an effective handler, a dog is capable of covering a relatively large segment of the search area. In

Dog Search in Avalanche
When teamed with an effective handler, a well-bred and well-trained dog can be a highly efficient search resource.

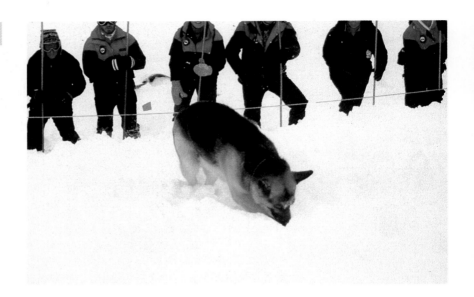

this way, the dog and handler team either locate the person or a clue or reduce the probability that the person is in that segment.

Human Trackers Persons trained to identify and follow the tracks and other signs left by a lost person can be highly effective searchers. One technique used by trackers is to create track traps. These are brushed out areas in trails or open areas to detect tracks left by someone passing through later. They also use a technique known as **sign-cutting**, searching along a feature such as a road shoulder or fence line to determine if someone has passed over the feature. Experienced and well trained searchers can be very effective in identifying clues that can be used to determine a direction of travel or to establish probabilities in the various search segments.

Helicopters Though dependent on terrain, vegetation density, and weather, helicopters can be very effective in searches because they can fly slowly and change directions quickly. However, it takes a great deal of practice to become effective as a spotter, or searcher, from a helicopter. Because intense concentration is necessary, persons usually are effective at searching from helicopters only for short periods of time. A new technique being used in helicopter searches is FLIR, forward looking infrared. FLIR units show an infrared scan of an area on a monitor screen. Originally designed for military and police work to spot "bad guys" trying to hide under plants, overhangs, and other natural cover, FLIR shows a living animal or subject as an infrared heat source even if the subject cannot be seen directly because of obstructing trees, vegetation, or overhangs (Figure 10.2).

FIGURE 10.2

Helicopter with Infrared Detection Device
The light colored device hanging from the center of this helicopter is an infrared detection device. When operated by trained observers, it can be used to help locate subjects on the ground.

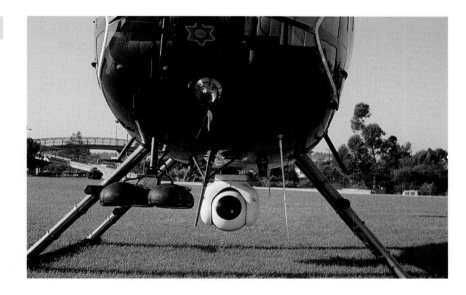

FIGURE 10.3

Map and Compass
In remote or roadless areas, searchers will use a compass and topographical maps to navigate.

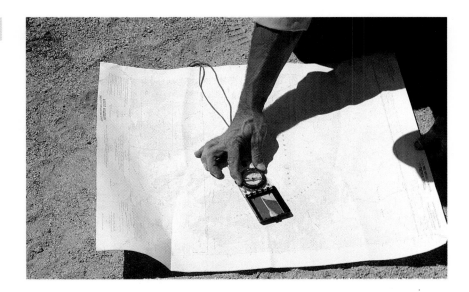

Map and Compass In remote or roadless areas, searchers have to navigate using a compass and topographical maps (Figure 10.3). These tools are necessary to find the missing person or clues and also to ensure that searched areas can be accurately identified. Good maps and a compass are necessary to ensure your well-being in remote locations. Topographical maps are important in order for you to report your position if you need assistance or need to direct other resources to your location, such as for patient transport. If you are not proficient with map and compass navigation, you must seek instruction and supervised practical experience in these skills before you travel into remote areas.

WATER SEARCHES

Situations involving a search for a missing person in water might take place in either moving or still water. The strategy and tactics of response are different in each case.

Initial Actions

If you are involved in the initial response to a water search, you should take several initial actions. You should assure that as much information has been obtained as possible about the circumstances involved. You should take some responsibility for those in the vicinity who might be interested in helping but who might not be competent to carry out a water search.

It is critical to establish the last known position of the subject. This point will be used by the incident commander to plan search actions that follow. If possible, you should identify, document, mark, and protect the last known position. You should keep witnesses at the scene for further investigation until a more highly trained individual relieves you of that responsibility.

While waiting for additional trained resources to arrive, you should initiate or coordinate a hasty search. Look along the shoreline for clues or to assure that the subject has not exited the water. Look down the current in moving water and all along the edge of the shoreline of lakes.

Refer to Chapter 6 for precautions related to carrying out a water-related rescue.

Strategy and Tactics

Take actions to exhaust all possibilities that the person is still alive somewhere. Continue shoreline searches until the person is found elsewhere or until you have checked out all possible locations where the person could have exited and you have considered all clues.

Trained dive rescue personnel have developed sophisticated methods and search patterns for both moving and stationary water. Highly competent rescuers and proper equipment are needed to search in swiftly flowing water for submerged victims who might be pinned against underwater obstacles. Similarly, special techniques and equipment are needed in deep, extremely cold, or murky water. Specialists are available in cave diving and in diving in contaminated water. During preplanning, the potential for these kinds of situations should be analyzed. When they are available, resources capable of responding should be identified, alerted, and response procedures determined.

Effective Resources

Highly trained dive rescue personnel are usually the most readily available and effective resources for underwater search operations. They usually have the equipment and knowledge necessary to undertake complex water searches. Normally, they will have trained for, or have specialists for, each specific environment, such as swift water, to which they might have to respond.

Air scenting dogs have become an increasingly effective resource in water environments. While they are searching along shorelines or from boats, dogs trained for this purpose have successfully picked up a scent rising to the surface from victims submerged in water. Successfully obtaining this kind of clue can help divers determine the most highly probable location to conduct an underwater search.

Technological equipment, such as "fish-finders" and other kinds of sonar-type and sound recording equipment, underwater cameras, and drag-lines, has also been successfully used to locate victims underwater.

STRUCTURAL FIRE, COLLAPSED STRUCTURE, AND DEBRIS SEARCHES

Searches for missing persons can occur in buildings that are ablaze, in structures that have collapsed from earthquakes or structural failure, or in debris resulting from such causes as floods, hurricanes, or tornadoes.

The search environment created by these conditions is among the most hazardous you can encounter. Because of burning conditions, toxic air, unstable footing, and potential for falling objects, you should *never* venture into one of these situations unless you have received proper training and are properly equipped.

Structural Fire

Initial Actions Members of a fire rescue team must quickly gather data, determine risks and strategies, and establish a plan of action. Information that is required for decision making in these incidents includes:

- How many people are inside the burning building?
- What are the age, size, and special problems of the persons in the building?
- What is the last known location or most likely location of the victim(s)?
- What is the building layout and the best and quickest way to access the subjects? What resources for search and rescue are available right now?
- What additional equipment and personnel are needed to conduct a safe rescue?

The actual search and rescue effort should be the result of a well established preplan or standard operating procedure (SOP). It is supplemented by the site and incident-specific information developed quickly from the answers to the above questions. The SOP should include priorities and specified tasks for each team member to maximize the rescue team's efforts. For example, normally if there are a number of victims, priorities might include direct initial rescue efforts for the victims in the most immediate danger. The largest group/ number of victims threatened by the fire is the second priority. Other persons in the immediate area of the fire are third priority. The last priority are the persons in the exposure areas.

Strategies and Tactics The search activities should follow specific protocols including:

1. Team makeup (number, skills, and expertise of the members)
2. Communications, verbal and nonverbal, to include: signals that may indicate distress; search patterns directions, such as, "I've found a victim;" and "Search complete"
3. Defined search patterns to provide reliable and thorough coverage of the search area
4. Methods for moving patients safely
5. Methods for marking searched areas
6. Methods for roll call and emergency recall of the search team

There are many search patterns (Figure 10.4). One effective tactic is to first make a perimeter search, moving around the wall of the room. Then, depending on the size of the search area and the time available, use a different search pattern such as the straight line pattern without using a line tender.

The straight line patterns can be used in almost all situations. This type of pattern requires the search team members to maintain their orientation within the room. If searchers become disoriented, valuable time is lost and there is a greater possibility of missing a victim.

The rope and tender technique may be difficult to use in structural search. However, if the area to be searched is not too cluttered, a tendered search can be very effective. Two tendered patterns that work in a structure search are the fan pattern and the circular/semicircular pattern.

The primary search usually is done before the fire is under control. If it cannot be completed according to established procedures, report this to the incident commander so he or she can include the area in the secondary search plan.

Sometimes the fire situation or resource limitations make it impossible to conduct a complete search. An example would be when the air in your self-contained breathing apparatus (SCBA) runs low. A hasty search pattern can be used in these situations. One method of hasty search in residential structures is for a team to enter the room, proceed directly ahead to the wall parallel to the entry door, and then turn to the left or right (according to a predetermined procedure) and move quickly around the perimeter. Frequent sweeps with a tool, leg, or arm to the middle of the room during the perimeter search will expand the search coverage.

To improve the search effort, keep these points in mind:

1. Be certain that you search under, behind, and inside closets, bathtubs, shower stalls, furniture, and other room furnishings. People tend to hide in an attempt to escape the smoke and fire.
2. Use your arms and legs to extend your reach under furniture or into other open areas.
3. Keep members of your search team within communications range of each other. Losing contact with other members causes team members to focus on contacting team members rather than on the search effort.
4. When possible, completely search one area at a time, leaving behind a predetermined sign that the area has been searched.

Effective Resources   A fire rescue requires a trained team to perform the rescue. The members must have prior working experience and frequently practice together under realistic conditions to sharpen and define group skills. A team cannot be efficient without the opportunity to work and solve problems together. Practice unifies the efforts of all involved.

Collapsed Structures and Debris

Search situations commonly result from the destruction caused by tornadoes, hurricanes, and earthquakes and from building collapses caused by structural failure. The potential of serious injury to rescuers from such hazards as sharp objects, unstable footing, falling objects, and entrapment makes this environment among the most dangerous of all rescue environments. You should *never* venture into debris or a collapsed structure unless you have had extensive training and are equipped to do so.

Initial Actions   The first action that should be taken is to make a quick survey of the affected area. Look for clues indicating the presence of victims, and listen for sounds that might indicate where entrapped victims are. Look for and mark openings that might later be used by searchers to get into the debris. Look for especially hazardous or precarious areas so that others can be warned about them. If possible, cordon off the area to keep others from entering without authority.

Then try to gather as much information as possible about the situation from witnesses, if any are available. They could provide clues about the numbers and locations of victims inside. Try to assemble witnesses in one location so that trained investigators can get detailed information when they arrive.

a.

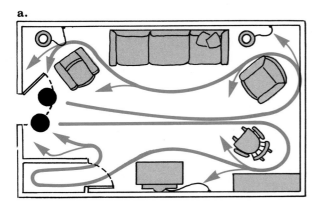

b.

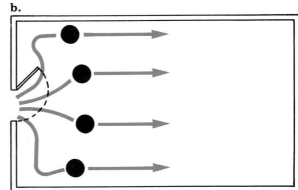

c.

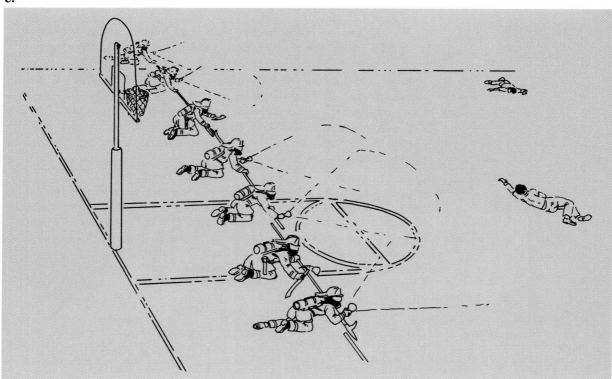

FIGURE 10.4	**Patterns for a Building Search**

Rescuers must use a systematic pattern when searching during a structure fire incident. A perimeter search (**a**), moving around the wall of the room, is made first. Depending on the size of the search area and the time available, a straight line search pattern without a tender (**b** and **c**) can be used. If the area is not too cluttered, a tendered search pattern is used. The semi-circular pattern (**d** and **e**) and the fan pattern (**f** and **g**) are two tendered patterns that work in a structure search.

d.

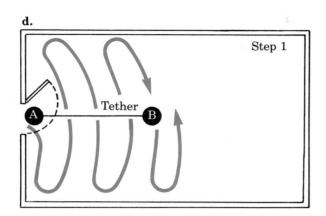

Step 1

Tether

e.

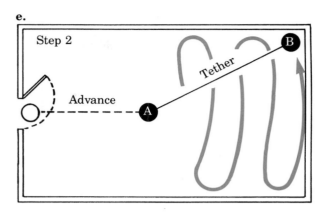

Step 2

Advance

Tether

f.

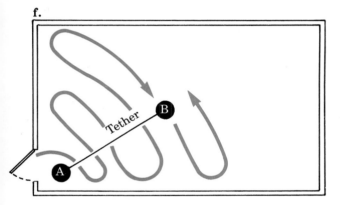

Tether

g.

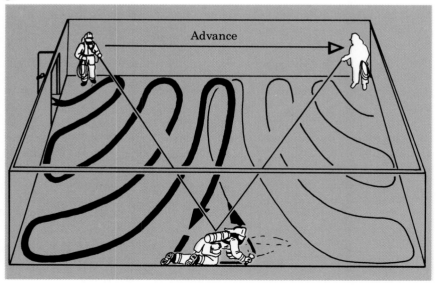

Advance

FIGURE 10.5

Camera Listening Device
Electronic equipment, developed originally for mine rescue, can be used to detect persons trapped in collapsed structure and debris.

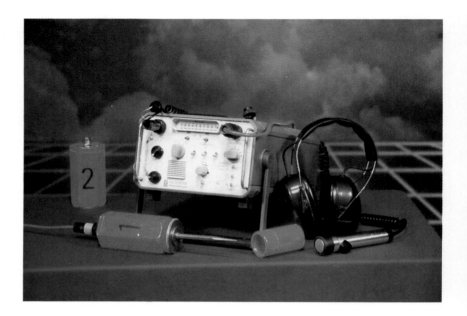

Effective Resources Air scenting dogs can be used effectively in rubble and debris searches. In some instances, they are able to enter areas that humans cannot or where it would be unsafe for humans to enter. Such dogs have been trained to inform their handlers, by alerting on scent, about the possible locations of victims. Some dog/handler teams are sophisticated enough that the handler can tell from the kind of alert the dog makes whether the victim is alive or dead.

Electronic equipment, developed originally for mine rescue situations, has recently been effectively applied to collapsed structures and debris. One example is a very small TV camera installed on a flexible tube. This device can be "snaked" into cracks and crevices to look for victims or to look for open areas in the debris where it might be possible for a victim to survive. Also, sophisticated sound recording and sound enhancement devices are being used to try to locate victims buried in rubble or debris. These devices might be important in identifying "high probability" locations in the search area in which to devote more extensive search efforts (Figure 10.5).

Trained "heavy rescue" specialists probably are the most important resources needed both to locate and access victims in collapsed structures and debris. This process often involves both moving debris and stabilizing or effectively demolishing the remaining parts of a structure to find victims and to make the area safe. The specialists need a high degree of knowledge, often including professional structural engineering information, and experience. They must have the ability to use specialized equipment, such as cranes, debris-moving heavy equipment, hydraulic tools, and high-powered saws to open spaces. They may even use explosives to move large pieces of debris.

SUMMARY

Rescuers trying to locate a lost, overdue, or missing person must understand that the nature of searches can vary greatly because of the environment in which the search occurs. Thus, it is important for you to be aware of the three main search environments—natural, water, and structural—and the types of response required for each one.

There are generic initial response actions, such as gathering information about the subject and interpreting clues in the area, that apply to the locate phase of any rescue situation. But the conditions in each search environment dictate the initial response actions in that environment. In addition, each environment determines the strategies and tactics that must be used for a successful outcome. Selecting the most effective search resources is also dependent on the situation in the search environment. Once you recognize the requirements of each search environment, you are better prepared to conduct a successful search and locate phase of the rescue mission.

ACCESS

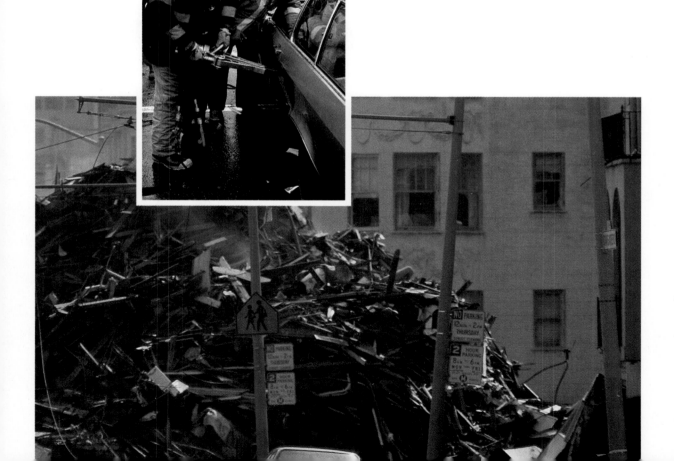

GAINING ACCESS IN AN URBAN SETTING

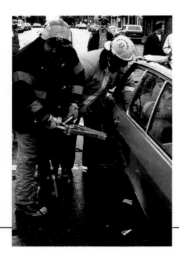

OVERVIEW

Access and rescue in the urban environment present many special conditions that a rescuer must be able to anticipate and manage. This chapter outlines these conditions and offers methods of avoiding or coping with problems.

Included in this chapter are discussions on accessing the scene on the road, at a civil disturbance, and in a mechanized environment. The chapter also explains the importance of avoiding hazards to rescuers and establishing safety zones in all of these situations.

OBJECTIVES

The objectives of this chapter are for the rescuer to describe:

- how to assess the scene and conduct a rescue at a vehicular accident.
- a safe and appropriate response to a civil disturbance.
- a mechanized environment rescue.
- a safety zone for each of these urban situations.
- rapid transport from civil disturbances.

Effective rescue is the organized effort of a team of personnel trained and equipped to manage the situation. Part of this effort is accessing the subject so you can assess his or her medical condition and provide appropriate assistance. The first step of access is securing the scene to protect the patient and the rescuers.

VEHICLE ACCESS

When you approach the scene, assess the situation, and select a safe site to park the rescue vehicle. Do not park closer than 50 feet from the emergency. If there are indications of chemical or fuel spills and/or fire, stop at least 100 feet away from the incident.

Determine if you need other agencies or resources such as utility companies, the public works department, specialized response teams, or special support equipment such as extra lighting. If needed, notify the dispatcher and arrange for their response.

When responding to an accident scene, plan at least one alternate response route. It is especially important to develop alternate routes during rush hour traffic and around road construction projects or detours, dense or special population areas such as hospital and school zones, frequently used railroad grade crossings, or other potential obstacles. You should carry area maps on all rescue vehicles to help locate alternate routes into accident sites.

Hazards to the Patient and the Rescuer

The first priority of all emergency responders is the safety of both rescuer and patient. All emergency responders must identify and control all safety hazards.

Fuel Hazards The fuel and the fuel systems of vehicles present a hazard to you and your patients throughout the duration of the incident. Gasoline, diesel fuel, and propane have different ignition and vaporization temperatures. But all fuels have the potential for ignition under the right conditions. If there is a known fuel leak, or if people are trapped in the vehicles, there must be adequate fire protection in position. This means that at least one charged 1½ inch diameter hose line is manned and ready for operation before beginning the rescue.

Because of pollution problems, it is no longer acceptable to routinely flush fuels or other spilled or leaking material into sewers or drainage ditches. Fuel and other spills require the response of specially trained and equipped personnel. Local protocols should detail the procedures for the callout and response of these special teams. If there is any question, it is best to ask for help from your local hazardous materials team to properly identify and manage spills and cargo losses.

Fire Hazards Fire must always be considered the rescuer's enemy. Almost all motor vehicle accidents pose the potential for fire, since there is fuel, air, and the potential for heat. Luckily, the risk of a vehicle fire is less than 0.05%. The incident commander should be notified of any potential or actual fire hazard. The incident commander should then assign available personnel for immediate fire protection (if equipped and trained to handle such an assignment) or request fire protection resources to respond.

If a fire is or has been present in a vehicle, you must use respiratory protection in addition to thermal protection. There are many toxic by-products in the smoke from vehicular fires. Use of full protective gear at accident scenes can reduce the risk to rescue personnel.

Flares Flares are considered essential tools by some rescuers. In the hands of an inexperienced user, however, they can be extremely dangerous. Because flares can be seen for long distances, they may be used to warn oncoming traffic of a hazard. Flares are used to route traffic into "safe" lanes and to alert the oncoming traffic to slow down.

The problems with flares include the facts that they are extremely hot and only burn for a limited period of time, 10 to 60 minutes depending on the wind. Flares are most dangerous during the lighting process. Following general safety guidelines when working with flares will decrease your risk of injury:

1. Do not set flares near flammable materials such as gasoline spills, open flames, or dry brush.
2. Extend flares outward toward oncoming traffic at least 15 to 20 feet apart.
3. Arrange flare patterns to direct traffic away from the scene yet keep traffic moving.
4. Stack several flares together so that as one burns out, another will ignite.
5. Put the end caps on the nonburning ends to keep the flares upright.
6. To avoid burns, do not hold on to or wave flares.
7. Do not extinguish flares. Let them burn out rather than risking splatter during extinguishment.
8. Light flares facing downwind. This will decrease the danger of burns and toxic fumes affecting you. Do not loiter in the roadway after lighting the flares.
9. If the road is two-way and only two-lane, place flares in both directions.

Since law enforcement personnel are trained in traffic control, they should assume responsibility for traffic control. They are better prepared to manage the risks and hazards of moving vehicles on open roadways.

Electrical Hazards Electrical hazards outside the vehicle may include both above ground and below-grade power lines or feeds. Overhead wires are usually a visible hazard. Many rescuers become too casual about electrical hazards at the emergency scene, because visible sparks and arcing are not always present in charged wires. The area around downed power lines is always a **danger zone** (Figure 11.1). This danger zone extends well beyond the normal accident scene. The utility poles supporting the broken lines should be used as landmarks for establishing the danger zone. The danger zone is a restricted area for all emergency personnel, equipment, and vehicles.

The hazard survey should include a visual inspection under, around, and above the involved vehicle. Below-grade power feeds supply power to street lights and residential housing, and can energize the ground around the vehicle along with the vehicle.

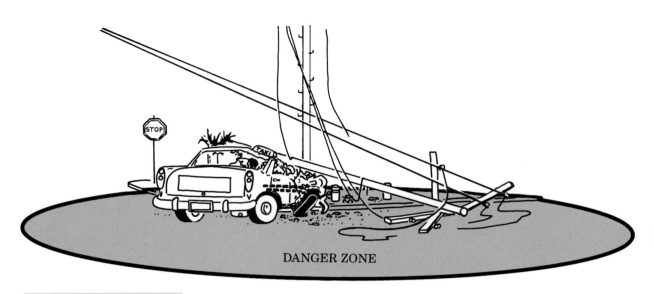

DANGER ZONE

FIGURE 11.1	**Downed Power Line**

The area around downed power lines is always a danger zone. The danger area extends to two poles on either side of the downed wire.

Rescue personnel are not trained or equipped to manage electrical hazards. When confronted with downed electrical power lines or below-ground electrical feeds, you must remember there is no way to tell the direction of travel of the electrical feed. Automatic devices in the electrical power system may energize wires or power feeds many times; therefore, one jolt does not disable the wire. All wires, utility pole support wires, and broken utility poles should be considered energized until qualified utility company personnel can verify otherwise. Remember that your normal protective clothing offers little protection against electrocution. All incidents involving power lines and feeds should be handled by trained utility company personnel.

Establishing a Safety Zone

The response to a highway emergency must include an initial hazard survey.

Make a visual inspection of the area upon arrival. First, assess the incident for risks related to traffic. Then, identify a safe parking area, and develop a traffic management plan if law enforcement personnel are not yet present. Traffic control must provide for the safety of the rescuers and the accident victims. Therefore, a safe working zone must include consideration of the traffic hazards.

There are three general methods to control traffic: stopping or blocking approaching traffic, redirecting traffic past the incident, or rerouting the traffic to a different road. The incident commander must have experience in vehicle rescue, a knowledge of the street/road conditions, law enforcement support, and the ability to anticipate the scope of the rescue operations.

Inspect the area around the incident for downed power lines, underground power feeds, fuel spills, smoke and fire, battery acid leaks, unusual sounds or odors, injured people, and vehicle instability. The incident commander should establish the **safety zone** by having two rescuers move around the incident in a circular fashion at least 15 to 20 feet away from the vehicle(s). With each rescuer moving in opposite directions, the safety zone is checked twice.

All hazards that are found must be reported to the incident commander. All emergency personnel operating on the scene must be warned of any hazard as soon as possible. The safety zone should be marked off with barrier tape or rope.

An equipment staging area should be set up on a tarp placed just inside or just outside the safety zone (Figure 11.2). All emergency equipment should be stored on the tarp when not in use. The staging tarp should also be used for final inventory checks before leaving the scene.

While the safety zone and equipment staging area are being set up, the incident commander should assign personnel to perform the close-up hazard survey. Again, two rescuers circle the vehicle(s) in opposite directions, closely watching for hazards directly related to the vehicle and the victims. This zone is known as the **action zone.** Only those personnel directly involved in patient care or extrication should be in the action zone. All nonessential personnel, loose vehicle parts, and unused rescue apparatus/equipment should be removed and kept out of this area.

As soon as possible after the safety and action zones are secure, the interior rescuer enters the vehicle and performs an immediate

FIGURE 11.2

An Equipment Staging Area

An equipment staging area at a traffic accident should be set up on a tarp placed just inside or just outside the safety zone. All emergency equipment should be stored on the tarp when not being used.

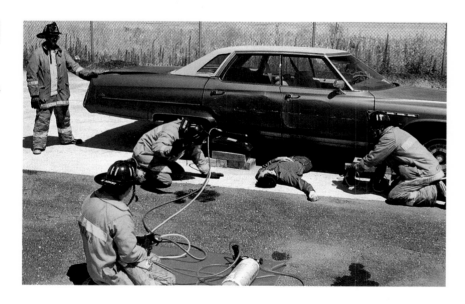

interior hazard survey. The primary mission of the interior rescuer is the immobilization and protection of the patient. The interior rescuer should not become involved in exterior extrication activities.

CIVIL DISTURBANCE ACCESS

Civil disturbances are incidents that cannot be handled with routine law enforcement resources. Such incidents include riots, strikes that turn violent, and large gatherings of hostile or potentially hostile people.

The hostilities and violence that these incidents generate may be directed at police and fire personnel and at EMS personnel, their patients, and other support personnel.

The most important concern in any civil disturbance is the safety of the rescuers and the safety of those they work with. Since these incidents are always multi-agency responses, everyone must know who is in command and from whom they will be taking orders.

Hazards to the Rescuer

Civil disturbances present risks to rescue personnel, including exposure to tear gas. Unprotected exposure can be destructive to lung tissue. In addition, high concentrations of tear gas can displace oxygen from a confined area and cause suffocation.

Tear gas is actually a fine powder. After the gas is released, the particles settle until movement resuspends them, or until they are removed by decontamination procedures. You can avoid secondary exposure by protecting your face with a gas mask, covering your arms and legs with close-knit material, and using proper footwear. You should wear gloves and cover all exposed cuts and injuries.

Once inside an area contaminated by tear gas, you should not move any items unless necessary. Fire service personnel can assist you with ventilation fans for air movement. After the incident, all exposed equipment and clothing must be thoroughly washed with soap and water for decontamination.

Secondary exposure may also occur when you treat people who have been exposed to tear gas. A patient's skin, hair, and clothing can all contain gas particles that may cause irritation when disturbed.

CS gas is the most common type of tear gas used in riot suppression. This type of gas causes temporary eye and skin irritation. The treatment for exposure to CS gas is to remove the patient from the gassed area. Then flush the eyes with copious amounts of water (Figure 11.3). The patient should then be moved into an area with uncontaminated air.

A less frequently used type of tear gas is **CN gas.** This type not only causes eye and skin irritation, but also stomach cramps and vomiting. The proper treatment for CN gas is removal of the patient from the exposed area and into clean air.

FIGURE 11.3

Treating for Tear Gas Irritation
To treat for exposure to CS gas, first remove the patient from the gassed area. Then flush the eyes with copious amounts of water.

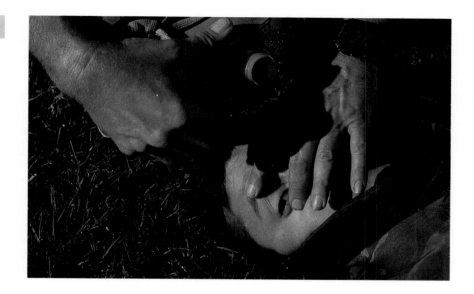

FIGURE 11.4

Types of Gas Masks
The two types of gas masks used by police agencies and the military are the M-17 (left) and the Grasshopper (right).

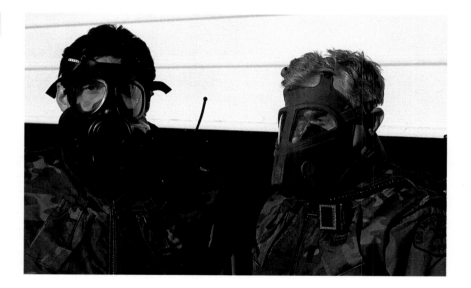

Both CS and CN gases will irritate open sores or freshly abraded skin, and the sweat glands, causing a burning sensation on all exposed skin areas. Therefore, it is important for you to cover all exposed skin. Tear gas irritations of the skin can be reversed by repetitive washings with uncontaminated cool water.

There are currently two types of gas masks being used by police agencies and the military (Figure 11.4). The Grasshopper is popular because it is small and easy to store. However, it limits visibility, and after long periods of using it, you may feel claustrophobic. The M-17 gas mask is larger, is easier to put on, and has large eye ports for increased visibility.

Establishing a Safe Zone

In a civil disturbance, *safe zones* are areas located away from the action. Buildings and other areas that would normally be considered safe can suddenly become the target of an enraged crowd, so safe zones may be temporary. A situation that moments earlier seemed safe can suddenly become a trap where a rescue team may be injured or held hostage and useless to those in need of their help. It is essential to be aware of the ever changing situation associated with a civil disturbance, especially areas being controlled by the adversary.

Escape routes should be planned and continually updated with the safety of the rescuers and patients in mind. The incident commander must plan for potential escape routes through areas that can be protected during use. Each individual member of a fire or rescue unit must also plan alternate escape routes for themselves.

During civil disturbances, a curfew, usually during the hours of darkness, may be ordered to prohibit movement inside the affected area. During such situations rescue personnel should stay within a safe zone for the duration of the curfew.

In most situations, it is not practical to have all personnel remain inside a safe zone at all times. Relief personnel must commute to and from their assignments through curfew zones. One solution is to use easily identified department or company vehicles to transport people in groups under escort. If privately owned vehicles must be used, car pooling and escorted convoys through restricted areas are preferred. Rescue personnel should wear their uniforms, and the vehicles should display identifying markings.

When rescuers respond to a civil disturbance, the logistics staff should plan the route of travel into and out of the involved area. The plan should consider the most direct route to the incident, with alternate routes to take responders clear of major traffic and crowd congestion. The route of travel must be protected. There have been numerous examples of those in uniform or in a marked vehicle being attacked because they seemed to represent the authorities.

Incidents involving special tactical teams may involve limited access in and out of hostile, life-threatening situations or environments filled with tear gas and smoke. This may require providing care while wearing a gas mask or working in the dark with only hand-held flashlights or headlamps for light. Rescuers must practice these kinds of operations under realistic conditions before attempting them during actual incidents.

Other Response Considerations

Preplanning Each agency, department, and unit responding to a civil disturbance should have its own action plan for the deployment of personnel and equipment within the overall incident action plan.

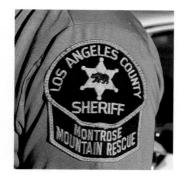

FIGURE 11.5

Distinctive Modes of ID
In a multi-agency response
to civil disturbances, distinctive badges and uniforms are
necessary to maintain
control and security.

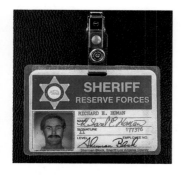

FIGURE 11.6

**ID Card for Rescue
Personnel**
Agency personnel who might
respond to a civil disturbance
should carry identification
cards with a color photo,
signature of the bearer, and a
control number. These ID
cards should be updated
yearly. Soft badges are used
during confrontations to
reduce risk of injury.

Before you respond to a civil disturbance, you should have had realistic training encompassing many of the elements that you may
face in an actual incident. These include working out-of-doors in
various types of weather; in the presence of a hostile and distracting
crowd; and with hazards such as smoke, thrown objects, and blocked
access. If possible, your training should include other units that will
respond. Such training should be conducted while you are wearing
full protective gear.

While administering emergency treatment to patients in a civil
disturbance, you must overcome many of the same problems found
in a natural disaster. These problems include confusion, chaos, large
numbers of victims, and environmental hazards. In addition, you may
have to contend with hostile, violent people potentially intent on
harming you and your patients.

Communication Communication during a civil disturbance is difficult when each agency involved uses its own radios and frequencies.
Therefore, there must be a single command radio net for the incident.

A second communication problem is the different radio terminology and codes. All multi-agency communications should be in
plain English. If codes must be used for tactical security, then the
use of coded messages must be uniform. Messages must be short,
concise, and necessary. There should be no idle chitchat.

Communication may be hindered by location or terrain, especially
if hills, large buildings, or high voltage lines are between your radio
and the command post. In these situations, radio relays or repeaters
may be necessary. Practice drills will help you expose communication
problems and their solutions.

Badges and Uniforms Response personnel must be able to identify themselves and each other instantly from a distance. Distinctive
types of identification include vests, colored hats, uniforms, or jackets
(Figure 11.5).

In an operation involving multiple agencies, distinctive badges and
uniforms are necessary to maintain control and security. Identification helps control the area of operation; prevents unauthorized
persons from entering the area; and, if a crime is involved, prevents
suspects from escaping. Identification cards, including a color photo,
the signature of the bearer, and a control number, should be issued
to all rescue personnel. The cards should be updated yearly (Figure
11.6).

Hard badges can be torn off during confrontations, causing possible
injury. If rescue personnel may be meeting rioters in a head-on con-
frontation, they should replace their hard badges and exterior identification cards with soft material such as patches.

Vehicles Marked vehicles should be used for emergency medical
service. In certain hostile situations, a vehicle distinctively marked
as a rescue or medical provider may be able to cross an area of unrest

relatively unmolested, while a police or fire vehicle could receive a barrage of abuse.

RAPID TRANSPORT

Under life-threatening conditions, such as civil disturbances, rapid extrication may take precedence over some medical assessment and stabilization protocols, including the ABCs (airway, breathing, circulation).

The methods for removing the patient from danger before treatment include Stokes litters, backboards, canvas burn packs, and the fireman's carry. If rapid spinal immobilization is required, the patient can be strapped to a backboard with the head taped to the board, and then placed and strapped into the Stokes basket. The patient may also be secured to only a backboard and then either carried or dragged to safety (Figure 11.7).

Conforming backboards can also be used. If a backboard is not available, the patient can be strapped into the Stokes litter and the head secured. If you do not feel comfortable removing a patient without back or C-spine precautions, you may have to ask law enforcement or military personnel to secure the scene before beginning treatment.

Nevertheless, if the situation is too dangerous to immobilize the patient before moving, grasp the patient's shirt, jacket, or vest at the top or back, below the collar, using both hands. Support the victim's head with your forearms as a cradle. Drag the patient backward, while maintaining alignment of the head, neck, and spine (Figure 11.8). Move the patient only the minimum distance necessary to reach safety. Then provide complete medical care to assess, stabilize, and protect from further injury.

When a call for patient transportation is received, there is the possibility you might respond to the scene of a hostile environment in which you could become a victim. In these cases, it is preferable to have the patient brought to your unit for treatment and transportation.

Rescuers may encounter patients with gunshot wounds, burns, and other major trauma at civil disturbances. You should plan to transport these patients to a trauma center. The medical coordinator should know which hospitals can receive victims of burns or trauma, including pediatric cases, and should direct the unit to the appropriate facility. Patients must be appropriately distributed among all available hospitals. Avoid overloading the closest facilities which will probably be inundated with "walk-ins" and private transports.

MECHANIZED ENVIRONMENT ACCESS

Extrication of a patient from a machinery entrapment often is a complex and challenging situation for rescuers (Figure 11.9). But an

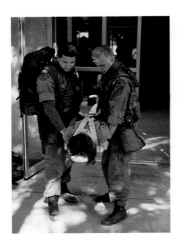

FIGURE 11.7

Moving Patient on a Backboard
When rapid spinal immobilization is required under life-threatening conditions, the patient may have to be secured only to a backboard and carried to safety.

FIGURE 11.8

Using Body Support for Patient Removal
If the situation is too dangerous to immobilize the patient before moving, grasp the patient's clothing below the collar using both hands. Support the patient's head using your forearms as a cradle. Drag the patient backward, keeping the head, neck, and spine as much in line as possible. Move the patient only the minimum distance necessary to reach safety.

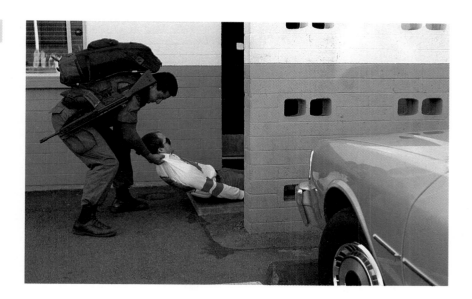

FIGURE 11.9

Hand Caught in Dough Rolling Machine
The extrication of a patient from machinery entrapment is often a complex and challenging situation. An organized, systematic approach permits the rescue team to deal with the problem safely and effectively.

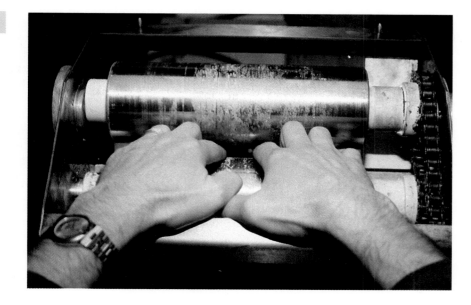

organized, systematic approach permits the rescue team to deal with the problem safely and effectively.

The steps for machinery entrapment are the same as for any rescue. Incident command should be established, the scene stabilized, and the safety zone established. The extrication/action zone should be identified, and an equipment staging area should be established.

Hazards to Rescuers

The vast array of machines and tools that may cause entanglement can overwhelm the rescuer. So you need a basic understanding of the principles and process of extrication from some common machines. This basic knowledge can be transferred to similar situations on other machines.

Size-Up

The rescue team responding to a machinery entrapment should begin size-up as soon as they arrive on the scene. The dispatcher should relay the initial information about the nature of the entrapment and the work environment to the rescue team. Incoming personnel should size up the building structure and layout for entrance and exit points, type of business, and general construction features. Because safety is the focus in all rescue operations, incoming rescuers should be aware of any hazards they may face and take appropriate precautions. Before entering the building, the rescue team should identify tools and medical equipment that may be initially needed.

Confirm the entrapment, and gather the preliminary data. Establish and notify all emergency agencies involved of the incident commander's identification and location. Quickly identify an in-house expert who has up-to-date knowledge about the equipment involved. This person is an important resource, providing critical information about the machinery and available resources in the building. The incident commander should keep the in-house expert close at hand during the extrication. Ask him or her numerous "what if" questions. For example, "What happens if that chain is cut?" or "What happens if that valve is opened?"

Establishing the Safety Zone

Assign at least two rescue personnel to establish the safety zone, removing all nonessential personnel and equipment from an area 15 to 20 feet around the entrapment. Meanwhile, assign one or two rescuers to perform the primary patient assessment. The ABCs (airway, breathing, circulation) take priority over extrication and treatment of an entrapped extremity.

When the safety zone is secured, rescue personnel must establish the *action zone* and a *staging area*. The staging area is a ground tarp to contain all the equipment brought into the building but not immediately being used in the extrication or patient care. The staging area should be set up just inside or just outside the safety zone and near the entry/exit point so that the safety zone will remain free of unnecessary traffic.

At the same time that the staging area is being set up, identify the extrication/action zone. Only those directly involved in patient care and extrication should be in the action zone. Rescue personnel should perform a second close-up survey of the entrapment looking for controls and hazards related to the specific machinery or equipment involved in the entrapment, such as controls or releases for electricity, air pressure, hydraulic pressure, and other drive mechanisms. Disengage the power source at this time, if that will not cause additional problems for the patient or rescuers.

This "walk around" is the time to identify hazards and secure the situation. Look for damage to machinery and to building structures. This is important even if no damage has been reported. Identify access, staging, and exit areas. Look for potential anchor points at ground level and above the entrapment area. Identify all sources of energy, including electricity, steam, and gas, and all chemicals in use or stored in the area. Assess floor stability and surface composition.

Extra lighting is frequently needed during the extrication process. Make the incident commander aware of all safety concerns and lighting and equipment needs. The incident commander should coordinate these requests with the in-house expert who may serve as an excellent resource for manpower, equipment, and trained technical personnel.

SUMMARY

Urban rescues may have mutliple agencies responding, which requires that a unified command approach be established and maintained.

A vehicle rescue is a common urban rescue environment. Rescue conditions and hazards vary, depending on the type of roadway and type of accident. You should know how to assess the accident scene for hazards such as a chemical or fuel spill or fire. In addition, you must determine if you need special resources, such as utility companies, public works departments, or specialized response teams.

Civil disturbances—including riots, strikes, and large gatherings of hostile people—are another kind of urban incident. You must remember that your primary goal in any civil disturbance is the safety of the rescue personnel. In addition, because these incidents are always multi-agency responses, you must know who is in command.

A mechanized environment response requires the same procedures as any rescue, beginning with the establishment of an incident command system. Rescuers then stabilize the scene, identify the extrication procedures, and set up an equipment staging area.

Size-up is important for the rescue team responding to a machinery entrapment. The size-up should indicate the nature of the entrapment and work environment, any hazards, and the tools and medical equipment that may be needed. The size-up should also identify an in-house expert with up-to-date familiarity with the equipment involved.

Safe zones located away from the action are essential in all urban rescue operations. In addition, it is often essential to have rapid transport away from life-threatening situations such as civil disturbances.

GAINING ACCESS IN REMOTE AREAS

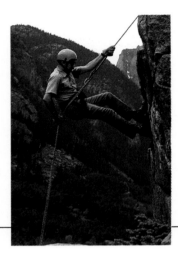

OVERVIEW

Securing the scene in remote areas requires that you be prepared for the environment into which you will be going. This chapter describes the conditions you may encounter in remote areas, including high altitude environment. The chapter also reviews the standard jurisdictional systems that have authority over different remote areas in the United States.

The chapter outlines the elements of a comprehensive preplan and stresses the importance of rescuers being familiar with compasses and topographical maps. In addition, there are sections on medical equipment and communications needs in remote areas.

Rescuers in remote areas must be well-trained in emergency services and in ways to avoid becoming victims of the environment they are entering. So this chapter describes the hazards facing the rescuers who access a patient in a remote area. The chapter also offers suggestions for preventing or combating those problems.

OBJECTIVES

The objectives of this chapter are for the rescuer to describe:

- the special response situations in a remote environment.
- the jurisdiction involved in each kind of remote rescue operation.
- a preplan for a remote rescue operation.
- the appropriate maps, compasses, and other equipment to locate the rescue site and avoid getting lost.
- medical equipment needs at a remote site.
- an effective communications system at a remote site where natural characteristics may impede communications.
- hazards inherent in remote environments that affect accessing the patient.
- ways of preventing dehydration in remote areas, especially high altitude environments.
- the effects of different air densities in remote areas.
- psychological threats during remote rescues.

Remote areas are known by a variety of terms including "backcountry" and "off road," as well as "remote." None of these terms is well defined. One will have one meaning to one person and something different to another person. Even the term "wilderness" has different meanings to different people. In the eastern United States, a "wilderness" may be an area that is recovering from lumbering and near civilization. In the west, it may indicate an untouched area that is remote from any settlements.

But whatever words are used to describe them, these areas have some common characteristics. You will be away from the comfort, convenience, and shelter of both buildings and vehicles. You will have to carry medical equipment and supplies, any rescue equipment, and any food and personal equipment with you. It means that any power source will have to be supplied by rescuers. And it often means that you will have to improvise medical equipment such as suction. And in these areas, you can expect a significant delay in providing patient care.

The high altitude rescue environment is characterized by extremes in temperature, wind, and other weather factors. It is complicated by travel through snow, ice, and rugged terrain of high angle relief, boulder fields, lakes, and streams.

Backcountry response requires that you be prepared for the environment into which you will be going. Without proper preparation, you can also become a victim.

JURISDICTIONS

Remote areas in the United States are under a variety of land ownerships. This means that there are different jurisdictions, rules, and regulations with which the rescuer must deal.

On most public lands such as those managed by the U.S. Forest Service, the Federal Bureau of Land Management, and many state agencies, emergency services, such as search and rescue, are usually under the jurisdiction of the county sheriff. The sheriff has primary agency responsibility for the protection of life and property. However, in an emergency on some of these public lands, the managing agency may be capable of assuming the lead role temporarily, if an immediate and quick response will reduce suffering or save lives. After transferring responsibility for the incident, the agency will fall back into a support mode and provide assistance.

The National Park Service has three primary types of jurisdiction (authority). *Exclusive* jurisdiction indicates that the Park Service has complete responsibility for emergency services and law enforcement. *Concurrent* jurisdiction means that these services are shared jointly with local authority. *Proprietary* jurisdiction means that emergency services and law enforcement are performed by the local authority, while the Park Service is concerned with certain resource protection statutes. The jurisdiction and preplan will define how the responsibilities for the response will be carried out by the agencies and responders involved.

The U.S. Congress has designated *wilderness areas* on federal public lands to be set aside for a minimum disruption by civilization. The Wilderness Act bans any roads, including temporary ones; motor vehicles; motorized equipment or motorboats; landing of aircraft or any other form of mechanical transport; and any structure or installation except ". . . measures required in emergencies involving the health and safety of persons within the area." The decision as to what constitutes an emergency is to be made by the administrators of the wilderness area.

PREPLANNING

One of the most critical aspects in planning an off-road rescue is determining how to get the rescue team to the site. The incident commander will need to determine how close to the site vehicles can get and what natural and man-made barriers, such as water, ridge lines, and locked gates, block access. Permission may also be needed for the rescue team and its equipment to access the site, and the preplan should outline how to obtain that permission.

Another consideration is the surface composition of the rescue site, which can create access problems. For example, in sandy areas, such as deserts and beaches, a rescue vehicle that goes off the road or pavement may become trapped in the sand. Gumbo, a clay soil in many of the prairie areas of North America, becomes extremely sticky after a rain or during spring thaws. The wet gumbo may mire vehicles or coat tires to the point that they jam against the body of the vehicle. Bogs and marshes may swallow any vehicle that does not float. During the winter months, many areas require over-the-snow machines for mechanized travel. If drifts of powder snow cause these machines to wallow and stall, travel by snowshoes or skis may be the only means of access.

Maps are extremely critical in evaluating the accessibility of an area. You should be familiar with a variety of maps. **Topographic maps**, published by the U.S. Geological Survey, accurately depict landforms, such as mountains and rivers, but may not contain up-to-date information on trails, roads, and airstrips (Figure 12.1). However, national forest maps usually have good depictions of access routes, such as roads and trails. County maps often provide accurate, up-to-date depictions of all roads in the county but usually do not accurately portray landforms.

A primary access consideration is how close to the incident site you can get your vehicle. Even though a map may indicate a road into the area, what constitutes a "road" changes from place to place, and may be open to interpretation. Road conditions may also vary significantly because of weather conditions and degree of use and

FIGURE 12.1

Topographic Map
Rescuers who might respond
to backcountry areas must be
familiar with a variety of
maps including topographic
maps.

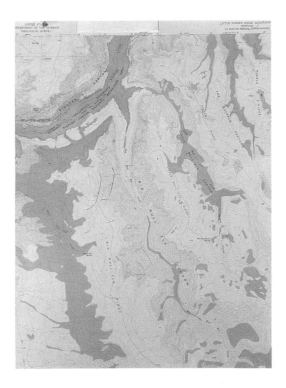

maintenance. Some backcountry roads may be blocked by fallen trees
or by snow well into the summer. Spring runoff or summer thunderstorms can wash out roadbeds.

Do not rely exclusively on maps to select access routes. Always
consult with someone with current local knowledge, such as a forest
service official, local state forester or ranger, game warden, hunting
guide, or sheriff. Such consultation should also help avoid any problems about taking vehicles into restricted "wilderness" or "primitive"
areas.

You should preplan decisions on as many predictable problems as
possible before a rescue incident occurs. The preplan should include
procedures for responding to the rescue, including an analysis of the
kinds of incidents in the area that may require rescue operations.
The preplan should also identify resources, both personnel and equipment including telephone numbers, radio or pager numbers, or other
means of contact.

MEDICAL EQUIPMENT

It is impossible to have every piece of medical equipment that you
could need in remote areas. A history of the accident will provide
clues to initial equipment needs. Meanwhile, a medical equipment

cache can be developed at the staging area of the rescue operation. Once access to the patient has been gained and equipment requirements are determined, equipment can be brought from the staging area. The equipment cache should be suited to the medical capabilities of the rescue team members and the history of actual rescue needs in the area. You should constantly update and inspect all rescue equipment.

COMMUNICATIONS

You should identify all communications needs in the preplanning process and outline them in the preplan to ensure that all units and agencies have compatible communications. You should also perform communications tests in those backcountry areas in which you will be working to identify and document problem areas or "dead spots."

Communication is a common problem in backcountry medical emergencies. Most emergency medical services (EMS) systems operate on the premise of readily available contact with medical control. Unfortunately, backcountry communications are often fragmented or nonexistent because of the distances between rescuers and base stations, the lack of repeaters, or terrain barriers blocking radio signals. Because of the potential problems with radio communications, rescue groups should consider written medical protocols. These protocols must be developed in cooperation with the medical control physician or medical center.

One solution to terrain problems is the use of communication relays. In the human relay, a person with a radio is stationed at a place where he or she can communicate with both the field team and the base station. This is often on an elevated point, such as a ridge line or a peak. The relayer then verbally passes along the message. Portable automatic relay stations are also available. In some areas, cellular phones are being used by emergency personnel.

Other problems that can impede communications are the lack of radios for all teams and dead batteries from extended operations.

HAZARDS TO THE RESCUER AND PATIENT

Rescuers going into the backcountry must be educated in emergency medicine and rescue techniques. But you also must know how to avoid becoming a victim of the very environment you are entering. Basic survival education topics include shelter building, food sources, wilderness travel, and map and compass navigation. You should participate in a regular program of aerobic exercise to develop the stamina needed for backcountry rescue.

You should carry a basic survival kit in case you become separated from your rescue team and must spend the night out away from resources. This would include a personal safety kit.

In addition, you are responsible for your own food and water supplies. There are often unexpected delays caused by such factors as changing weather conditions or complications in the rescue effort. Because it is common for rescuers to be delayed in leaving the backcountry, your self-sufficiency in food and water supplies must be not only for the planned time in the backcountry but for the potential time of stay. If there is a chance that the mission may be delayed overnight, then your personal supplies should be adequate for a minimum of 48 hours.

Weather

Weather in the backcountry, particularly in mountainous areas, may change suddenly, affecting the conduct of the rescue and, perhaps, threatening the lives of the rescuers. Persons who travel into the mountains may leave good weather in the lowlands and encounter raging blizzards at the upper elevations. Mountains make their own weather, and often it is the worst kind. Winds at higher altitudes are usually stronger. There is often greater precipitation than at lower altitudes. Temperature decreases about 3°F for each 1,000 feet of elevation change. If you are traveling into higher altitudes, you must be prepared for the worst kind of weather with appropriate food, clothing, and shelter.

You must determine the type of clothing, shelter, and sleeping bags you should carry depending on weather conditions; the rescue equipment you need; and the techniques you will use. Weather will profoundly affect the use of aircraft. It may determine the approach and evacuation routes used. The sudden passing of a weather front may mean that you must delay your mission, particularly if the patients are safely sheltered and stable. You should begin monitoring National Weather Service channels and other available local forecasts as soon as you receive the report of a mission. Accurate weather forecasts are an essential part of the mission planning.

You must be able to adapt the materials available—clothing, sleeping bags, shelters, and patient packaging equipment—to provide a comfortable environment for the patient based on weather and transport conditions. Wind chill charts, barometers, and environmental thermometers can increase your ability to meet the changing needs of you and your patients.

Dehydration

For a combination of reasons, many individuals traveling in the mountain environment become dehydrated. Most high altitude environments have drier air, so there is more water loss than at lower altitudes. Furthermore, because persons traveling in the mountains are hiking uphill or climbing, usually with a heavy pack and often not acclimated, they must work harder. This causes increased water loss through perspiration and respiration. Since it is colder, there may be less feeling of thirst and, therefore, less water intake. There also may be less water available, particularly in the winter when the only source may be melting snow. Decreased urinary frequency and a dark yellow urine are signs of dehydration. You must maintain fluid intake for your patient and yourself to avoid dehydration.

Air Density

As you move to a higher altitude, there is decreasing barometric pressure. This means there is less pressure to force oxygen into the lungs, which leads to lower blood oxygen levels. This results in less available oxygen for body use, which decreases work efficiency. For anyone not acclimated to the altitude, each task becomes harder.

Altitude also makes a critical difference for aircraft such as helicopters. At higher elevations, the air is less dense. The helicopter rotor blades cannot create as much lift as at lower elevations. As a result, the helicopter engines must work harder, and the aircraft cannot carry loads as heavy as they can at lower altitudes. This means that you must be particularly careful when using helicopters at higher altitudes. The power margins on some helicopters are so critical that at higher altitudes, they are unable to take on additional persons or cargo. In the summer, or over lakes, the effects on aircraft of altitude density become more severe. When the air is warm or humid, it is even less dense which further decreases aircraft performance.

Psychological Threats

Many backcountry emergencies involve psychological components. Some of the more common psychological problems you may face are fear of isolation and abandonment, anxiety and panic, reactions to dead bodies, and fear of animals (both small and large). Such psychological problems are contagious and can quickly overcome rescuers. Dealing with psychological problems requires that a rescuer who is not overcome with the problem take charge, gain the patient's confidence and trust, and defuse the problem. It is important that the patient not be lied to or misled. You also need to discover the cause of the psychological problem because once the cause has been discovered, it can be dealt with effectively.

SUMMARY

While securing the scene in a remote location, you will be away from buildings and vehicles and will have to personally transport any equipment or supplies needed at the rescue site. You may have to provide a power source and improvise medical equipment. And there may be a delay in transporting patients to medical facilities. High altitude environments present challenges in terms of weather extremes and traveling conditions. You must be prepared for these conditions lest you become a victim yourself.

Another important consideration for rescuers in remote areas is the jurisdictional authority over the rescue site. In addition, within these agencies there may be various types of jurisdiction. Therefore, you should know what type of jurisdiction is involved before responding to a remote area operation.

The jurisdictional authority should be spelled out in the preplan. The preplan should also outline how you can gain access to the site and can determine if permission from the jurisdictional authority is necessary for your team, vehicle, and equipment to approach the site. The preplan should also identify resources, both personnel and equipment, and list communication needs.

Transporting medical equipment into remote areas can be difficult. Therefore, it may be more efficient to develop a medical equipment cache at the staging area until access to the patient has been attained and equipment requirements are determined. At that time rescuers can carry equipment from the staging area.

Communication needs should be predetermined, and communication methods should be pretested. Radio communications are a common problem in remote areas because of distances, terrain barriers, or lack of radios. You can overcome terrain barriers by using a human relay system; a person with a radio is stationed at a point, usually elevated, from which he or she can communicate with both the field team and the base station. Portable automatic relay stations are also available. If neither of these systems works, rescuers may have to use pre-approved written medical protocols.

You should anticipate the hazards to you and your patient. Such hazards include changing weather conditions, the risk of dehydration at high altitudes, change in air density, and psychological threats.

STABILIZE

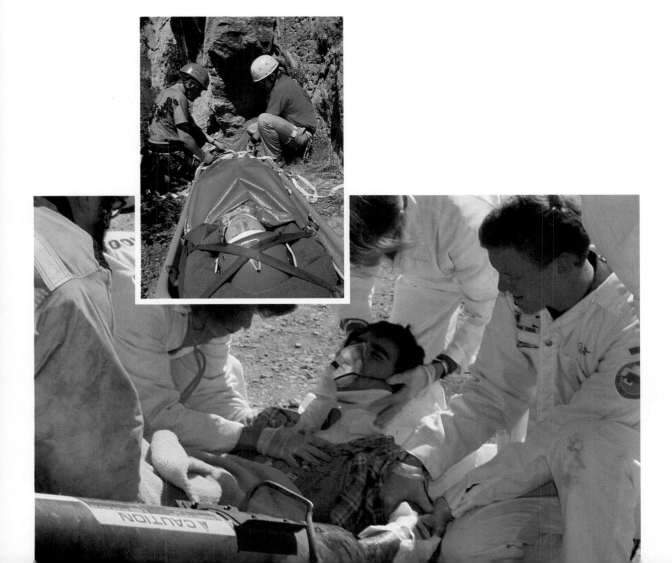

MEDICAL CARE IN THE RESCUE SETTING

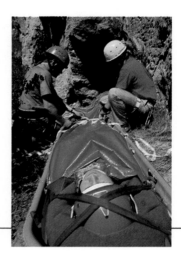

OVERVIEW

This chapter reviews common medical problems that rescuers encounter and basic emergency medical procedures that rescuers may perform during rescue operations. It emphasizes the steps that need to be taken in every rescue situation. In addition, rescuers will read about a number of specific medical problems and treatments illustrating how the extended incident aspects of emergency care differ from conventional rapid transport or "street" emergency care. Many of the more practical, action-oriented steps are highlighted here. But the greater the rescuer's understanding of anatomy, physiology, and basic emergency medical care, the more effective he or she will be as a rescuer.

OBJECTIVES

The objectives of this chapter are for the rescuer to recall:

- the common medical problems encountered during rescues.
- the basic medical procedures performed during rescue operations.
- the effects of extended transport.
- the information gathering process during a rescue.

- rescue safety.
- medical communications during a rescue.
- requirements regarding deceased persons.
- that rescuers must not perform procedures or use equipment that is not in their scope of practice.
- that rescuers must operate under medical control.

This medical section is presented assuming that you have a basic knowledge of conventional rapid transport emergency medical care, and basic life support procedures such as cardiopulmonary resuscitation (CPR). It is impossible to completely review all the aspects of emergency medical care in this section. For additional specific information and review, you should refer to *Emergency Care and Transportation of the Sick and Injured,* and *Save a Life,* both published by The American Academy of Orthopaedic Surgeons; and *Standards and Guidelines for Cardiopulmonary Resuscitation,* published by The American Heart Association.

There are important distinctions that set rescue emergency care apart from conventional, ambulance-based, rapid transport, emergency medical care. Rescue emergency care will place greater demands on you in terms of your medical training, individual responsibility, and your ability to assess situations and make decisions on your own. In many situations, rescue emergency care occurs in incidents in which you face a substantial time interval from injury to definitive care because of an extended response or patient transport time. You may be required to improvise equipment or use medical procedures that differ from what you would use in conventional rapid transport situations.

RESCUE AND MEDICAL CARE

In the rescue environment, there must be cooperation between the rescue and emergency medical care providers. That is, during the rescue you and your team must simultaneously rescue the patient and provide medical care. Furthermore, each rescue technique must be evaluated for its effect on the patient's medical outcome. There may be times when you must assign a priority to either a rescue technique or to a medical technique. For example, are the dangers so great that the patient must be moved to a safe area before any medical care is provided? Should IV lines be started before or after the patient is extricated? Is the patient protected from the hazards of the rescue operation?

The LAST acronym describes the four phases of rescue:

L   Locate
A   Access
S   Stabilize
T   Transport

The stabilize phase includes providing medical care to the patient. However, medical care will often begin *before* the stabilize phase and must continue *after* it.

During the transportation of a rescued patient, the stabilize or medical phase continues. Basic life support and all other treatment procedures initiated during the stabilization phase must continue. You must judge all transport techniques on their effect on the patient's medical condition.

The primary objective during transport is maintaining a stable patient. Therefore, you must monitor the patient's physical and mental status during transport. This cannot be overemphasized. To do this effectively, one person must be assigned responsibility for monitoring the patient during transport.

EXTENDED TRANSPORT

Conventional, rapid transport emergency care based on the U.S. Department of Transportation curriculum assumes a quick response, speedy access to the patient, expeditious assessment and stabilization, and rapid transport to definitive care. During rescue incidents, however, the transportation of a patient to definitive medical care may be delayed or may take place over an extended period. Depending on the specific incident, it may be hours or days before you deliver the patient to definitive medical care. This extended time frame may be caused by patient entrapment, difficult patient access or extrication, travel time to and from the incident site, or environmental conditions such as weather. Whatever the reason, an extended incident means that you must care for your patient differently than you might for a patient with similar problems during a conventional rapid transport.

Extended incidents are situations in which the time from the initial injury to definitive care will be greater than two hours. The following are a few examples of rescues that may require you to provide medical care during an extended incident. Note that extended incidents are not always in remote or wilderness locations:

- Entrapment in machinery, motor vehicle collision, or rockfall
- Confined spaces
- Hazardous materials incidents
- Storms or hazardous wintertime conditions
- Long rural ambulance runs
- Vessels at sea
- Backcountry/wilderness
- Civil disturbance/hostage/terrorist incidents
- Natural disasters such as earthquakes or flooding
- Structural disasters such as a building collapse or cave-in
- Underground mine or cave rescue
- Downed aircraft in remote locations
- Rafters or boaters on wild rivers
- Wildland fire fighting
- Train or bus wrecks
- Expeditions and treks
- Difficult terrain
- Insufficient number of personnel to transport patient

The ways in which extended transport may affect you as a rescuer include the need for:

- Assuming additional patient care responsibilities.

   Instead of a brief period of responsibility for patient stabilization during a quick run to the hospital, you may have to provide some of the medical assessment and care that might ordinarily be done at the hospital. During a rescue, there may be prolonged periods without direct communication with medical control or others having higher level skills. You must rely entirely on your training and experience.

- Additional definitive assessment skills and perspectives.

  You must develop your assessment techniques and skills so you may detect the subtle, hidden, or late-appearing signs and symptoms that indicate serious medical management problems not commonly seen during rapid transport.

- Anticipating problems.

  During extended incidents, you will see patients progress to more severe levels of medical problems than would normally be seen during a rapid transport. You must detect immediate medical problems and anticipate those that may develop. By knowing what problems may occur, you can attempt to prevent or delay them.

- Improvising equipment.

  In most extended rescue incidents, your equipment will be limited. At remote rescue sites with difficult access, it is not possible to carry enough equipment to meet every possible medical need. You must be able to improvise equipment and solutions. You and the other rescuers must use a small amount of equipment that can serve many different purposes.

- Basing patient assessment on clinical signs and symptoms rather than on readings of diagnostic equipment.

  During a rescue, you may have limited equipment to aid in patient assessment. The environment may prevent your using routine diagnostic tools. You must learn to use your senses of sight, hearing, touch, and smell to detect the often subtle changes in the patient's condition.

- Extending the "golden hour".

  The **golden hour** is the period after an injury in which the patient's body is able to compensate and remain relatively stable. After this period, morbidity and mortality increase tremendously as the patient becomes increasingly unstable. This period of danger does not end until definitive medical care such as surgery is provided. You must learn those techniques within your scope of practice that will allow you to extend the patient's "golden hour." These may include the use of a pneumatic anti-shock garment (PASG) or advanced life support techniques such as intravenous (IV) fluids, intubation, or medications.

- Coping with increased stress on rescuers.

  Extended incidents put you at greater risk for emotional stress from greater patient care responsibility and fatigue. You will also face the psychological stresses that result if patients in your care suffer or die despite your best efforts. It may be difficult for you to face long-term exposure to dead bodies.

- Attending to basic personal needs of the patient (nursing care).

  During extended incidents, you must provide the patient with food and water, physical comfort, emotional support and reassurance, shelter, and personal hygiene. You must assist the patient in urination and defecation. You must prevent the patient from becoming chilled, overheated, or dehydrated.

- Modifying rapid transport procedures and techniques.

  During the longer time periods of extended incidents, the patient's illness or injury may evolve beyond conditions normally found in conventional rapid transport situations. The rescue environment may alter the patient's response, or severe environmental conditions may affect the manner in which you can care for the patient. Examples of modifications in conventional procedures and techniques that may be required for extended incidents include when to cease CPR, the realignment of certain types of dislocations, management of open wounds, and removal of impaled objects.

  REMEMBER: YOU MUST NOT PERFORM PROCEDURES OR USE EQUIPMENT THAT IS BEYOND YOUR SCOPE OF PRACTICE. YOU MUST OPERATE UNDER LOCAL MEDICAL PROTOCOLS APPROVED BY YOUR MEDICAL CONTROL.

INFORMATION GATHERING

Rescues are often hampered by missing, incomplete, or unreliable information. This may occur because communications are difficult or impossible. The reporting party may be excited, confused, or frightened. Or a reliable observer cannot reach the scene to confirm the facts.

When receiving the initial report of an incident, you must gather as much information as possible, particularly:

- Description of the incident
- Potential hazards to rescuers or patient
- Condition and number of patients
- Potential required equipment, both for the rescue and emergency care

The information gathering process should continue even as the rescue team responds to the scene. As additional information becomes available on the true nature of the incident, you must be prepared to adapt to the changing conditions. The dispatcher should continue gathering information regarding the incident and advise you of any significant changes.

PERSONAL SAFETY OF THE RESCUERS

The most important aspect to any rescue is your personal safety as well as the safety of everyone else involved in the rescue. It is essential that you avoid becoming a victim of the incident yourself. If you are injured, there is then a greater burden, and thus additional risk, to all others involved in the rescue effort.

The first step in rescue safety is to *evaluate the scene.* This begins when the first notice is received. The person taking the call must ask the caller about any local hazards. Before leaving for the scene, you must be equipped for protection against any local hazard and against other general or long-term threats such as the weather.

Upon arriving at the scene you and the other rescuers must evaluate the site before entering it. If the scene is unstable or threatening, you and the other rescuers must stabilize it before entering, no matter what the condition of the patient is. If you and your partner enter a silo filled with silo gas without proper breathing apparatus to rescue a patient, most likely the local media will report three deaths rather than one.

After entering the scene, you must also protect the patient from further harm from threats that could include hazardous materials, falling objects, or extremes in weather. This may require moving the patient before treatment. You must also protect the patient from any dangers inherrent in the tactics used in the rescue operations, such as flying debris, fire, or falling.

Before transporting the patient, you must evaluate the evacuation route, pinpoint potential hazards, and take appropriate precautions or actions to neutralize the hazards.

You and the other rescuers must also constantly evaluate one another's mental and physical states. Overexcited or fatigued rescuers are a danger to themselves, other rescuers, and the patient.

COMMUNICATIONS FOR RESCUE EMERGENCY CARE

Accurate and definitive communications between the rescuer and a medical facility are important for good patient care. When the transportation of the patient is extended, you may need additional guidance or instruction from medical control on the care of the patient as the medical or rescue conditions change. When this communication is possible, you must be able to describe accurately, intelligently, and precisely, the medical condition of the patient to medical control. During extended incidents you must also provide dependable, concise follow-up assessments, describing changes in the patient's status over time.

A second reason for accurate and definitive communication is to obtain assistance in the field, such as higher-level medical expertise; additional skilled rescuers; more physical help for transporting patients or equipment; specialized rescue equipment or transportation, such as helicopters; and relief for fatigued rescuers. Good communications also prepares the receiving medical facility for your arrival.

In accurately communicating the patient's condition, you provide yourself an additional advantage in a rescue. To communicate the patient's medical condition precisely, you must accurately assess the patient. A comprehensive medical communication system helps you discipline yourself to perform the accurate, comprehensive patient assessment so necessary in extended incident rescue situations.

Before communicating the patient's condition, you must write the information to be communicated down in a systematic way. This will provide a check that nothing is missed. Then you can effectively and efficiently communicate your message. There is one additional advantage: you have created a record of your assessment and planned treatment that provides **documentation**.

The Form for Communications: Subjective, Objective, Assessment, and Plan

The use of the SOAP format is a logical and efficient method of communicating patient information that will improve your communication discipline. It is commonly used by all levels of medical personnel to communicate patient information in a logical sequence. You subjectively and objectively describe the patient's condition, your assessment of the problems, and your planned medical management (Figure 13.1).

FIGURE 13.1

SOAP Form
The SOAP format is a logical and efficient method of communicating patient information. It organizes patient information in a logical sequence to describe the patient's condition, assess the problems, and plan medical management.

S Subjective
O Objective
A Assessment
P Plan

S Subjective
A listing of the patient's *symptoms and history* (what the patient or bystanders have told you).

O Objective
Results of the *patient exam and vital signs* (what you have found from your observations and examination of the patient).

A Assessment
A list of problems and anticipated problems that you develop using your training and experience to assess the subjective and objective data you just collected.

P Plan
Your treatment plan for each listed problem or anticipated problem.

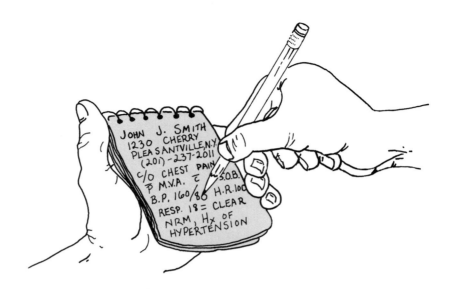

FIGURE 13.2

Street Card
During rescue operations you must write down everything you find during your initial patient assessment.

Communications Discipline

During rescue incidents, you should use your radio only to report your initial assessment of the patient, changes in the patient's condition, and the status of the rescue operation or to request assistance. Stay off the air unless you have new information to transmit. Following these guidelines, you maintain a professional demeanor, decrease your workload and that at the receiving facility, keep the frequency clear for other radio traffic, and save your batteries.

DOCUMENTATION

During rescue operations you must be as diligent in your documentation of patient care as is expected in conventional rapid transport emergency care. There is increasing litigation in rescue emergency care even for those rescuers who are volunteers. Your memory is not dependable. *Everything* that you find during your patient assessment and everything that you do for or to the patient must be written down. In a legal sense, *if you did not write it down, you did not do it.* Although you may use your state's model ambulance run sheets for documentation in a rescue situation, you may find it more convenient to use a smaller, modified form that prompts you to collect all the essential information (Figure 13.2).

In extended incidents, your careful documentation will improve continuity of patient care when additional rescuers relieve you and when the patient arrives at the receiving medical facility.

DECEASED PERSONS

For deceased persons, you must follow your state's legal requirements applicable to all other medical providers. These statuatory requirements relate to such actions as declarations of death and the removal of dead bodies. In some rescue environments, the officials normally responsible for declaring death or giving permission to remove a body may not be able to reach the scene. In some of these cases, they may verbally give permission to the rescuer to do so. When you are given such permission, you must document, such as in a log, that they have done so. However, the best approach is to establish written protocols on handling the deceased before the incident occurs.

Before removing a body, you should completely document the scene and situation with photographs, sketches, and a written description.

SUMMARY

There are basic steps that must be taken in every rescue situation. An extended rescue, however, presents unique problems that the rescuer must address.

In an extended rescue operation, you must continue to give medical care until the patient arrives at a medical facility. Because of the extended times, the patient may develop more severe medical problems than would be seen during a conventional, ambulance-based rapid transport. You will need assessment skills for long-term evaluation of a situation.

Anticipating problems, improvising equipment, and managing stress are essential skills for rescuers in an extended rescue. In addition, gathering information, evaluating rescuer and patient safety, and establishing accurate communications are necessary components of any rescue. But they are especially crucial in an extended rescue operation. You must also understand legal requirements pertaining to deceased persons.

PATIENT ASSESSMENT IN RESCUE MEDICAL CARE

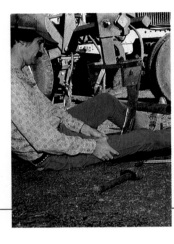

CHAPTER OUTLINE

Patient assessment in an extended incident is critical for identifying active medical emergencies and anticipating and managing any medical problems that may develop during a lengthy rescue operation.

This chapter explains the seven-step Patient Assessment System (PAS). Each step, which includes specific procedures for assessment and reassessment, is described in detail. In addition, a sample case history illustrates the development of a problem list with its accompanying management plan that addresses each real and potential problem.

The objectives for this chapter are for the rescuer to describe:

- the importance of patient assessment in an extended incident emergency care.
- the Patient Assessment System.
- common procedures that a rescuer should use to evaluate and reevaluate the patient's condition.
- methods of identifying problems and developing a plan to manage current or potential problems.

Patient assessment is the critical first step in any emergency medical situation. But in an extended incident rescue situation it is even more important that you do a thorough patient assessment. You will be responsible for the patient for a longer period of time. In addition to current problems, you must anticipate and be thoroughly prepared to manage any medical problems that may develop while the patient is in your care.

Your assessment does not end with your initial examination of the patient. In an extended incident, patient assessment is an ongoing process that continues for as long as the patient is in your care. Even with a stable patient, reassessments should be done at least every 15 to 20 minutes. The more severe the injuries or potential injuries, the more frequently you must reassess the patient.

THE PATIENT ASSESSMENT SYSTEM

To ensure that no critical aspect of the patient's condition is missed, you must consistently use a methodical, step-by-step system during your patient assessment. One such assessment method is the **Patient Assessment System (PAS)**. The PAS is a seven-step system based on the widely used SOAP scheme (See Chapter 13). The initial four steps of the PAS are

1. Scene survey
2. Primary survey
3. Secondary survey (physical exam and vital signs)
4. Patient history

These steps develop the database used for steps 5 and 6, the assessment and planning phases of SOAP (See Chapter 13). Step 7 is the continuing reassessment of the patient.

The use of PAS provides a framework for many of the activities involved in emergency medical care including patient triage, assessment and management, patient monitoring and reassessment, communication discipline, and records/documentation. (Figure 14.1)

Scene Survey

Hazards Your first assessment step is to survey the incident before entering the scene. The safety of all those involved in a rescue—both rescuers and patients—is your primary concern during any rescue operation. A survey of the scene may take a little extra time but may prevent additional injuries or death and avoid complicating the rescue. You must survey the scene for any threats or hazards to you or your patient's safety. Such threats might include unstable objects or unsecured vehicles, fires, downed electric wires, poisonous gas or other hazardous materials, and unsafe human situations such as civil disturbances.

You should not enter a rescue scene until all the threats and hazards have been stabilized, neutralized, or secured. Do not approach or enter a rescue scene unless you have the appropriate protective clothing, equipment, and training. And when you have identified threats or hazards at a rescue scene you must notify all other rescuers about their existence.

Mechanism of Injury/Illness As you enter the rescue scene, you should briefly survey the area for indications of the mechanism of injury/illness. If you have some knowledge of the factors involved in producing the injury/illness, then you will have a better idea of the nature and extent of the potential injuries to the patient. Knowledge

FIGURE 14.1

Patient Assessment Survey Form

To ensure that you miss no critical aspect of the patient's condition, you must use a methodical, step-by-system during patient assessment and to record your findings.

Woodbury Rescue
Patient Assessment Summary

Location:_____ Date:_____ Time:_____
Rescue Team: _____
Name:_____ Age:_____ DOB_____
Address:_____
SUBJECTIVE
History:_____
_____
_____
_____
Complaints:_____
_____
_____
Meds:_____
Allergies:_____
OBJECTIVE:_____

Time								
B/P								
Pulse								
Resp								
Eyes/AVPU								
Skin								
Temp								

Exam:
   General: _____
   Head: _____
   Eyes: _____
   Ears: _____
   Nose: _____
   Mouth/Throat: _____
   Neck: _____
   Chest: _____
   Back: _____
   Abdomen: _____
   Pelvis/Genitals: _____
   Buttocks: _____
   Neuro: _____
   Arms: _____
   Legs: _____

ASSESSMENT	PLAN
Current Problems:	Management:
_____	_____
_____	_____
_____	_____
_____	_____
_____	_____
Potential Problems:	_____
_____	_____
_____	_____
_____	_____

of the mechanism of injury/illness will also assist hospital personnel in treating serious injuries. The typical mechanisms of injury that suggest major trauma include falls of more than 15 feet, motor vehicle incidents with the death of another occupant, ejection from a vehicle, falling objects, and crush injuries.

Some typical injuries that might be revealed by knowing the mechanism of injury include spinal injuries caused by falls or blows to the head and chest, or abdominal injuries caused by blunt trauma to the patient's body.

Primary Survey

The **primary survey** covers immediate life-threatening conditions that affect the three major body systems—circulatory, respiratory, and central and peripheral nervous systems. These are the ABC standbys—airway, breathing, and circulation. You must also add "D"—disability—which includes conditions such as spinal injuries that could lead to disability.

You can perform the ABCD elements of the primary survey in sequence or simultaneously. But you must cover all of the ABCDs before beginning the physical exam. You continue with your physical exam if you find no problems ("normal exam"), but you must stop and treat any problem found in the primary survey ("red flags") as you find it.

Normal Exam	Red Flags
A Airway	
The patient's airway is clear so that he or she can breathe.	Air is not moving in or out (the airway is obstructed).
B Breathing	
The patient is breathing, and the ventilation is adequate.	The patient is not breathing, and/or the ventilation is not adequate.
C Circulation	
1. The patient has a carotid pulse, and 2. There is no severe bleeding.	1. The patient has no carotid pulse, and/or 2. There is severe bleeding.
D Disability	
1. There is no mechanism for possible spine injury, and 2. There is no obvious spine injury, and 3. The patient has a normal pain response, and 4. The patient's AVPU status is alert (see page 228).	1. There is a mechanism for spine injury, and/or 2. There is an obvious spine injury, and/or 3. The patient has an altered pain response, and/or 4. The patient's AVPU scale is V, P, or U.

Basic Life Support (BLS) and Advanced Life Support (ALS) are procedures that you perform when you find problems in the primary survey. Local protocols, your scope of practice and level of training, and available resources will determine the level of care you may provide in a given circumstance as you strive to maintain the circulatory, respiratory, and nervous systems.

Secondary Survey

Physical Exam Complete the head-to-toe exam of the patient before you begin any treatment other than BLS or ALS. Avoid focusing in on a dramatic injury, such as a fracture or skull laceration. Otherwise you may miss other injuries that might be more serious, such as spinal injury or blunt trauma and internal injury to chest or abdomen. You must visually inspect the site of any injury. To do this you may have to pull or cut clothing away from the injury site. But in severe environments, such as cold, avoid long exposure that could worsen the patient's condition.

To ensure that you do not omit or miss anything, you must consistently conduct the exam in a logical order. The following is one example of a area-by-area exam. You may change the order, but make certain you do so in a way that prevents you from overlooking a potential injury.

Head	Pelvis
Eyes	Genitalia
Ears	Legs
Nose	Arms
Mouth/Throat	Neurological
Neck	Back
Chest	Buttocks
Abdomen	

Once you complete the entire exam, you may need or want to return to an injured body part for further inspection.

Vital Signs

Your attention to changes in a patient's vital signs over a period of time can give you important clues about the patient's progress or deterioration. You must be cautious about relying on only one set of vital signs or a single exam or test to indicate that a patient is doing well. For example, low blood pressure may be a *late sign* of shock. When a patient's blood pressure begins to drop, he or she may already be in a great deal of trouble. A rising pulse rate might have provided a you an early warning of impending shock. What is more important is the *change* and *pattern of change* in vital signs over time. If the patient transport will be extended, you must continue to monitor the patient's status throughout the transport. Frequent reassessments will allow you to recognize clinical patterns such as volume shock as they develop.

Time Every time that you take a set of vital signs, you must document the time and values. A series of vital signs has no meaning unless you record the time.

Blood Pressure (BP) If possible, record both systolic and diastolic blood pressure, since in some medical conditions the relationship between systolic and diastolic is important. However, some environmental conditions or lack of equipment may prevent you from recording the diastolic pressure.

A significant change in blood pressure will usually result in changes in the pulse rate. If the patient is alert and oriented, and the pulse rate is steady and normal, then it may not be necessary to continually recheck the BP with each reassessment. This can be an important practical matter during an extended or difficult evacuation.

Pulse (P) Record the pulse according to the rate. Use terms such as "regular" or "irregular" that have meaning to other people. Avoid terms such as "weak" and "thready," which are subjective and only have meaning for yourself.

Respiration (R) Record the respiration rate and describe it in terms like "regular" or "irregular," or "easy" or "difficult." If your patient is able to speak to you without difficulty, he or she probably is not experiencing any respiratory difficulties.

Level of Consciousness (LOC) Describe the patient's level of consciousness in as precise terms as possible. Avoid vague descriptions such as "semi-conscious." One commonly used measurement of level of consciousness is the **AVPU scale**:

A *Alert.* The eyes open spontaneously. The patient answers questions in a clear and appropriate manner. They know the date, where they are, and their own name. They are oriented.

V Responds to *Verbal* stimulus. The eyes do not open spontaneously. The patient is not oriented to time, place, and person. There is some manner of response when spoken to.

P Responds to *Painful* stimulus. The patient does not respond to verbal stimuli, but does move or cry out in response to pain.

U *Unresponsive* (unconscious). The patient does not respond to any stimulus.

You can further describe "alert" patients by their behavior, such as hysterical, disoriented, frightened, relaxed, calm, or cooperative.

Temperature It is important to know the body core temperature of a patient, particularly in environmentally-caused illnesses such as hypothermia and heat exhaustion. Oral and skin temperatures are not always an accurate measurement of the patient's temperature. The most accurate method is with a rectal thermometer. But conditions may not permit you to use it. If you are unable to take a rectal temperature, then estimate the patient's temperature by clinical signs and history.

Skin Color/Temperature/Moisture The skin condition, along with the appearance of the nail beds, are an indication of blood perfusion to the skin and extremities, the body's shell. The change in color in the lips, for example, is particularly prominent with decreased perfusion, because the color changes from deep red to pale. Skin color is not a reliable indicator of core temperature, nor is it a reliable indicator in parts exposed to the cold.

History

The patient history is recorded using the acronym AMPLE

    A   Allergies

    M Medication

    P   Pertinent Past Medical History

    L   Last Meal

    E   Events (what happened to the patient?)

The patient's history should include any preexisting illness or significant previous injuries, particularly to the same body parts.

Assessment

After collecting the database information in the scene survey, primary and secondary assessments, and history, you will use the information you have gathered to assess the problems and potential problems facing your patient. You should develop a list of all the problems or anticipated problems that you have determined from your evaluation of the database.

Plan

After you have developed your problem list, you must plan your management for each problem that you have identified. You must also plan how you will manage any anticipated problems that you anticipate might arise.

The following is an example of a SOAP format PAS problem list for a 30-year old, insulin-dependent diabetic hiker who has fallen 20 feet, sustained an open, mid-shaft fracture of the tibia and fibula, and had a witnessed 30-second loss of consciousness (LOC) that was resolved by the time the rescue team arrived (Figure 14.2). Vital signs are stable.

FIGURE 14.2

Completed Patient Assessment Summary Forms

Your findings are recorded in SOAP format, on the PAS.

Woodbury Rescue
Patient Assessment Summary

Location: HEADWALL 2½ M. N OF COWSKIN CREEK RD.   Date: 8/17/83   Time: 1030
Rescue Team: RYAN, THOMAS, KALLI, LYNN, M. MAULY, B. MAULY, G. MAULY, KING, S. McPHERTENS, J. McPHERTENS
Name: ROBERT S. THOMAS   Age: 30   DOB 5/23/53
Address: 1323 HACKETT, SOMERSET COVE

SUBJECTIVE
History: 30 YO INSULIN DEPENDENT CLIMBER, ANCHOR FAILURE DURING RAPPEL, PT. FELL ~30', LANDED FEET FIRST, 30 SEC POSITIVE K.O. PER FRIENDS ATE BRKFST @ 0730, FELL ABOUT 0900 HRS

Complaints: C/O PAIN (R) TIB/FIB, NO LOSS OF SENSATION, NO BACK PAIN, SLIGHT HEADACHE → IMPROVING

✱ WEATHER: HIGH WINDS Ē FOG/LOW CLOUDS, BAROMETER FALLING. BELOW MINS FOR HELI
Meds: INSULIN 200 NPH QAM-TJOR AT 0800   NOT EXPECTED TO CLEAR
Allergies: ∅ FINGERSTICK GLUCOSE 100 AT 0800

OBJECTIVE: ✱ START TRANSPORT   TR. TO SEDGWICK EMTS ⌐

Time	1200	1220	1225	1245	1300	1310	1330	1400	1415
B/P	120/78	130/80	134/80	130/78	140/80	130/74	130/80	134/78	134/80
Pulse	80	84	84	80	84	76	80	76	76
Resp	12	13	14	12	14	13	13	13	12
Eyes/AVPU	PERLA/A →	→	→	→	→	→	→	→	
Skin	WM/PK/DRY →	→	→	→	→	→	→	→	
Temp	98⁴	—	98⁴	—	—	—	—	—	

Exam: GCS   16   16   16   16   16   16   16   16

General: WDWM MOD. PAIN ORIENTED X3 NL PAIN RESPONSE
Head: 3" CONTUSION ABOVE (R) EYE, NO PALP. DEFORITIES, MINOR SWELLING
Eyes: PERL
Ears: CLEAR & DRY
Nose: CLEAR & DRY
Mouth/Throat: CLEAR
Neck: NON-TENDER NL ROM
Chest: CLR, NON-TENDER, BREATH SOUNDS CLEAR
Back: NON-TENDER SOFT, NL BOWEL SOUNDS ERROR S.K.
Abdomen: NON-TENDER SOFT, NL BOWEL SOUNDS ALL 4 QUADS
Pelvis/Genitals: NL TO EXAM, NO PAIN Ē COMPRESSION
Buttocks: NL TO EXAM
Neuro: ORIENTED X3, NO LOCALIZING SIGNS, NO AMNESIA
Arms: WNL
Legs: PUNCTURE WOUND Ē BONE PROTRUDING MID (R) TIBIA, GOOD DISTAL PULSE, MIN BLEEDING

ASSESSMENT	PLAN
Current Problems:	Management:
1) DIABETES	OBSERVE
2) L.O.C. Ē CHT - RESOLVING	OBSERVE
3) OPEN (R) TIB/FIB FT	IRRIGATE TO CLEAN, DRY STERILE DRSG OVER WOUND LONG LEG BOARD SPLINT REPEAT CMS V'S
4) TRANSPORT → BAD WEATHER - NO AIR EVAC.	LITTER TO FLINT OAKS TRAIL, USE BEARTOOTH'S 4×4 TO GET TO AMB AT JUNE Ē CTY W.
Potential Problems:	
1) INSULIN REACTION	WATCH GIVE GLUCOSE IF DEVELOPS.
2) CHT - UNKN SEVERITY	WATCH NEURO & NUPV, WATCH FOR ↑ IN, CP
3) NEUROVASCULAR COMPROMISE (R)	MONITER DISTAL CMS, LOOSEN DRESS. IF CHANGES
4) HYPOTHERMIA	KEEP WARM & DRY ADDITIONAL COVERS, IF RAINS

SUMMARY

Patient assessment is an important first step in an extended rescue operation. During such a rescue, patient assessment is an ongoing process, and you must be prepared to manage any medical problems that arise.

You may wish to use a seven-step system called the Patient Assessment System (PAS) to assess patients. The seven steps are:

1. Scene survey
2. Primary survey
3. Secondary survey
4. Patient history
5. Assessment
6. Planning
7. Reassessment

Each step has established procedures that enable you to make a thorough evaluation of the patient.

INDICATIONS AND TREATMENT OF COMMON MEDICAL CONDITIONS AND INJURIES

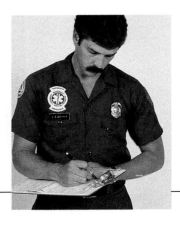

OVERVIEW

The ability to recognize and treat common medical conditions and injuries is an important skill for rescuers who work in any environment. Rescuers need to be able to manage illnesses and injuries during a rescue operation.

This chapter examines some of the more common medical conditions and injuries and their management. The conditions are discussed in relation to mechanisms of injury, assessment, and treatment.

OBJECTIVES

The objectives of this chapter are for the rescuer to describe:

- the mechanisms of injury for common medical conditions and injuries encountered during a rescue operation.

- assessment of common conditions encountered during rescue.
- treatment of common conditions encountered during rescue.

The following sections describe some of the medical conditions that rescue personnel may encounter. This list of conditions does not cover all situations, but is meant to examine some of the more common problems and their management.

SHOCK

Used in a strict medical context, **shock** is the acute loss of capillary blood perfusion that results from a loss of pressure within the cardiovascular system. There are various degrees of severity of shock. Severe shock will often result in death if not reversed. In rescue situations, shock always indicates a serious threat to life that requires aggressive treatment by you. Unfortunately, field treatment for shock is limited to measures that may briefly extend the time available to evacuate the patient to definitive medical care.

Mechanisms of Injury

Shock results from three basic mechanisms: fluid loss, failure of the heart to pump effectively, and dilation of the blood vessels. Whatever the mechanism, the common element is loss of perfusion pressure.

You will frequently encounter patients with shock during serious incidents such as major injuries, accidents, and heart attacks. Regardless of the circumstances, however, there are three basic mechanisms that can be involved in shock:

- **Hypovolemic shock** Loss of blood/fluid depletes the vascular system volume to the point that it is insufficient for perfusion. The volume loss may be the result of internal or external bleeding. But the loss may also occur as a result of dehydration secondary to diarrhea or vomiting.
- **Cardiogenic shock** The heart muscle is damaged so that it is unable to pump the blood volume effectively. Perfusion pressure is lost even though blood volume is normal. Common mechanisms for cardiogenic shock include myocardial infarction, cardiac ischemia, tamponade, contusion, arrythmia, and electrical shock.
- **Vascular shock** Normally, a large percentage of the blood vessels in the body are partially constricted. If all the blood vessels dilate, then the blood within them, even though it is of normal volume, is insufficient to fill the system and provide perfusion pressure.

There are generally two basic causes of vascular shock:

- Mechanical (spinal shock). Injury to the spinal cord causes loss of autonomic control over blood vessels. This results in vasodilation in all parts of the body.
- Chemical (anaphylactic shock). This is an allergic reaction that results in a generalized vasodilation—dilation of all the vessels in the body—and subsequent loss of perfusion pressure to the body tissues.

Assessment

The effects of all three mechanisms of shock are identical. There is insufficient blood perfusion through the tissues to provide adequate nutrition and oxygen and to carry away waste. All local body processes are affected by shock (Figure 15.1).

One of the dangerous aspects of shock is that the patient's body may try to compensate for the loss of perfusion. This may hide the signs and symptoms of shock until it reaches a dangerous level. You must anticipate the possibility of shock developing based on the history, mechanism of injury/illness, and physical findings. You must watch for the subtle warning signs of impending collapse of the cardiovacular system before it reaches a dangerous level. The signs and symptoms of hypovolemic or cardiogenic shock include:

FIGURE 15.1

Signs of Shock
You must anticipate the possibility of shock developing in a patient based on the medical history, mechanism of injury, and the physical findings during the assessment.

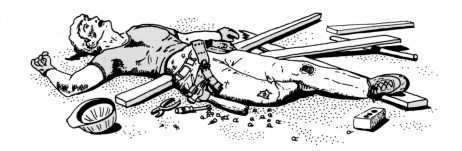

- Agitation, anxiety, or a feeling of impending doom
- Increased pulse rate
- Pale, ashen, cool, or moist skin
- Diminished urinary output
- Gasping for air, "air hunger"
- Falling blood pressure (often a late sign)

These signs and symptoms are the result of the body's compensation mechanisms that decrease blood perfusion in the extremities or body "shell" to provide additional perfusion to the brain and other vital organs of the body "core." These clinical patterns will not be seen in vascular shock, since the peripheral vessels are dilated and unable to constrict and transfer the blood volume to the core.

One or more of the signs of shock listed above may be present in situations involving severe blows to the head or body, massive external or internal bleeding, fractures and broken bones, an acute abdomen, stab or puncture wound, gunshot wounds, spinal injury, severe infection, or poisoning. Regardless of the cause of shock, it is essential that you anticipate its development based on the history, mechanism of injury, and physical exam. You must promptly recognize the early signs of impending shock, take immediate measures to delay its onset, and rapidly transport to definitive care.

General Treatment of Shock

- Oxygen. Give high flow oxygen if available. This increases the oxygen content of the limited blood perfusion to body tissues.
- Position. Position the patient flat with legs slightly elevated to help perfuse the body core. This treatment is helpful but has limited effect.
- Temperature. Maintain normal body temperature. This is particularly important for any patient who is seriously injured, exposed to the environment, or unable to move and maintain body heat. This also applies in hot environments where increased temperatures can increase peripheral vasodilation and aggravate the shock.

Specific Treatment for Hypovolemic Shock

- Stop the bleeding. Use direct pressure for external bleeding. PASG may help stop bleeding in the pelvis and upper legs. To stop most internal bleeding, surgery is generally required.

- Administer IV fluids. If *within your scope of practice*, replace fluids via IV using the "3 : 1" rule: 300 ml of electrolyte solution for every 100 ml blood loss. Blood replacement is generally required after 2,000 ml of blood loss. Fluids taken orally are usually not absorbed fast enough to replace severe losses and must not be used in patients with suspected internal injuries or diminished level of consciousness.
- Apply PASG. This may increase fluids available to the patient's core. To avoid injury to muscles and nerves, do not keep PASG inflated for more than two hours.

To treat hypovolemic shock, you must stop or slow the flow of blood. You must apply sufficient pressure to external bleeding points. You must splint major long bone and pelvic fractures properly to minimize internal bleeding. You must also monitor the patient's vital signs and urine output. Remember that field management of hypovolemic shock is your attempt to provide a little extra time to get the patient to definitive medical care, which usually requires surgeons and an operating suite.

If you are adminstering IV fluids for the management of shock during an extended incident, you should carefully monitor urine output. This is done preferably with a Foley catheter, if *within your scope of practice and authorized by medical control.*

Specific Treatment for Cardiogenic Shock

- Medication. Certain medications can decrease the workload of the heart, restore normal heart rhythm, increase pumping strength of heart muscle, and reduce ischemic pain.
- Defibrillation. Defibrillation restores normal pumping rhythm.
- IV fluids. If *within your scope of practice*, start an IV, and infuse fluids as slowly as possible to avoid adding additional workload to the heart. The IV line will be used primarily as an access route for medication administration according to your local protocols or at the hospital. It generally is easier to get a line started as early as possible before decreasing perfusion makes it even more difficult to locate an accessible vein.

Treat and transport patients with cardiogenic shock in the position in which they can breathe most easily. Monitor vital signs and urine output. If available and if feasible, *within your scope of practice*, use portable cardiac monitors.

Specific treatment for vascular shock is as follows:

1. Spinal shock
   - IV Fluids—as for hypovolemic shock
   - PASG
2. Anaphylaxis
   - Medication—epinephine by injection and oral or injectable antihistamines if *within your scope of practice*

- IV fluids—as for hypovolemic shock
- PASG
- Airway managment—high flow oxygen, ventilatory assistance as needed, and possible intubation if *within your scope of practice.*

Autonomic Stress Reaction (Psychogenic Shock)

There is also a reaction sometimes known as psychogenic shock, a misleading term. This condition is different from true shock in that it is usually temporary and not life-threatening. It will generally resolve with minimal intervention. The term **autonomic stress reaction (ASR)** is a better term for this parasympathetic reaction. ASR is commonly associated with emotional situations such as fear, bad news, good news, the sight of an injury or blood, the prospect of medical treatment, severe pain, and anxiety. ASR results from a temporary reduction in perfusion of the brain as blood momentarily pools in dilated vessels in other parts of the body and the heart rate suddenly slows. ASR is usually self-correcting since the patient usually ends up horizontal, thereby restoring the blood flow to the brain. If you suspect ASR, have the patient lie down to improve blood flow to the brain. If ASR causes the patient to fall, the fall may cause other injuries, especially in an older patient. Therefore, it is important to check for such injuries. Where psychogenic shock involves an injury to the head, it is important to stabilize the patient; place the patient in a secure, supine position; and transport immediately.

Nausea, vomiting, confusion, fainting, and disorientation are common ASR responses to severe injury or stress. ASR can be a problem in rescue situations because it may cause confusing symptoms and mask real injuries. ASR can be confused with shock, though it may also coexist with shock. But ASR tends to improve spontaneously, while true shock does not. ASR can affect you as well as patients.

ASR can have a positive effect on patient survival, and there have been numerous cases where severely injured persons have performed heroic acts while under the influence of ASR. ASR tends to diminish with time and reassurance. It is important when you suspect that a patient has ASR that you reevaluate that patient at regular intervals to ensure that ASR is not masking serious injuries.

HEAD INJURIES

Increased Intracranial Pressure

The terms "closed head trauma" (CHT) or "head injury" are inexact but usually imply injury to the brain. It is important to distinguish CHT from "head wounds," which are scalp or facial soft tissues injuries without injury to the brain.

The brain is enclosed in a rigid skull that prevents any expansion of brain tissue. Thus, any bleeding or swelling of the brain may result in increased intracranial pressure (IICP). Unless corrected quickly, IICP will result in permanent neurological damage or death.

Mechanism of Injury Trauma is the most common mechanism of IICP seen in rescue situations. Lacerations, tears, or contusion of the brain or vessels within the skull may cause bleeding and/or swelling, resulting in increased pressure.

Much less frequently, you may see IICP as a result of cardiovascular accidents (CVAs or "strokes"). These are localized infarctions that cause cell death within the brain and may result in bleeding or swelling. In addition, cardiac arrest or cardiogenic shock decrease brain perfusion resulting in IICP from edema, that is, extra fluid in and around the cells of the brain due to cell death.

You may also see edema formation as a result of the vascular changes of hypoxia at high altitude. This is called high altitude cerebral edema (HACE), a form of acute mountain sickness.

Assessment Whatever the cause, IICP presents a relatively constant clinical pattern. Determine the patient's history. Has the patient received a blow to the head or suffered a cardiac arrest or CVA? Is the patient at high altitude?

With a positive mechanism of injury and an altered level of consciousness, you must assume CHT with IICP. Monitor and record the progression of the vital signs and other signs and symptoms. They may be helpful in predicting the outcome of the injury.

The following signs and symptoms will help confirm the assessment:

- Blood pressure—will increase in a severe head injury.
- Pulse—will decrease in severe CHT.
- Respiration—altered breathing patterns are common following head injuries. Some patients may breathe more deeply or more rapidly than normal following head injury. Do not assume that head injury automatically means lower respiration. If the injury is severe, the breathing may be irregular or absent.
- Temperature—will be variable.
- Skin—will be variable.

Level of consciousness and mental status are the most sensitive indicators of a change in status of the patient. In the early states, the patient may exhibit restlessness or signs of being intoxicated or combative. If severe, there will be a decreased level of consciousness as measured by the AVPU scale (Table 15.1).

Assessing the overall level of consciousness is a crucial step in evaluating a patient with a head injury. You should determine the level of consciousness immediately after completing the primary survey of the patient. The level of consciousness is generally determined using the AVPU scale.

The initial level of consciousness should be determined and the time noted. The level of consciousness should be rechecked every ten minutes and documented. Any change in the level of consciousness,

TABLE 15.1   AVPU Scale

Alert	The patients' eyes open spontaneously, and they will answer questions in a clear and appropriate manner. They know the date, where they are, and their own names. They are oriented.
Responsive to verbal stimulus	The patients' eyes do not open spontaneously. They are not oriented to time, place, and person. But they do respond in some manner when spoken to.
Responsive to pain	The patients do not respond to verbal stimuli but do move or cry out in response to pain.
Unresponsive	The patients do not respond to any stimulus.

either positive or negative, is significant in a head injury patient. The level of consciousness may fluctuate—improving, deteriorating, then improving again over time. On the other hand, a progressive deterioration in the patient's response to stimuli usually indicates serious brain damage requiring prompt surgical treatment. Physicians need to know when loss of consciousness occurred and what the patient's responses have been, if any, during the rescue and transport phases of tactical operations. Your neurological evaluations will be compared with the neurological evaluations obtained when the patient reaches an emergency facility. Therefore, it is critical that you obtain the baseline evaluation as soon as possible during the rescue process.

Headache is an early sign of IICP but may be confused as pain associated with trauma to skull or neck. Vomiting is often also seen in early stages of IICP. Late signs include seizures, unequal pupils, and paralysis, which may be localized to one side of the patient's body.

Decorticate or decerebrate posturing are always signs of very serious CHT with high IICP (Figure 15.2).

The CHT patient with increased intracranial pressure does not generally present a typical clinical picture for shock. If the patient does exhibit a pattern of shock, look for additional injuries that might cause internal bleeding.

Treatment In cases of patients with IICP, you must arrange transport to definitive medical care (surgery) as soon as possible. Like those for shock, field treatment options are limited and have little

Decerebrate and Decorticate Posturing
Decerebrate, or extensor, posturing (left) and decorticate, or flexor, posturing (right) are signs of severe closed head trauma with increased intracranial pressure.

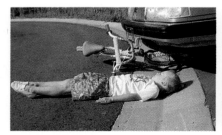
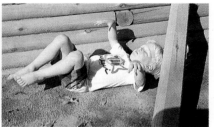

effect on patient survival. In these patients respiratory failure often occurs before cardiac failure.

It is critical that patients with IICP be given high flow oxygen and be hyperventilated to reduce the intracranial pressure.

Since spine injuries are often present in patients with closed head trauma, you must protect the spine.

Concussions

Injuries to the brain have a broad band of severity and do not always result in increased IICP. Concussions are generally minor injuries. They range from temporary memory loss or confusion to a temporary alteration in the patient's level of consciousness. No treatment is indicated for a concussion. Patients should be monitored carefully for possible IICP. They should not be allowed to return to activities where they would be at risk of additional CHT until evaluated by a physician. All neurologic changes from a concussion will resolve within a few minutes. Therefore, if your patient shows any neurologic abnormalities lasting more than a few minutes, they should not be attributed to a concussion. You must then look for another cause for the changes. Severe concussions may result in loss of consciousness for 15 to 20 minutes. Such injuries indicate a more severe brain injury that may require aggressive medical intervention. If your patient's confusion does not clear completely, that is also a sign of a more severe injury requiring medical evaluation and intervention.

Contusion

Contusions are bruises to the cortex of the brain asssociated with severe concussions. They are characterized by longer periods of confusion, memory loss, or loss of consciousness. Contusions may result in focal neurologic defects if the area of contusion is in a sensory or motor area of the cortex. Coup contusions occur directly under the point of impact. Contrecoup injuries occur opposite the point of impact and occur as a result of a bounce phenomenon. Bleeding into contused areas can result in a major neurologic injury from a mass effect. Contusions require evaluation by a physician.

Intracranial Hemorrhages

There is no typical picture for intracranial hemorrhage because of the great variation in location, size, and rapidity of bleeding that may occur. Patients with an intracranial bleed may show focal neurologic defects and deteriorate rapidly. They require rapid evacuation for medical evaluation and intervention.

Scalp Lacerations

Because the face and scalp both possess a rich blood supply, significant amounts of blood may be quickly lost even from small lacerations about the head, neck, and face. In rare cases, blood loss from a scalp laceration may be severe enough to cause hypovolemic shock.

Treatment Bleeding from scalp lacerations can almost always be controlled by direct pressure with a dry sterile dressing applied to the wound. Apply firm compression for several minutes in order to control the bleeding. Avoid applying pressure to underlying skull fractures and increasing the injury to the brain.

In circumstances involving triangular or square flaps of skin protruding from the scalp, the flap of skin should be folded back down onto its bed before the compression dressing is applied. If it becomes saturated with blood, a second dressing may be applied over the first one to reinforce it. Manual pressure should be continued until the bleeding is controlled (Figure 15.3).

Skull Fractures

Skull fractures can result in serious injury to the brain and result in IICP. It is important to protect the skull from further injury during evacuation and transport.

Assessment All patients with skull fractures need to have their cervical spine totally immobilized because of the risk of associated spinal injury. One indication of skull fracture is the appearance of clear or pink watery fluid dripping from the nose, the ear, or from an open scalp wound. This fluid is cerebrospinal fluid, which leaks to the outside only if the dura (covering of the brain) and the skull have both been penetrated. This indicates serious injury. Do not attempt to pack the wound, the ear, or the nose. Such packing of the draining site could block the escape of fluid and cause additional pressure on an already damaged brain. The presence of the so-called grey matter of the brain in an open skull fracture is obviously a poor prognostic sign.

Treatment Simply cover the wound with a sterile dressing to prevent further contamination and infection, but do not bandage tightly.

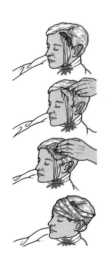

FIGURE 15.3

Scalp Laceration
When a laceration involves flaps of skin hanging from the scalp, the flap should be folded back down onto its bed and a compression dressing applied.

CLOSED SOFT TISSUE INJURIES

Closed soft tissue injuries are either contusions or hematomas. However, contusions may also exist with open wounds such as lacerations and abrasions. Contusions may be minor, or they may be severe, such as in the brain with increased IICP or in the abdomen with a ruptured spleen, liver, or kidney.

a.

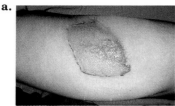

b.

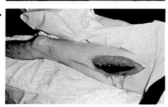

c.

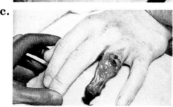

d.

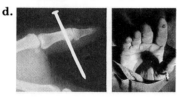

FIGURE 15.4

Types of Wounds
a. Abrasion, a shallow wound where the skin is rubbed or scraped against a rough or hard surface.
b. Lacerations and incisions where the skin is cut or torn, exposing underlying tissues and structures.
c. Avulsion in which a segment of tissue is torn completely loose from its attachment or left hanging as a flap.
d. Puncture, a wound that penetrates into underlying tissue with a minimum of skin disruption.

A **hematoma** is a localized collection of blood beneath the skin that occurs from the rapid bleeding when larger blood vessels tear. The progression of swelling is the greatest during the first 6 hours following injury and continues for up to 24 hours. A hematoma can also occur following fractures or when the blood vessels to any organ in the body are damaged. In the instance of the fracture of a large bone such as the femur or pelvis, large hematomas may form and contain more than a liter of blood.

Assessment and Treatment The most important part of assessing a closed injury is the examination for injury to underlying organs and structures. During extended transport, additional bleeding and swelling may cause problems, so repeat examination is necessary.

Small bruises in most soft tissue injuries require no special emergency medical care and generally heal on their own. With more extensive closed injuries, swelling and bleeding beneath the skin can be extensive and may even result in hypovolemic shock.

Treatment during the initial 24 hours is intended to minimize the swelling by following the acronym RICE:

R   Rest the injury by splinting the affected extremity and limiting its use.

I   Ice applied as tolerated during first 24 hours. Do not expose the skin directly to the ice, or frostbite may result.

C   Compress the injury and distal extremity. Isolated proximal compression can obstruct circulation to the extremity distally.

E   Elevate the affected part above heart level to reduce bleeding and promote drainage.

If there is potential for underlying damage and further bleeding, monitor vital signs and urine output.

WOUNDS

Wounds are injuries that disrupt the skin. Wounds may involve the underlying **soft tissues** such as fat, muscle, and connective tissue between the skin and underlying bones, joints, and organs as well as the small vessels and nerves (Figure 15.4). Wounds are quite common in accidents and range from simple abrasions to serious lacerations, impaled foreign objects, gunshot wounds, and other more serious injuries. The three goals of wound management are:

1. Control bleeding
2. Prevent or control contamination and infection
3. Protect the wound from further damage

Types of Wounds

Abrasion An **abrasion** is a shallow wound that occurs when the skin is rubbed or scrapped against a rough or hard surface. Blood may ooze from the injury, but the abrasion normally does not penetrate completely through the dermis.

Lacerations and Incisions In a **laceration** or an **incision** the skin is cut or torn, exposing underlying tissues and structures. A laceration may leave either a smooth or a jagged wound through the skin. Bleeding and injury to the underlying structures will vary with the wound.

Some lacerations present a high risk of serious infection. These include:

- Animal or human bites
- Dirty or contaminated wounds or those likely to get dirty or contaminated
- Ragged, crushed, or contused tissue, such as a chain saw wounds or power takeoff injuries
- Injuries to a bone, joint, or tendon
- Wounds that are not immobilized

Puncture Wound A **puncture wound** penetrates into underlying tissue with a minimum of skin disruption. Typical puncture wounds result from a penetration with a knife, ice pick, splinter, bullet, or with any other pointed object. External bleeding from puncture wounds may not be severe, but internal bleeding may be significant. Puncture wounds carry a high risk of infection, especially if they cannot drain.

Avulsion An **avulsion** is an injury in which a segment of tissue is torn completely loose from its attachments or is left hanging as a flap.

Amputation In an amputation, a segment of an extremity (finger, arm, leg) is completely detached. In some amputations, bleeding may be severe. With your careful preservation, the amputated part often can be reattached at the hospital.

Preserve the amputated part by placing it in a sterile dressing moistened with sterile saline. Place the part and moist dressing in a container, preferably sterile. Place the container in another cool container containing ice and water. Do not allow the amputated part to freeze.

Near amputation refers to a segment of an extremity that has been severed except for a small flap of skin. Other than trying to maintain the attachment of the distal part, near amputations are managed as amputations.

Assessment and Treatment Assess potential injuries to underlying organs and structures, and evaluate for continuing blood loss. Determine if the injury is at high risk of infection.

Well-positioned direct pressure will stop most bleeding within 15 minutes as normal clotting mechanisms are activated. Since direct pressure requires that you see the wound, you may be required to cut hair or remove clothing.

If bleeding persists, it may be the result of inadequate pressure or pressure not applied directly to the source of bleeding. For a rapid transport, it is generally better to widen the pressure dressing to attempt to more accurately cover the point of bleeding. In an extended incident or transport, the original, ineffective dressing should be removed to examine the wound. Then reapply pressure directly to the bleeding site(s).

During short transports, PASG can provide direct pressure to multiple bleeding sites in the patient's lower extremities. Air splints may be used for upper extremity injuries. When the patient is moved to a warmer or cooler environment or is evacuated by air, you must carefully monitor the pressure being applied to the extremity by any inflatable device.

Monitor the circulation, sensory, and motor status in the affected limb. If it is diminished, loosen the pressure dressing as long as bleeding does not restart. Loosen dressing, but do not remove it in case the bleeding recurs.

Control bleeding by elevating the affected limb and splinting, preventing motion that might loosen clots or cause addition injury. Splinting also increases patient comfort and may make it easier to maintain elevation to decrease the swelling. Use ice in addition to direct pressure.

The use of arterial pressure points to control bleeding is rarely effective. Do not use hemostats outside the operating room to control bleeding. You should use tourniquets only as a last resort, and only if approved by your medical control.

In instances of avulsion injuries, gently irrigate the wound to remove debris, then carefully fold the soft tissue onto the wound if possible.

If a flap of tissue has been completely amputated, collect it and take it to the emergency department. It is often possible to reattached these totally avulsed tissues. The most effective way of transporting the part is to wrap it in sterile gauze, moistened with sterile saline, and place it in a plastic bag that, in turn, should be placed in a cool container. Do not allow the tissue to freeze.

In the extended incident setting, open wounds, especially if contaminated with foreign matter, should be gently cleansed. Irrigate them with sterile fluid if it can be done without restarting bleeding. Local medical protocols may instruct you to use an antibiotic solution for the final rinse, or to use an antibacterial dressing.

Impaled Objects

Your objective in treating an impaled object wound is to reduce injury from further movement. In a rapid transport situation, the impaled object should be stabilized in place unless it is obstructing the airway.

If the impaled object prevents safe and effective patient packaging or transport, in an extended transport situation it is sometimes best to remove the impaled object if removal is simple, safe, and easy. Removal of any impaled object by rescue personnel must be done only in special circumstances by trained personnel under direct orders of the medical control physician

Gunshot wounds are a special form of puncture wounds with unique characteristics that require special prehospital care. Gunshot wounds frequently are multiple, so you should inspect the patient carefully to identify the number and sites, including exit wounds.

BURNS

Burns are among the most serious, painful, and dangerous of all injuries. They occur when the body receives more thermal energy than it can absorb without injury. The sources of this energy are generally heat, but may include toxic chemicals, electricity, and nuclear radiation.

The four major concerns with a burn patient are:

- Volume shock. The clinical pattern will begin within minutes or hours after the patient suffers the burn injury.
- Respiratory burn or irritation. Swelling occurs during the first 24 hours after the patient suffers the burn injury.
- Infection. Signs of infection in the burn patient usually begin to appear several days after the accident. But the degree of infection and the outcome are affected by the way you handle the patient and early treatment.
- Pain. The pain the patient suffers may be severe, but it often diminishes over several hours after the accident.

Assessment Make certain that the scene is secure and that you are not threatened by burns from live electrical wires, toxic fumes, exposure to radioactivity, or outbreaks of fire and explosion. When the scene is secure for you, stop any further burning process. Move the patient from the burning area, and remove any smoldering clothing. If the skin and clothing are still hot, they should be immersed in cold water or covered with a wet, cool dressing.

As in any other emergency medical response, always do the ABCDs. Check for respiratory burn as indicated by singed facial hair or skin or soot in nostrils. If there is any possibility of respiratory burn, continue to monitor the airway. Respiratory burns generally cause problems 4-6 hours after injury as swelling in the airway develops.

If the burn is the result of electrical contact, including lightning, monitor for cardiac arrhythmias.

Perform the body exam. Do not let the burn injuries distract you from the possibilities of other injuries the patient may have suffered at the time of the burn accident. For example, the injured person may have sustained fractures as the result of falling or thrashing around, especially following an electric shock.

Estimate severity of the burn. The actual depth of the burn and the surface involved are calculated together to determine the seriousness of the burn. There are three categories of burns (Figure 15.5). First-degree burns are those in which only the superficial part of epidermis has been injured. The skin may turn red but does not blister or actually burn through. A sunburn is an example of a first-degree burn.

In second-degree burns, the epidermis and a portion of the dermis are burned without destroying the entire thickness of the dermis. A second-degree burn is commonly characterized by the formation of blisters.

Third-degree burns extend through the dermis into or beyond the subcutaneous fat. The area becomes dry, leathery, and discolored with a charred, brown, or white appearance Clotted blood vessels may become visible under the burned skin, or the subcutaneous fat itself may be visible. In severe third-degree burns, superficial nerve endings and blood vessels are destroyed, leaving the burned area without feeling, although the surrounding areas will be extremely painful.

Estimate the area burned by the **rule of nines.** (Figure 15.6). Five factors determine the seriousness of a thermal burn:

FIGURE 15.5

Categories of Burns

The three categories of burns include first-degree burns, in which only the superficial part of epidermis has been injured; second-degree burns, in which the epidermis and a portion of the dermis are burned without destroying the entire thickness of the dermis; and third-degree burns, in which the burn extends through the dermis into or beyond the subcutaneous fat.

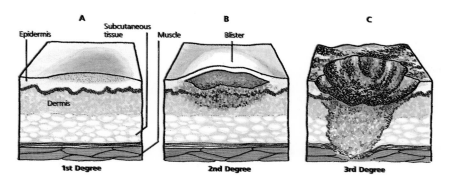

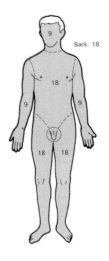

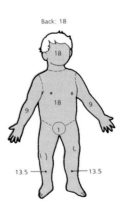

FIGURE 15.6

The Rule of Nines
The percentage of body surface affected by a burn is estimated by the rule of nines. In the adult, most areas of the body are divided roughly into multiples of nine. In the small child, relatively more area is taken up by the head and less by the lower extremities.

- The depth (first-, second-, or third-degree)
- The amount of body surface area (BSA) involved (rule of nines)
- The involvement of critical areas (hands, feet, face, or genitalia)
- The patient's age
- The patient's general health, especially if there are other injuries or illnesses present

Critical burns include any third-degree burns that involve the hands, feet, genitalia, or face, or any third-degree burns involving more than 10 percent of the body surface. All burns complicated by fractures or any degree of respiratory injury are considered critical. Critical burns also include any second-degree burns involving more than 25 percent of the body surface or any otherwise moderate burn in an elderly or critically ill patient.

Moderate burns are less serious than critical burns. But they are dangerous and susceptible to infection and other complications. Moderate burns include third-degree burns involving 2 to 10 percent of the body area and second-degree burns involving 15 to 25 percent of the body surface. First-degree burns, including sunburn, involving 50 to 75 percent of the body surface can also be characterized as moderate burns.

Minor burns include third-degree burns that involve less than 2 percent of the body surface area or second-degree burns involving less than 15 percent of the body surface area.

In children, a second-degree burn of more than 20 percent of the body surface is considered a critical burn, and a second-degree burn of 10 to 20 percent of the body surface would be considered a moderate burn as would any first-degree burn. Any third-degree burn in a child is considered a critical burn.

Treatment Continue to monitor the patient's airway for signs of respiratory distress. A developing cough suggests impending airway problem. Give oxygen according to local medical protocol.

Perform initial cooling with sterile dressings soaked in water to reduce injury to tissues and relieve pain. To avoid hypothermia in patients with greater than a 10 percent BSA burn, limit cooling to several minutes on each area.

Apply dry, sterile dressings to prevent contamination and relieve pain. Treat any associated injuries. If the area of burn is extensive, you should begin IV fluid replacement if *within your scope of practice.*

Treatment for Extended Transport In extended incident transport, continue soaks to areas less than 10 percent BSA as long as pain is evident. Cleanse the burn as you would an abrasion. After the wound has been cooled and cleansed, apply an antibacterial dressing if instructed to by your medical control physician.

IV Volume Replacement During extended incidents of second- and third-degree burns of greater than 20 percent BSA, begin IV volume replacement if *within your scope of practice* and ordered by medical control. The Brooke formula for fluid replacement, using Ringer's lactate or normal saline, for burn patients is

$$2\text{--}4 \text{ ml} \;\times\; \text{Kg body} \;\times\; \% \text{ burn} = \frac{\text{estimated fluid}}{\text{needs for 24 hours}}$$

Give half the estimated fluid requirement in the first 8 hours. The remaining half is given over the next 16 hours. This guideline is an estimate only. Adjust the actual volume and rate according to the patient's vital signs and urine output. Use the same standards as for volume replacement in shock. Monitor urine output using a Foley catheter, if *within your scope of practice and training*, and if ordered by medical control. Refer to local medical protocols for specific clinical standards regarding the treatment of burns during extended incidents.

MUSCULOSKELETAL INJURIES

Musculoskeletal injuries are among the most common problems seen in rescue work. Effective emergency care of musculoskeletal injuries decreases immediate pain, reduces the possibility of nerve or vessel injury, and improves the patient's chances for a rapid recovery with early return to normal activity.

Mechanisms of Injury   In general, any incident in which the body has been thrown against a barrier, fallen on a hard surface, or been struck by a moving object has the potential to cause a fracture, dislocation, or sprain.

Extremity Fractures

Fractures result in unstable bone fragments with sharp ends that can cause injury to adjacent structures such as nerves, blood vessels, and muscle. Fractures result in internal bleeding because bones have a rich blood supply. Severe bleeding may be associated with fractures of the pelvis and femur. But if your fracture patient shows signs of impending shock, do not assume that the fractures are their only source of bleeding (Figure 15.7). Assess your patient for internal injuries and bleeding.

Open fractures may be caused by sharp fragments of bone protruding through the skin from the inside. They may also result from penetrating injuries through the overlying soft tissues to the bone such as a gunshot wound. Open fractures are at high risk for serious infection. Larger wounds, contamination, and associated soft tissue and vascular injury all increase the risk of infection.

Unstable bone fragments also cause pain in the periosteum, the membrane that covers the bones. This pain often produces an autonomic stress reaction (ASR) in patients, resulting in decreased blood pressure and pulse, clammy skin, and fainting.

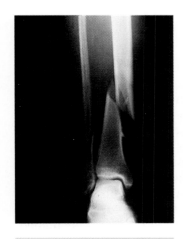

FIGURE 15.7

Fractures
Fractures can result in
unstable bone fragments with
sharp ends that can cause
injury to adjacent structures
such as nerves, blood vessels,
and muscle.

The instability of long bone fractures is increased by movement of the joints at either end of the affected bone. Muscle imbalance and spasm may also cause significant movement. Fractured long bones are generally most stable in their normal "in-line" anatomical position where the muscle pulls are balanced. Stability is also improved when splints control the joint at both ends of the fractured bone.

Bleeding and swelling increase at the fracture site for the first 24 hours, with most swelling occurring during the first 6 hours.

One critically dangerous result of fractures is **ischemia** or reduced perfusion of the extremity distal to the fracture. Ischemia may occur because of swelling or angulation at the fracture site or injury to the vessels at the time of fracture. Ischemia can also result from movement during the reduction or splint application or movement allowed by improper splinting. A tightly secured splint may also reduce circulation. If the ischemia is prolonged, generally greater than two hours, it may lead to **tissue necrosis**, death of the ischemic tissue. Severe tissue necrosis may require amputation of the limb. This is why you must frequently monitor the distal circulation of a fractured extremity. If circulation decreases, you should loosen all dressings and splints on the injured extremity.

Assessment The objective of fracture assessment is to indentify any potentially unstable injuries or injuries that have the potential to damage adjacent structures. Without X rays, the assessment of *fracture,* is essentially the same as *possible fracture.* In the field fractures and possible fractures are treated the same.

$$\begin{array}{ccccc}
\text{positive} & & \text{positive} & & \text{fracture or} \\
\text{mechanism of} & + & \text{signs and} & = & \text{possible} \\
\text{injury} & & \text{symptoms} & & \text{fracture}
\end{array}$$

$$\begin{array}{ccccc}
\text{positive} & & \text{negative} & & \\
\text{mechanism} & + & \text{signs and} & = & \text{no} \\
\text{of injury} & & \text{symptoms} & & \text{fracture}
\end{array}$$

Positive signs and symptoms
Non-specific:

a. Pain
b. Tenderness and/or point tenderness
c. Swelling

Specific:

a. Inability to move/use/bear weight immediately following injury. (Remember that even if the patient can move or use an extremity, it may still be fractured.)
b. "Snap" or "crack" at time of accident.
c. Obvious deformity or angulation.
d. Crepitus—grating sound when the moving ends of a fractured bone rub against each other.

Treatment The three phases of fracture management are:

1. Traction in position (TIP).
2. Hands-on stable.
3. Splint stable.

Traction in position. Fractures of long bones are most stable when in their normal anatomic alignment. The distal blood supply is also generally best maintained in this position. Stabilize the proximal part of the fractured bone. Apply gentle, steady traction to the distal part in the position found. While maintaining traction, slowly and smoothly bring the distal part into its normal anatomic position.

Fractures that involve joints are generally not improved by repositioning. The exceptions include fractures with loss of distal circulation or a severely rotated or deformed joint. In these cases, apply gentle traction, and attempt to move the joint to its normal anatomic position For most joints, this is the "mid-range" position, mid-way between flexion and extension.

Discontinue TIP and stabilize the injured extremity in the position found if:

1. TIP causes a significant increase in *pain.*
2. Movement of the distal part is met by *resistance.*

You can use TIP on open shaft fractures that have protruding bone ends. Before applying traction, gently cleanse the exposed bone ends by irrigating with a sterile solution. Then apply a dry sterile dressing. The bone ends will often retract beneath the skin surface when traction is applied. Do not attempt to prevent this from happening. Be sure to report to the receiving medical facility that the bone ends were protruding before you applied the traction.

Hands-on stable. Use hands-on stability of the fractured limb to control unstable injuries if the patient or injured limb must be moved before you apply a splint. Situations where hands-on stability might be helpful include lifting a leg to apply a splint or making a rapid emergency extrication from a hazardous location. Hands-on stability will also help you stabilize an injured part while you assess or treat associated wounds. To understand hands-on stability, imagine that you are moving a chain while you keep all the links in line with one another.

Stabilize shaft fractures of long bones by maintaining position in the normal axis of the bone. Stabilize fractures involving joints in the position that is most comfortable for your patient. This is generally in the "mid-range" position. The stability of joint fractures is usually not improved by traction along the axis of the limb. Release hands-on stabilization only when the injured part is stabilized by a splint.

During patient movement, the rescuer who is stabilizing the most unstable or serious injury coordinates the actions of other rescuers.

Splint stable. In the **splint stable** phase, a splint replaces hands-on stability to maintain the fracture in position and minimize additional injury and pain.

After splinting, you must monitor ischemia in the distal extremity by checking circulation, sensation, and movement (CSM). This is particularly important during extended incidents because of swelling that occurs with time.

C   Circulation
- Pulse
- Capillary refill (warm conditions only)

S   Sensation
- Numbness
- Tingling
- Severe pain

M   Movement
- Ability to move fingers or toes

General Principles of Splinting

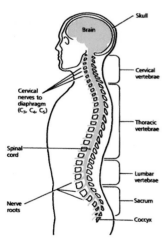

FIGURE 15.8

Spinal Column
The spinal column protects the delicate nerve tissue of the spinal cord. Unstable spine injuries may damage the cord that the spine normally protects, and result in permanent paralysis.

- Always perform the ABCDs and a secondary assessment of the full body exam before beginning treatment for fractures.
- Always check CSM before and after applying splints
- In cases of injury around the joint, make certain that the splint immobilizes the bone above and the bone below the injured joint.
- Use "sandwich splints" — splint material applied on both sides of the injured part for stability and comfort.
- Pad all splints to prevent deformity of unstable bone fragments in a straight splint and to prevent pressure injury, particularly during extended incidents.
- Monitor splints frequently, particularly during extended transport.
- Check CSM at regular intervals, again particularly during extended incidents.
- Document the CSM as you would the vital signs.

FRACTURES OF THE SPINE

The spinal column protects the delicate nerve tissue of the spinal cord. Unstable spine injuries may damage the cord that the spine normally protects (Figure 15.8). Fractures and disruptions of the soft tissues, tendons, and ligaments that hold the vertebral bodies in alignment present similar patterns of injury. They all will be considered under the heading of fractures. Such injuries are extremely serious because they can result in permanent paralysis. Major cervical injuries generally result in quadraplegia, complete or partial paralysis of all four extremities. Thoracic and lumbar injuries may result in paraplegia, a partial or complete paralysis of the lower extremities. Up to 20 percent of all cord injuries occur after the initial injury.

This additional damage to the cord is caused by movement of the unstable spine during extrication, treatment, or transport.

The field treatment of spine injuries is similar to that of other fractures, but there are important differences. The long-term consequences of spinal injuries are much more serious than those of other fractures. During field management of spinal injuries, you must exercise even greater care.

Another concern in spine injuries is **spinal shock.** This may result from an injury to the spinal cord causing loss of the autonomic nervous system's control of dilation and constriction of the blood vessels. This loss of autonomic control results in a generalized vasodilation below the level of the cord injury. The resultant pooling of blood in the involved extremities results in a loss of perfusion pressure and decreased perfusion of the body core.

Mechanisms of Injury Spine injuries may result from direct trauma to the spine such as being crushed by a falling beam. Or they may result from indirect trauma such as the fractures of the thoracolumbar junction seen in a patient who falls 20 feet and lands on his feet. Cord injuries result when the stablility of the spine is disrupted to the point that it can no longer protect the cord.

A *positive mechanism of injury* is any mechanism of injury capable of causing a fracture to the spine. Examples include any head or facial injury, a direct blow or impact on the neck or back, a fall of greater than 15 feet, or a shallow water diving injury.

Assessment Rapid transport. If the mechanism of injury suggests a possible spine injury, you must assume there is a spine injury. Treat the patient with full spinal immobilization. A person's pain response is usually abnormal immediately following a significant or major injury. So the signs and symptoms may be an unreliable indicator of injury. In conventional rapid transport EMS, it is not usually a problem to immobilize a patient for a short trip to the hospital. Sufficient resources are usually available to load and transport the immobilized patient without danger to the patient or you.

Extended incident. During extended incidents, your ability to provide full spinal immobilization can range from difficult to impossible. It can even be dangerous in certain severe environments or when using improvised equipment. During extended incidents, you will have the opportunity to repeat surveys and observe changes in the patient's condition. If approved by your medical control physician, there may be circumstances in which it is appropriate to manage your patients without full spinal immobilization.

To determine whether your patient requires full spinal immobilization, you must assess for a positive mechanism of injury, and for signs and symptoms that suggest spinal injury. Then you must determine if the patient's response to pain and the examination is normal and reliable.

Positive signs/symptoms include:

- Spine or neck pain
- Spine or neck tenderness/point tenderness
- Abnormal motor or sensory function

A normal response to pain or examination assumes the patient is cooperative, alert, calm, oriented, and sober. Possible causes of an abnormal pain response or abnormal response to examination include:

- Alcohol/drug intoxication
- Severely altered mental status or reduced level of consciousness
- Brain injury (concussion/increased ICP)
- Severe multisystem injuries
- Autonomic Stress Response (ASR)—sympathetic type with pain masking

Patients with a positive mechanism of injury, without signs or symptoms, and with a normal pain response may be treated without full spinal immobilization, if approved by your medical control physician. Since cervical spine injuries may show few signs or symptoms initially, these patients should still be treated with an extrication collar.

Negative signs and symptoms may not be accurate under conditions that might give an altered pain response or response to examination. Patients with a positive mechanism of injury and a potentially abnormal pain response are treated as possible unstable spine injuries. Remember that negative signs/symptoms are dependable only in the context of normal pain response.

$$\begin{array}{ccccc} \text{positive} \\ \text{mechanism} & + & \begin{array}{c}\text{positive}\\\text{signs/}\\\text{symptoms}\end{array} & = & \begin{array}{c}\text{possible}\\\text{unstable}\\\text{spine injury}\end{array} \end{array}$$

$$\begin{array}{ccccccc} \text{positive} \\ \text{mechanism} & + & \begin{array}{c}\text{negative}\\\text{signs/}\\\text{symptoms}\end{array} & + & \begin{array}{c}\text{abnormal}\\\text{pain}\\\text{response}\end{array} & = & \begin{array}{c}\text{possible}\\\text{unstable}\\\text{spine injury}\end{array} \end{array}$$

$$\begin{array}{ccccccc} \text{positive} \\ \text{mechanism} & + & \begin{array}{c}\text{negative}\\\text{signs/}\\\text{symptoms}\end{array} & + & \begin{array}{c}\text{normal}\\\text{pain}\\\text{response}\end{array} & = & \begin{array}{c}\text{no}\\\text{reasonable}\\\text{possibility}\\\text{of unstable}\\\text{spine injury}\end{array} \end{array}$$

Cervical Spine Injuries

The cervical spine is the most commonly injured area of the spine because it is the most mobile area of the spine and may be affected by blows to the head. Injuries to the cervical spine have a higher potential for more generalized damage to body function than other areas of the spine. The action of the diaphragm is controlled by the phrenic nerve arising from the third, fourth, and fifth cervical levels

(C_3, $_4$, and $_5$). Injuries to the cervical cord at or above these levels will result in respiratory failure and arrest. Injuries to the cervical cord may result in paraplegia, the loss of use of the lower extremities. But they are more likely to result in quadriplegia, the loss of function in all four extremities.

Thoracic Cord Injury

The area of the thoracic cord is the most stable area of the spine. Injury here is less common than in the cervical spine. Injury to the spinal cord at a thoracic level may result in paraplegia, but the upper extremities will be spared.

Thoracic spine injuries may be seen in motor vehicle incident patients who were incorrectly wearing their shoulder harnesses under their arms. These patients have a high incidence of abdominal injuries from their improperly positioned restraints as well.

Lumbar Injury

The lumbar spine is more mobile than the thoracic spine, so injury here is more common, though less common than in the cervical area. Injuries at the thoracolumbar junction are frequently seen in deceleration injuries such as falls from a height. This is because of the relatively fixed thoracic spine and the stiffness of the large vertebral bodies in the lower lumbar region. Severe injuries may result in paraplegia.

Assessment Check for:

- Loss of motor and sensory function below the site of injury
- Spinal shock
- Priapism in males, a sustained erection that often occurs with spinal cord injury
- Respiratory distress or failure from a cervical or high thoracic injury causing paralysis of the chest muscles

You must remember that not all cord injuries result in a complete injury to the cord. Some patients will have an *incomplete cord injury* and show signs of partial paralysis and partial loss of sensation below the injury site. You must repeatedly reassess these patients for possible progression or resolution of their symptoms. Report any changes to medical control and the receiving medical facility. You must also ensure that your management of such a patient does not result in further injury that converts a partial cord injury into a complete one.

Treatment The principles of treatment of suspected spine factures are essentially the same as those for any long bone/joint fracture:

1. Traction in position (TIP)
2. Hands-on stable
3. Splint stable

Traction in position. The principles of spinal TIP are the same as TIP for long bones and joints. The injured spine is most stable in the normal anatomic "eyes forward" position. Transporting a patient with an injured spine that is out of normal anatomical position is often impractical and may increase the risk of additional injury. Discontinue TIP and stabilize in the position found if:

- TIP causes a significant increase in pain.
- You feel resistance to movement of the distal part.

Hands-on stable. Hands-on stability applies to all unstable fractures, including fractures to the spine. When done correctly, log rolling and patient lifting are hands-on stable procedures to control an unstable spine during patient movement before immobilization. A spine injury is more important than an extremity injury. You must provide the maximum stability to the spine when moving the patient. If a spine injury is suspected, stabilizing the head and neck coordinates patient movement.

Splint stable. Apply splints to all unstable fractures, including fractures of the spine. Spine boards are splints applied to the spine to hold it in a normal anatomic position. Short boards are splints applied to aid in patient extrication. They provide partial immobilization of the cervical and thoracic spine. Patients on short boards should be secured to a long spine board after extrication. Long spine boards also provide immobilization for the lumbar spine. They may be used to provide immobilization to the pelvis and lower extremities as well.

Lifting, Extricating, and Moving Patients with Spine Injuries

The principles involved in accessing, stabilizing, and transporting a spine injury patient are identical to those involved in managing unstable fractures of the extremities:

- Traction in position (TIP)
- Hands-on stable
- Splint stable

For example, to splint a thoracic spine injury, immobilize the thoracic spine. Include the cervical spine and lumbar spine, pelvis, and femurs. The legs should also be immobilized because the pelvis cannot be immobilized effectively if the legs are free.

In a patient with multiple injuries, the spine injury is more important than an injury to any extremity. If you suspect a spine injury, spine immobilization takes precedent over control of the extremities.

You must refer to your local protocols for the specific clinical standards to follow in assessing and managing spine injuries during extended incidents.

DISLOCATIONS

A **dislocation** is a disruption of a joint. Such a disruption occurs when the supporting ligaments and capsule of the joint tear and allow

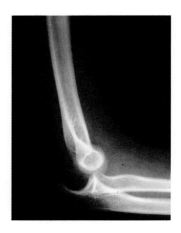

FIGURE 15.9

Dislocations
A dislocation occurs when
the supporting ligaments and
capsule of the joint tear and
allow the bone ends to separate completely.

the bone ends to separate completely (Figure 15.9). In some cases, a dislocation may be accompanied by a fracture. The term for this injury is a **fracture-dislocation.**

Because the surfaces of joints have sensory nerve fibers similar to those found in the periosteum, dislocations can be painful, especially when muscle spasms cause movement across unstable joint surfaces. Muscle spasms and pain will increase with the length of time the joint is dislocated.

Dislocated joint surfaces can injure adjacent structures by direct impact that causes a contusion. Dislocations can also obstruct vascular circulation by compression. Direct compression of nerves may result in permanent loss of nerve function. The effect on adjacent structures increases with the length of time the joint is dislocated.

The joint cartilage has no direct blood supply but depends on the synovial fluid within the joint for nutrition. Without this nourishment, injury to the cartilage of the joint surface increases with the length of time the joint is dislocated.

Mechanisms of Injury The are two basic mechanisms for dislocations. In a *direct injury*, the force is applied directly to the joint area. This separates the bone ends within the joint. An example of a direct injury would be a patient falling directly on their shoulder causing it to dislocate. A direct injury is often associated with the more serious fracture/dislocation-type injury.

An *indirect injury* occurs when the force is applied to the extremity distal to the joint. The dislocation results from a leveraging force at the joint. An example of an indirect injury would be the knee striking the dashboard. The force travels from the knee up the femur and levers the hip out posteriorly.

Assessment You should direct your field assessment of dislocations toward simple dislocations from indirect force. Base your assessments on the mechanism of injury or the patient's history of previous dislocations. The presence of *minor* associated fractures should not change your treatment plan.

Treatment Rapid transport. In conventional rapid transport, stabilize all dislocated joints in the position found. Transport the patient to definitive care. Use traction in position (TIP) to attempt to reposition dislocations anatomically *only if distal circulation is impaired.*

Extended incident. Refer to local medical protocols for specific local clinical standards regarding the assessment and treatment of dislocations during extended incidents. Dislocations associated with direct force that could also cause severe fractures should be treated as joint fractures. Splint or stabilize in the position you find the joint.

If you have been properly trained in the procedure, you may consider an attempt at reducing a *simple dislocation* if an extended

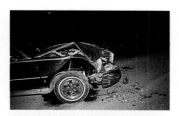

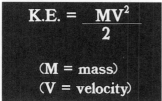

$$K.E. = \frac{MV^2}{2}$$

(M = mass)
(V = velocity)

FIGURE 15.10

Kinetic Energy
You must be able to predict
the type and severity of injuries by using your knowledge
of mechanism of injury.

transport time is expected. Do not attempt reductions unless you
have been trained and authorized to perform the procedure by your
medical control physician and the procedure is *within your scope of
practice*. Simple dislocations include:

Shoulder—indirect injury

Patella—indirect injury

Digits—direct/indirect injury

Discontinue any attempts at reduction if pain is significantly increased, or if you encounter resistance to movement. In these cases,
splint the joint in the injured position for transport.

After reduction, recheck circulation and nerve function. Splint in
anatomic position for transport.

TRAUMATIC INJURIES

Most of the patients you encounter in rescue situations will be suffering from some form of traumatic injury. To understand why particular injuries occur in certain instances, you must have a knowledge
of the laws of physics as well as anatomy and physiology. You must
be able to predict the type and severity of the injuries you see based
on your knowledge of mechanisms of injury. By using this knowledge,
you will be able to anticipate the potential complications of the injuries you find while you assess the patient.

Traumatic injuries are the result of forceful movement of an object
into the body, or forceful movement of the body onto an object.
*Trauma is the transfer of this energy of movement to the body tissues,
which result in injury.* To understand trauma, you need an understanding of the laws of motion and **kinetic energy**, the energy of
motion (Figure 15.10).

In physics, energy cannot be created out of nothing, and existing
energy cannot be destroyed. Energy simply changes form.

Example 1: A falling rock (kinetic energy) strikes a person climbing
on a mountain. The energy of the falling rock does not disappear but
is converted into the deforming force that crushes soft tissues and
breaks bones.

Example 2: In an automobile, gasoline (chemical energy) causes
the engine to run (mechanical energy) which moves the vehicle (kinetic energy). If the automobile hits a bridge abutment at 60 miles
per hour, the kinetic energy is converted into a force that crumples
the car. If the driver is unbelted, then he is still traveling at 60 miles
per hour. He then strikes the dash and steering wheel. His kinetic
energy is transformed into a crushing force that fractures ribs and
sternum and crushes organs in the chest and abdomen.

This example also demonstrates the second law of physics. A body
in motion (the driver) will continue in motion until acted upon by
an outside force (the steering wheel).

To estimate the degree of trauma, you must understand the relationship between kinetic energy and the mass of the moving object and its velocity. The mathematical formula for this relationship is:

$$\text{kinetic energy} = \frac{\text{mass} \times \text{velocity}^2}{2}$$

In simple terms, if you double the mass involved in a collision, you will double the amount of energy that can cause tissue damage. That is why there is more damage when you are hit by a semi than when you are hit by a half-ton pickup truck. But if you double the velocity of the object, you quadruple the energy that can cause tissue damage. That is why there are a lot more broken parts when a pedestrian is hit by a car traveling 30 miles per hour, than when hit by one traveling only 15 miles per hour (Figure 15.11).

Mechanism of Injury Trauma usually results from two types of forces, **compression** and **deceleration**. The mechanism of compression injuries is obvious: tissue gets crushed between two objects— for example, a hand caught in a punch press. Deceleration injuries occur when the body stops suddenly but organs or tissues within the body continue until they strike another object. An aortic tear caused by a fall from a height is an example of a deceleration injury. Most injuries you see will be a combination of these two forces, such as the ruptured spleen that occurs in the unrestrained driver whose automobile was traveling at a high rate of speed until it was stopped by a bridge abutment.

FIGURE 15.11

Kinetic Energy Table
These calculations approximate kenetic energy and illustrate that changes in mass have a smaller effect on kenetic energy than do increases in velocity.

Assume a 155 pound (70 kilo) object traveling at 30 mph, the kinetic energy (KE) would be:

$$\text{kinetic energy} = \frac{\text{mass} \times \text{velocity}^2}{2}$$

$$\text{kinetic energy} = \frac{(155) \times (30)^2}{2}$$

$$\text{kinetic energy} = 69{,}750$$

For comparison, look at what happens with changes in mass and velocity:

	155 lb (70k)	165 lb (75k)	200 lb (90k)
30 mph	69,750	74,250	90,000
40 mph	124,000	132,000	160,000
60 mph	279,000	297,000	360,000

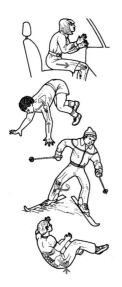

FIGURE 15.12

Mechanisms of Injury
Different mechanisms of
injury often produce different
kinds of injuries.

Compression injuries are frequently classified as blunt and pene-trating trauma. In **blunt trauma**, the kinetic energy is spread over a greater area of the body. This compresses the soft tissues and ruptures or breaks underlying organs and bones. To understand how a direct impact on "solid" organs such as the spleen, liver, or kidney can cause lacerations and contusions leading to internal bleeding, remember that the "solid" organs are filled with fluid (blood). They behave much like a well filled water balloon on impact. An example of a blunt injury is the ruptured spleen resulting from the handlebars of a dirt bike impacting the abdomen.

The hollow organs, such as the stomach and intestines, tend to be moved aside by an impact. So they are often not seriously disrupted. They may also pop like a balloon if severely compressed while fully inflated. The bladder will behave like a hollow organ when it is empty, but like a "solid" organ when full. Rib fractures can injure the lungs. Lungs may also "pop" if compressed while the patient was inhaling.

Penetrating trauma is the result of a localized application of force that drives an object through the skin, injuring the underlying tissues. High velocity penetrating injuries may have a zone of injury beyond the area of direct contact with the object such as the cavi-tation effect of a high velocity gunshot wound. Do not rely on the size of the surface wound to assess the extent of injury in penetrating trauma.

A **rotational injury** is an indirect injury caused by twisting forces transmitted to a distant body part such as when a skier catches a ski tip on a tree. The ski tip rotates externally, which results in a torque injury to the medial structures of the knee.

A **levering injury** occurs when a lever effect disrupts structures at a distance from the point of impact. An example of a leverage injury is when a person falls from a bicycle onto an outstretched arm, which forces the shoulder to dislocate anteriorly.

Anticipating Problems

First survey the scene to determine a mechanism of injury and es-timate the kinetic energy available to cause tissue damage. Then use your knowledge of anatomy and physiology to anticipate the type and severity of injuries the patient might have sustained (Figure 15.12). Also anticipate the complications that might develop while the patient is in your care. For example, a lumberjack is pinned by a six-foot diameter tree trunk falling across his lower abdomen, pelvis, and legs. Anticipated injuries would include a pelvis fracture, lumbar spine fracture and cord injury, femur fractures, and abdominal organ ruptures (liver, spleen, kidney, and bladder). Additional injuries might include crush injuries to the soft tissues of the buttocks and thighs. Anticipated complications would include respiratory com-promise resulting from abdominal compression and hypovolemic shock occuring when the tree trunk is lifted for extrication.

In conventional rapid transport, ambulance-based EMS in which the patient can be quickly stabilized and transported to a hospital

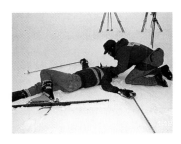

FIGURE 15.13

First Response
Extremes in the environment and difficult terrain can complicate the field management of trauma.

within the "golden hour," management of trauma is often relatively predictable and controlled—"scoop and run." On the other hand, field management of trauma under rescue conditions or in extended incidents often occurs in situations that are difficult at best.

Because of the circumstances of the incident, the patients may be hysterical, uncooperative, withdrawn, disoriented, aggressive, rude, intoxicated, or otherwise difficult. Because serious injury generally comes as a surprise, the patient's realization and adjustment to what has happened takes time. At or around the time of injury, patient behavior is rarely normal. Bystanders, especially family, can compound the problem by being difficult or by behaving erratically.

Environmental extremes such as heat or cold, rain, blowing snow, high winds, high altitude, icy water, and darkness will increase the difficulty of the field management of trauma (Figure 15.13). Extremes in heat and cold can also affect the nervous system as well as sensitive higher functions such as judgment, problem solving, and even consciousness. They can make trauma assessment and treatment more difficult for both you and the patient.

The location or terrain where the incident occurs may also complicate patient management. Confined spaces, rough seas, falling rock, hazardous materials, live electrical wires, piled up vehicles, collapsed buildings, icy slopes, swift water, and vertical terrain make patient assessment, stabilization, and transportation difficult. They also pose hazards for the rescuers. Before you can begin treatment, the patient may require extrication from a collapsed building, avalanche, tangled vehicle, top of a tree, or bottom of a well.

Time is your major enemy in the management of serious trauma. Urgent conditions require that you make important decisions with limited information. In many situations, seconds count in saving lives or preventing serious long-term injury. Equipment may be limited or unavailable. You must frequently improvise.

You may become "stressed out" in situations involving trauma. Even experienced rescuers may be emotionally overwhelmed at the sight of severe bleeding, crushed body parts, starkly angulated fractures, grossly deformed faces, or other serious wounds. Under such circumstances, it is important for you to stick to your training and basic knowledge rather than attempt to recall obscure or complex information. You must understand the basic mechanisms and principles of injury and their management to perform effectively under stress.

Associated Conditions

There are many situations in which trauma occurs simultaneously with other medical problems. Alcohol intoxication and drugs are major contributing factors to much of the trauma you will see. In addition, alcohol and drugs will complicate your assessment and treatment. Intoxicated patients are often abusive, uncooperative, or outright hostile.

Trauma may occur in patients with chronic medical problems or even be caused or aggravated by chronic medical problems. For example, diabetics with open wounds have poorer wound healing and higher risks of infection. Patients with chronic heart disease have less cardiac reserve. Therefore, they are at greater risk of cardiac failure or collapse. Chronic heart disease may also result in heart attacks as a result of traumatic stress.

Very young or very old patients have lower tolerances for trauma. In children, a small blood volume creates a lower tolerance for acute fluid loss. At the same time, their proportionately greater surface area to body weight results in more rapid heat loss. The body tissues of the elderly are less elastic. Therefore, they are more susceptible to a variety of injuries including broken bones and torn aortas. They also have an increased incidence of complicating chronic disease.

Assessment Trauma has two components:

- What you see (external)
- What you do not see (internal)

External injury may be difficult to manage but is relatively easy to assess. Internal injuries are generally more serious than external problems. Internal injuries are more difficult to assess. They usually require surgical intervention for definitive management.

Management of Internal Injury To manage internal injury effectively, you need a solid understanding of the following:

- Anatomy. You must have a three-dimensional, perspective of the human body to know what organs and structures underlie the site of the injury and therefore might be affected by the injury.
- Kinematics. You need to know how kinetic energy (the energy in motion) is transformed into tissue damage, and the reaction of body tissues to those damaging forces.
- Mechanisms of injury. If you know how the trauma occurred, you should be able to predict the type of injuries the patient may have. For example, you would be highly suspicious that a shallow water diving accident would result in a cervical spine injury.
- Anticipated problems. It is easier to find something if you know what to look for based on your knowledge of anatomy, mechanism of injury, and injury patterns. After your inital assessment of the patient's injuries and condition, you should also be able to anticipate potential problems that might develop during your stabilization and tranportation of the patient.
- Signs/symptoms pattern recognition. You should understand how these reflect the mechanism of injury. It is easier for you to find something if you know what it looks like—for example, the pattern of volume shock and its progression.
- Patient Assessment System (PAS). You should use a system to reevaluate the patient at intervals. PAS will help you find problems even if you forget to look for them. For example, the regular use of PAS may show the patient developing a volume shock pattern.

Polytrauma

Trauma often results in injury to more than one system or body part. Patients with multiple system involvement are referred to as **polytrauma** patients. This distinguishes them from incidents in which there are two or more patients, called **multiple trauma**.

On initial evaluation, all injuries may not be be equally apparent. You should avoid focusing on the most obvious injuries. You must complete an initial assessment, even if you find significant problems part way though the assessment. Stop only to treat immediately life-threatening problems found during the initial assessment. After completing the secondary assessment, begin management of the problems found in their order of importance. In situations involving trauma or serious injury, you must reassess the patient continually. Identification of some injuries become apparent only after a span of time:

- Injuries may require time to develop. Examples include bleeding into a body cavity or soft tissues from blunt injury, or respiratory swelling from smoke inhalation.
- Autonomic stress reactions can cause "pain masking," which diminishes with time. An example is pain and tenderness in the spine that becomes apparent during an extended incident but was not apparent during the initial exam of a confused, disoriented patient.
- Patients often focus on one injury at a time. An example would be a patient who complains loudly of pain in an open femur fracture but whose dislocated shoulder might go unnoticed for several hours.

THE BIG NET PRINCIPLE

In assessing trauma in the field, you may find that in the same patient you will find different clinical problems that have varying degrees of seriousness. The problem for you is that it may be difficult or impossible for you to determine if the overall clinical picture of the patient is caused by a more serious problem or possibly by a less serious problem. Some examples of this dilemma would be:

- Case One: Is the patient's abnormal behavior due to a head injury or hypoxia or is the patient intoxicated?
- Case Two: A patient complains of pain and tenderness in the neck following a 15-foot fall. Are these signs and symptoms due to a muscle strain or could they be caused by a potentially unstable spine injury?

In some cases, an event can have more than one possible result. During your initial field management, it is often impossible to determine the final outcome. Some examples would be:

- Case Three: The signs and symptoms of coral snake envenomation can be delayed for several hours. Has your patient been envenomated?

- Case Four: A construction worker has fallen 20 feet into an excavation. He is confused and anxious, appears pale and sweaty, and has a pulse of 120/minute. Is his condition due to ASR or volume shock? Will he get better or worse with time?

In the hospital, it would be easier to get answers to these questions. While keeping the patient alive with advanced life support equipment, you could observe the patient over time. But in the field, you have none of this available. The patient may continue to deteriorate. So, in the field, it is best for you to assume that Murphy's Law is operating. In other words, assume the worst possible case, and plan your patient management on that assumption. If the patient's condition improves with time, you can modify your treatment plan. If you overtreat an injury, you will rarely cause harm. But if the worst case proves correct, you have anticipated the problems and you are ready to manage them correctly. This method of anticipating the worst case scenario to avoid overlooking injuries or complications is known as the "big net principal."

Treatment There is a saying in trauma care: "Speed saves." Patients with major trauma are saved by definitive treatment within the first or second hour after the injury, also known as the "golden hour." The "golden hour" refers to the initial period after a traumatic injury when a patient's body is able to compensate for his or her injuries. During the golden hour, the patient's condition remains relatively stable. After that initial period, patient mortality and morbidity rapidly rise unless definitive trauma management has been successfully instituted.

The "golden hour" begins when the patient is injured. It does not end when you reach the patient and begin your assessment and treatment. Nor does it end when the patient is put into an ambulance. It does not end when the patient goes through the doors of the emergency room. The "golden hour" ends only when the patient has received definitive trauma care in the surgical suite.

Less severely injured trauma patients may have four to six hours to be saved by definitive treatment. For effective treatment of serious trauma, rapid transport to a trauma center is imperative.

Ideal trauma management is rapid stabilization of the patient and immediate transport to definitive medical care. Unfortunately, in rescue situations, definitive medical care is not always nearby or easily accessible. Even if access, stabilization, and/or transport are extended, the medical objectives and the treatment principles are the same. And though your situation may go beyond the "golden hour," there are holding actions that may extend the time available for you to maintain your patient. Such actions include PASG and Advanced Life Support techniques such as IVs and fluid therapy and advanced airway techniques if they are *within your scope of practice*.

Patient Control

Patient care during extended incidents involves other areas of care, such as "bedside manner" and "TLC," that are as important as medical skills and procedures. These skills are less definable yet still important to your patient's well-being. Patient comfort and reassurance are important components of any medical treatment but are especially important in trauma care.

Because of the excitement, surprise, anger, stress, and pain that occur with injury, patients often become their own worst enemies. Fear or confusion may be translated into "uncooperative behavior" such as sudden, dangerous movements. Therefore, it is important for you to establish a trusting relationship and working rapport with your patients.

A relaxed patient with a positive attitude will make treatment and evacuation easier for you. And it will also provide the patient with a better chance at survival and recovery.

SUMMARY

Rescuers often encounter certain medical conditions and/or injuries during a rescue operation. Therefore, it is important that the rescue team members be able to recognize, assess, and treat the more common medical conditions they face.

Some of the more common conditions include shock, head injuries, wounds, burns, musculoskeletal injuries, fractures, dislocations, and injuries caused by trauma. Some of these conditions, such as shock, indicate a serious threat that requires immediate treatment. Others, such as concussions, may be minor and simply require monitoring for change during the rescue operation.

It is important that rescuers are able to assess patients, looking for signs and symptoms of a medical problem. A careful assessment allows rescuers to differentiate among potential problems or injuries and indicates the seriousness of any possible medical condition.

For a rescue involving medical conditions and/or injuries to be successful, rescuers must be familiar with appropriate treatment measures for conditions commonly encountered. This is especially true for those conditions that require immediate and aggressive treatment measures.

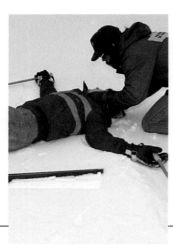

INDICATIONS AND TREATMENT OF ENVIRONMENT-SPECIFIC MEDICAL CONDITIONS AND INJURIES

OVERVIEW

Many medical conditions encountered by rescuers are specific to the environment in which the rescue is taking place. For example, the environment may contain toxins, or the rescue may occur in frigid water where there is a danger of hypothermia.

This chapter discusses environment-specific medical conditions. The conditions are viewed from the perspectives of mechanisms of injury, assessment, and treatment.

OBJECTIVES

The objectives of this chapter are for the rescuer to describe:

- medical conditions that are specific to or caused by the environment in which the rescue is taking place.

- the mechanisms of injury in environment-specific medical conditions and injuries.
- assessment of environment-specific medical conditions.
- treatment of environment-specific medical conditions.

TOXINS

Toxins are any substances that have an abnormal effect on the body. Toxins may be ingested, inhaled, injected, or adsorbed. They may act systemically, locally, or as a combination effect.

Assessment When assessing for toxins, you need to obtain as much information as possible at the scene of the incident. You need to answer three basic questions:

- What was it?
- How much?
- When?

If possible, obtain a sample of the substance. If none is available, then obtain the container that held the substance, and question witnesses at the scene.

Treatment Most toxins are excreted or metabolized by the body over time. Your initial treatment is to support body systems using routine BLS/ALS procedures. Treat clinical signs and symptoms until the toxin is removed, excreted, metabolized, or neutralized by an antidote. Use this basic approach when toxins are mixed or unknown.

Effective antidotes are not always available. Consult your medical control physician for specific antidote treatment. Poison Control Centers are a national information network available by phone 24 hours a day. You should have your local Poison Control Center number readily available.

Treatment for all toxins is to *remove and dilute.* For ingested toxins, the treatment specifics depend on patient condition and the type of toxin that has been ingested. As a general rule, after you have determined that the patient has ingested a toxin, your first step is to dilute the agent in the stomach. Load with water or milk. If authorized by medical control or local protocol, you may induce vomiting under the following conditions:

- The toxin is noncorrosive or not petroleum-based
- The patient is alert and oriented

Induced vomiting is most effective within the first hour but may be effective for up to six to eight hours. Induce vomiting by oral administration of syrup of ipecac (one to two teaspoons for children under one year of age, three teaspoons for older children and adults), followed by a glass or two of water. When the vomiting stops, give one tablespoon of activated charcoal suspended in a glass of water.

Do not induce vomiting if:

- The patient is unconscious, semiconscious, or having a convulsion.
- The toxin is a corrosive, such as a strong acid, lye, or drain cleaner, or has caused obvious burns around the mouth.
- The toxin contains any petroleum product such as kerosene, gasoline, lighter fluid, or clear furniture polish.

In a rescue involving inhaled toxins, you must first *protect yourself.* Avoid inhaling the toxin. First, ventilate the area before entering. Then wear protective clothing. Use equipment such as breathing apparatus. Move the patient into fresh air. Then provide supplementary oxygen and basic life support.

The initial management for injected or adsorbed toxins is to use BLS/ALS techniques to support body functions. If possible, obtain samples of the toxin while taking care not to expose yourself. For toxins being adsorbed through the skin, try to dilute the toxin by

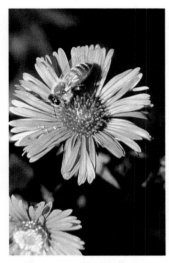

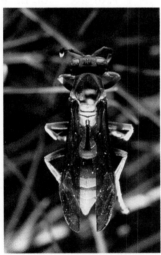

FIGURE 16.1

Stinging Insects
One common cause of
anaphylaxis is the venom
injected by stinging insects.

irrigating the area with copious amounts of water or neutralizing solution. Follow this with a thorough cleansing with soap and water. This treatment is most effective if done within an hour of exposure to the toxin. If the eyes have been exposed, irrigate them with large volumes of fluid.

Refer to local medical protocols for specific clinical standards regarding the assessment and treatment of toxins during extended incidents.

ANAPHYLAXIS

Anaphylaxis is a widespread vasodilation that causes swelling of all body surfaces including the pharynx, respiratory surfaces, gut, eyes, and skin. During anaphylaxis, the onset of vascular shock can be sudden and severe. In severe reactions, death can result in a matter of minutes.

Mechanism of Injury Anaphylaxis can be caused by a foreign material that enters the circulating blood, including food, drugs, or venom from stinging insects. One aspect of anaphylaxis that makes it so dangerous is its rapid onset and course. For a sting or injection, this onset may occur within 5 to 15 minutes (Figure 16.1). The onset for antigens in ingested food may be delayed until the food is digested, which can be up to one hour.

Assessment The history of an anaphylactic patient can vary. Anaphylactic reactions to a specific antigen may develop over time. Some patients have no previous history of anaphylaxis. On the other hand, many anaphylactic patients have a past history of a systemic reaction to a specific antigen and will know about their sensitivity. The severity is also variable. For example, a repeat exposure may result in a severe reaction, even though the first one was mild. Use the big net principle and consider any immediate systemic reaction to a sting or injection to be anaphylaxis.

The signs and symptoms of anaphylaxis include:

- "Hot, burning," itching skin from cutaneous vasodilation
- Nausea, vomiting, and diarrhea from gut surface vasodilation
- Labored breathing from respiratory surface vasodilation
- Profound weakness from loss of perfusion pressures

On examination you may find swelling of the face, eyes, tongue, pharynx, and skin (hives). The patient's skin is usually flushed. They may be itching, and sweating. The patient may have an increased respiratory rate with wheezing. The pulse is increased. If the ana-

FIGURE 16.2

Bee Sting Kit
Prescription insect sting
treatment kits contain
epinephrine injections to
reverse severe anaphylactic
reactions.

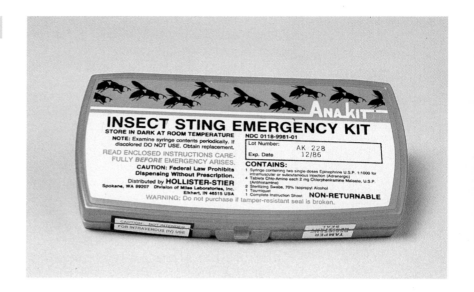

phylaxis is severe, the blood pressure may be decreased to the point
of shock.

Treatment—General

- Basic Life Support (BLS)
- Advanced Life Support (ALS) (if *within your scope of practice*)
- Oxygen
- PASG (use limited to two hours)
- IV fluids to expand volume (if *within your scope of practice*)

Treatment—Specific Specific treatment is usually required to reverse severe anaphylactic reactions. Treatment will be most successful
if started early, before the reaction has progressed to a critical condition (Figure 16.2). If *within your scope of practice*, and if authorized
by medical control, consider:

1. Epinephrine injection.
2. Antihistamines.

Monitor the patient closely. Rebound reaction can occur in several
hours. A second exposure to the same antigen can cause a severe
reaction.

HYPOTHERMIA

Hypothermia is the progressive cooling of the body core that occurs
when passive heat retention and active heat production are overwhelmed by the cold challenge. The body can tolerate a drop of a

few degrees of internal body temperature. However, when the temperature of the heart, lungs, brain and other vital organs—the core temperature—falls below 95° F (35° C), the body functions slow down, and survival becomes threatened. If nothing is done to reverse the lowered temperature, death will ultimately result. The hypothermic patient requires special medical and rescue care. The mishandling of an acutely hypothermic patient can result in that patient's death.

Hypothermia is usually classified into one of two types, depending on core temperature:

- Mild — core temperature above 90° F (32° C)
- Severe — core temperature below 90° F (32° C)

Mechanisms of Injury   Hypothermia is found in one of three clinical states, which generally reflect its rate of onset. Acute hypothermia is usually associated with immersion in water. Its onset is relatively short, ranging from minutes to a few hours. Sub-acute hypothermia has a longer onset, usually hours or days. It often occurs in outdoor situations, such as the backcountry or on a mountain. Chronic hypothermia may have a very slow onset. It is usually found in urban situations, associated with the elderly. It may result from inadequate heat in living quarters. It may be compounded by inadequate nutrition.

Hypothermia often coexists with other problems such as trauma, intoxication, drowning, and chronic illness. Hypothermia may contribute to a person's ultimate death from other mechanisms such as drowning. This is because hypothermia can lead to impaired judgment and cause the person to lose coordination in the water.

Hypothermia may also be a major problem for both patient and rescuers in extended incidents in cold and/or wet environments.

The **metabolic icebox** refers to severe core cooling in which all body systems slow down to a state that resembles death. This situation can protect body systems. Patients have regained normal health and function following hours in a hypothermic state without pulse or respiration. This situation is a challenge for you since the patient appears dead. But with proper care the patient sometimes may be resuscitated. In caring for the hypothermic patient, remember: "You're not dead until you're warm and dead."

Assessment   Signs and symptoms of mild hypothermia include:

- Cyanosis and pale, cool skin
- Cold diuresis (excessive urination)
- Mild to severe shivering
- Reduced dexterity because of shivering or alteration of peripheral nerve function
- Mild to moderate changes in personality
- Mild to moderate changes in higher level mental processes. These changes might include lethargy and withdrawal from the group,

increased irritability, and loss of problem-solving ability and judgment
- Core (rectal) temperatures ranging from 90° to 95° F (32° to 35° C)

Patients with severe hypothermia may show:

- Severe changes in mental status that may include:
  Bizarre personality changes
  Hallucination, severe confusion, disorientation, memory loss
  Antisurvival actions—undressing in the cold, sleeping in the snow
  Decreased AVPU rating that closely follows the severe mental
    status changes
- No shivering
- Core (rectal) temperature below 90° F (32° C). A special thermometer is required for reading temperatures below 94° F

Treatment Mild hypothermia can be effectively treated with field rewarming. Three basic techniques for rewarming are available to you. You can use them alone or in combination.

- Change the environment. Reduce the cold challenge to the patient by providing shelter from the wind and wetness.
- Add heat. Actively rewarm the patient with fire, sun, warm bodies or other methods. Shivering also adds heat.
- Retain heat. Help the patient with heat retention or passive rewarming. Put the patient into warm, dry clothing or a sleeping bag.

In addition, you can help the patient develop his or her own heat production,through increased metabolism, such as exercise. However, exercise is only effective in rewarming if sufficient calories are available as fuel for the increased metabolism. Therefore, encourage the alert, cooperative patient to eat foods that are readily converted to available calories. Hypothermia patients are often dehydrated because of cold diuresis. If they are conscious and alert, you should encourage them to drink plenty of warmed fluids.

Severe hypothermia is a serious, life-threatening condition. Severely hypothermic patients often die during the rescue effort. It is extremely important to handle a hypothermic patient gently without sudden changes in temperature or body position.

If you have rapid transport capability, transport the patient as quickly as possible to a medical facility that has the equipment, knowledge, and experience to rewarm severely hypothermic patients. Handle the patient gently to prevent ventricular fibrillation. Keep him or her lying down. Insulate the patient to avoid further heat loss, but do not actively rewarm with external or internal heat sources.

Follow local BLS/ALS protocols for severe hypothermia patients. Chest compressions in a severe hypothermic patient with a heartbeat may cause ventricular fibrillation. If a patient with severe hypothermia has a pulse, it will be extremely low and faint.

In an extended incident, the goal is to maintain the protective effect of the "metabolic icebox" and to quickly and gently transport the patient to definitive medical care. Field rewarming of the severely hypothermic patient can be dangerous and is usually ineffective.

During transport, handle the patient gently. Do not allow the patient to exercise or walk. Do not jostle the patient. DO NOT perform chest compressions if any functional cardiac activity is present. Avoid further heat loss through passive rewarming Remove wet clothing. Place patient in dry clothing and a sleeping bag, or cover with warm, dry blankets.

Heated, humidified air or oxygen will prevent further heat loss through respiration. If spontaneous respirations are absent, positive pressure ventilation by bag-valve-mask or pocket mask is generally safe and effective. Add oxygen to inspired air, but make sure that the oxygen bottle is warm so you do not cause additional heat loss by administering cold oxygen.

If it is *within your scope of practice,* consider expanding the patient's volume using IV fluids. The initial expansion should use 300 to 500cc of normal saline. Adjust the subsequent rate according to vital signs and urine output. You may give calories via IV. Give oral calories only if the patient is conscious, alert, and able to swallow.

FROSTBITE

Frostbite is the actual freezing of body tissues from severe cold. This freezing of tissue occurs more readily when local circulation is reduced by such factors as:

- The body's activation of its "cold response" to decrease perfusion to the body shell in order to maintain the core temperature
- Clothing or boots that constrict circulation
- Vasoconstrictors, such as nicotine

Tissue damage resulting from frostbite occurs during both the freezing and thawing phases. Even solidly frozen tissue can often recover with the proper treatment. Severe damage to frostbitten tissue occurs when the affected area is refrozen after being thawed, is improperly rewarmed, suffers trauma after rewarming, or experiences prolonged freezing.

Frostnip is the earliest stage of ice crystal formation in tissues. It occurs before the more serious condition of frostbite. Prompt intervention by rewarming at this stage generally causes no serious disability or tissue loss.

Assessment Before rewarming an affected part, determine if it is:

- Soft (frostnip)—will be stiff but pliable. Skin moves over joints and tendons.

- Solid (frostbite)—will be hard and frozen solid (like a piece of frozen chicken).

The most reliable indicator of early frostnip is numbness when the temperature is below freezing. The normal sensations of pain and cold are replaced by a loss of sensation. Immediate treatment at this point usually prevents further complications.

Evaluate the severity of the injury after rewarming:

- First-degree—redness, swelling, no blisters
- Second-degree—swelling, flesh-colored blisters
- Third-degree—blood blisters, proximal blisters
- Fourth-degree—few blisters, minimal swelling

Frostnip, when the tissue is still soft, can result in significant tissue damage if allowed to remain for an extended period. However, serious tissue damage can be prevented if frostnip is identified and treated early enough by field rewarming. If treated early enough, frostnip does not result in blisters. If it is identified and treated late, frostnip can be associated with rewarming blisters.

The presence of blisters after rewarming usually indicates significant tissue damage and potential for loss of tissue. Field treatment at this point becomes complex and difficult. It is especially important to avoid refreezing or causing additional trauma to the injured part during the evacuation and transport of the patient to definitive medical care.

Treatment For frostnip, begin field rewarming immediately at the first sign of numbness. Use any method of rewarming that does not cause burns (such as radiant heat) or tissue damage (such as rubbing with snow or any other material). Remove constricting materials, such as watches, rings, or boots, before rewarming

The most practical rewarming techniques for frostnip are skin-to-skin contact, arms in axilla, feet on abdomen. If available you may try immersion in water heated to 105° to 108° F (40° to 42° C). Because the affected parts may have no sensation, take care to avoid burns.

If rewarming does not produce blisters, further tissue damage is unlikely, though there may be pain and swelling. The affected part will, however, be more susceptible to further cold injury. If rewarming produces blisters, further tissue damage is possible. Prevent further trauma by preventing further use as much as possible. Treat frostbite blisters the same as abrasions or minor burns.

Improper rewarming of frostbite can result in tissue damage. The rewarming of a frostbitten extremity will severely restrict the use of that part. Consequently, it is generally best to keep a solidly frostbitten part frozen during evacuation to definitive care if the evacuation will last less than 24 hours.

If evacuation to definitive medical care is going to take more than 24 hours, then consider rewarming the affected part. Rewarm with water heated to 105° to 108° F (40° to 42° C). Keep the affected part immersed completely until the tissues are warm and soft. This will usually take about 30 minutes. Avoid damage from burns and from rubbing the affected area. After rewarming, avoid refreezing and prevent further trauma, by preventing further use as much as possible.

HYPERTHERMIA

The opposite of hypothermia, **hyperthermia** results when the body is exposed to more heat than it can handle. **Heat exhaustion**, also known as heat prostration or heat collapse, is the most common heat-related illness. It is really a volume loss problem. It occurs when the body loses enough water and electrolytes through heavy perspiration that fluid depletion (hypovolemia) occurs. Patients who have developed heat exhaustion show a clinical pattern that is similar to mild hypovolemic shock.

Heat stroke is a less common but more serious illness caused by heat exposure. Untreated or improperly treated heat stroke will result in death. Heat stroke is the result of the body's core temperature rising to dangerous levels when the body is subjected to more heat than it can handle. This overwhelms the normal mechanisms for getting rid of the excess heat.

Assessment   Heat exhaustion appears as mild, compensated, hypovolemic shock (dehydration). Blood pressure is normal or slightly decreased, while the pulse is increased. Respiratory rate is increased as well. The patient's skin may be flushed or "clammy" and sweating. Core temperature is normal or moderately elevated but below 105° F (40° C). The patient may be vomiting. There will be decreased urine output. The significant clinical aspect that sets heat exhaustion apart from heat stroke is that the patient's mental status is normal. There are no motor or sensory changes in heat exhaustion.

In heat stroke, the patient will have an increased pulse with a variable blood pressure. Respirations are increased. Body core temperature is significantly elevated over 105° F (40° C). The patient will have significant alterations in mental status that precedes deteriorating AVPU levels. The patient will usually have decreased urine output.

The significant clinical aspects of heat stroke relate to the nervous system. Any motor/sensory changes, severe changes in mental status, signs of increased intracranial pressure, and seizures occurring under a heat challenge should be treated as heat stroke.

Treatment   For heat exhaustion, the basic treatment is replacement of fluids. If the patient is not vomiting, fluids may be given by mouth. Reduce the heat challenge by having the patient rest in a cool, shady area (Figure 16.3). Radical cooling is not necessary.

FIGURE 16.3

Heat Exhaustion
Treat heat exhaustion by
having the patient rest in a
cool, shady area. Replace
fluids lost through perspiration.

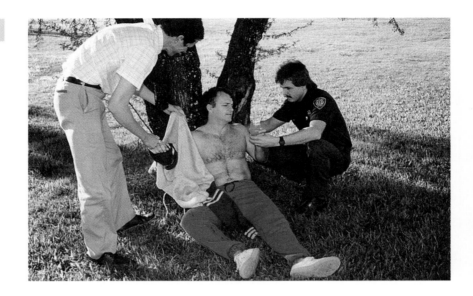

Heat stroke is an emergency that can quickly lead to brain damage or death. Immediate field treatment with radical cooling, such as immersion in cold or iced water, is imperative. Monitor core temperature to prevent hypothermia. If *within your scope of practice*, replace volume with IV fluids as authorized by medical control. Provide BLS/ALS as necessary.

ACUTE MOUNTAIN SICKNESS

Acute mountain sickness (AMS), also known as altitude sickness, occurs most commonly in people climbing in the mountains. It may appear in others who venture to high altitudes, such as at ski resorts. AMS usually occurs only at altitudes greater than 12,000 feet. But it has been reported at altitudes as low as 7,500 feet. It rarely occurs after five days at altitude, unless precipitated by a stress such as hypothermia or a respiratory infection.

AMS is probably the result of vascular changes resulting in edema in the lungs and the brain. The clinical patterns of AMS are usually classified into three groups according to severity: mild, moderate, and severe. Severe AMS usually manifests itself as high altitude cerebral edema (HACE) and high altitude pulmonary edema (HAPE).

Assessment The patient with mild AMS will have nausea with little or no vomiting, dizziness, loss of appetite, a mild headache that may be relieved with pain medication, and mild fatigue at rest. The feeling of a mild hangover is common.

Patients with moderate AMS will be suffer from nausea and vomiting, a feeling of moderate fatigue, along with shortness of breath on moderate exertion, and a severe headache unrelieved by pain medication. A particularly significant aspect of the condition is any sign of early changes in coordination.

In severe AMS, the patient's condition has progressed to the point of having HAPE or HACE. There will be **ataxia** (failure of muscular coordination), altered mental status or consciousness, cyanosis, extreme weakness, dyspnea at rest, increased pulse rate, rales in the chest, and a productive cough.

Treatment For mild AMS, over-the-counter pain medications can be taken for the headache. If *within your scope of practice* and authorized by local medical protocols, give acetazolamide (Diamox) 500 mg a day. The patient should avoid alcohol and other sedatives, which act as respiratory depressants. If symptoms do not resolve after a night's sleep, the patient should descend to a lower altitude or spend rest days at the same elevation for acclimatization. If symptoms increase, descend to a lower altitude immediately.

Treatment for moderate AMS is the same as for mild AMS, plus descent to a lower altitude. The descent should be to below 10,000 feet, but must be at least 2,000 feet below the altitude at which symptoms began. You should observe the patient closely for increasing symptoms. It is best to descend early before the patient has to be carried to the lower altitude.

Severe AMS is a medical emergency. The most productive and important action is immediate descent by at least 2,000 feet. Oxygen may be helpful, but is not a substitute for descent. If *within your scope of practice* and authorized by local medical protocols, consider giving systemic steroids for HACE.

DROWNING/NEAR-DROWNING

Drowning refers to death by respiratory failure in a liquid. The term near-drowning indicates at least temporary survival.

Mechanisms of Injury Respiratory failure in drowning or near-drowning occurs through one of two mechanisms. In wet drowning, the alveoli, air sacs in the lungs, are filled with water from aspiration. Wet drownings occur in about 85 percent of the patients. In dry drowning, laryngospasm from cold water causes an upper airway obstruction. The laryngospasm is triggered when the larynx suddenly contacts the cold water. Though the laryngospasm obstructs the airway, it can protect the patient by keeping water out of the lungs, and increasing the chances of survival if rescued. A laryngospasm is ultimately relaxed as the patient's level of consciousness decreases, and eventually the lungs will fill with water.

Acute, or immersion, hypothermia is often the direct cause of near-drowning. A person loses coordination and slips underwater. But, if rescued, the protective effect of hypothermia may increase the patient's chances of survival.

Assessment   For the field rescuer, there are no practical differences in assessment and field management of saltwater and freshwater near-drownings.

Note the length of time that the patient was under water and the temperature of the water. Respiratory arrest usually occurs before cardiac arrest. The pulse may be difficult to detect under field conditions. In cases of near-drowning, immersion hypothermia is common. Check for associated conditions common to water accidents, such as cervical spine injuries and intoxication.

The inhalation of water may also result in delayed edema that resembles the irritation that comes from inhaling smoke. This effect can be delayed, with symptoms usually appearing within 24 hours after the incident.

Treatment   If a positive mechanism of injury (such as diving) is present, protect the spine during rescue and during treatment.

Give oxygen, and use suction. Clear the airway of vomit and debris. Provide "aggressive" ventilatory support (Figure 16.4).

During extended incidents, observe the patient for the delayed effects of pulmonary edema. The onset is usually within the first 6

FIGURE 16.4

Artificial Ventilation
When rescuing a near-drowning patient, clear the airway and provide aggressive ventilatory support as soon as the person's head is above water. If there is a positive mechanism of injury, protect the spine during rescue and treatment.

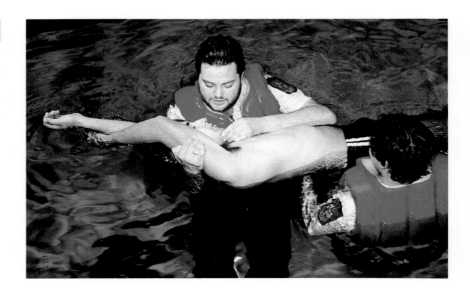

hours but is often delayed for 24 hours. Rarely it may be delayed for up to 72 hours.

Recovery with normal neurologic function following near-drowning in cold water has occurred in patients who have been submerged for up to one hour. Follow aggressive BLS/ALS procedures, and transport as quickly as possible to definitive medical care. Although near-drowning and hypothermia often occur together, your priority should be treatment of the near-downing.

DIVING MEDICAL EMERGENCIES

Two types of SCUBA diving emergencies need to be mentioned. The first is known as air embolism. This occurs when a diver holds his or her breath during a rapid ascent. The air pressure in the lungs remains at a high level, while the external pressure on the chest decreases. This causes the air inside the lungs to expand rapidly and rupture the alveoli (air sacs) in the lungs. When the alveoli rupture, the air that is released can cause internal injuries. These include bubbles of air in the bloodstream that prevent the normal flow of blood and oxygen to a specific part of the body.

The second major type of diving emergency is decompression sickness, often called the "bends." This also results from a too rapid ascent from a dive. In decompression sickness, bubbles of nitrogen form in the blood vessels and joints when the diver ascends rapidly. These bubbles of nitrogen cause the same problem that occurs in air embolism, including blockage of the blood vessels that deprives parts of the body of the normal blood supply. The bubbles in the joints expand, resulting in significant pain. The pain often causes the diver to bend over—a reaction from which the condition got its name.

Assessment Both air embolism and decompression sickness have similar signs and symptoms:

- Blotching of the skin
- Froth, often pink or bloody, at the nose and mouth
- Severe pain in muscles, joints, or abdomen
- Dyspnea (shortness of breath) and/or chest pain
- Dizziness, nausea, and vomiting
- Dysphasia (difficulty in speaking)
- Difficulty with vision
- Paralysis and/or coma

It is often difficult to distinguish between air embolism and decompression sickness. As a general rule, air embolism occurs immediately upon return to the surface, while decompression sickness may not appear for several hours. Emergency treatment is the same for both: BLS followed by recompression in a recompression chamber.

Treatment You should follow these steps:

- Remove the patient from the water, and try to calm him or her.
- Administer oxygen.
- Begin BLS/ALS, if necessary.
- Place the patient on his or her left side with the patient's head lower than the feet. This decreases the chance of an air embolus traveling to the brain.
- Listen to the chest carefully for absent or decreased breath sounds that would indicate a pneumothorax.
- Transport the patient promptly to the nearest recompression chamber for treatment (Figure 16.5). You should know the location of and best access to recompression chambers in your region. To avoid the additional decompression that occurs at altitude, do not transport the patient by air.
- Continue to administer oxygen while transporting the patient to the chamber.
- Obtain a history of the duration and depth of the dive. If appropriate facilities are available, have the patient's SCUBA tank transported so it can be analyzed for the amount of air remaining, and its carbon monoxide content.
- Assess and monitor the patient's level of consciousness using the AVPU scale.

The objective of recompression treatment is to restore the body to a high pressure environment. This will redissolve the bubbles of gas, whether air or nitrogen, and equalize the pressures inside and outside the lungs. Once the pressures are equalized, gradual decompression proceeds under controlled conditions.

FIGURE 16.5

Recompression Chamber In preplanning for diving emergencies, you should know the phone number, location, and best access to recompression chambers in your area.

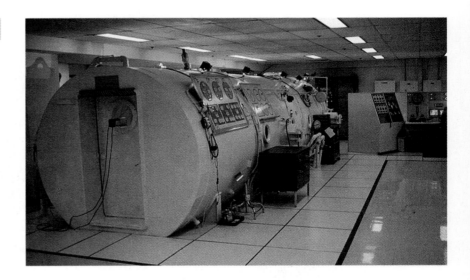

SUMMARY

Certain environments or environmental conditions can threaten patients and rescuers alike. It is vital that rescuers understand the impact of each environment on everyone involved and be able to recognize, assess, and treat conditions caused by the environment in which the rescue operation is taking place.

Some of the more common environment-specific conditions include exposure to toxic substances, anaphylaxis, hypothermia, frostbite, hyperthermia, acute mountain sickness, and water problems such as near-drowning and diving emergencies.

Rescuers must be able to assess patients to evaluate the signs and symptoms of a potential problem. They must also understand the mechanisms of injury and the impact of the environment on the patient and the situation. Finally, rescuers must be equipped and prepared to treat an environment-specific condition encountered during a rescue. The rescue team must familiarize itself with treatment measures that reduce or eliminate the effects of the environment in which the rescue occurs.

TRANSPORT

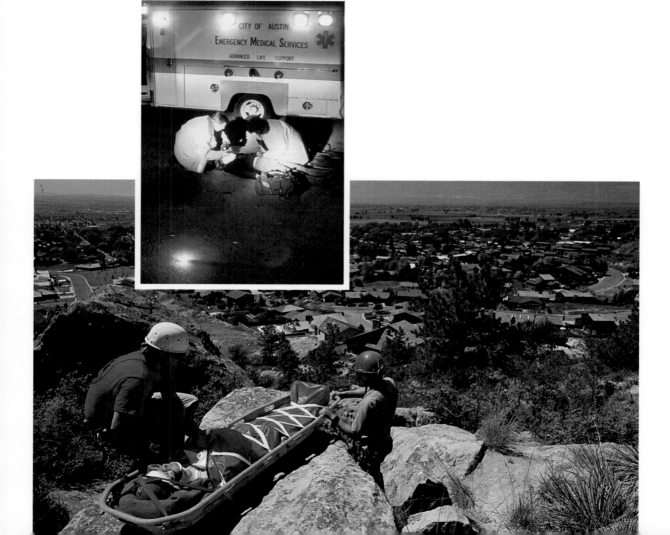

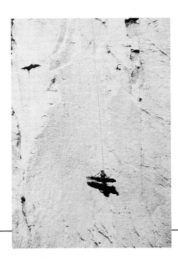

CHAPTER

17

PATIENT PACKAGING AND LITTER EVACUATION

CHAPTER OUTLINE

OVERVIEW

Knowing how to package and transport patients in a safe and efficient manner is crucial to the successful outcome of a rescue. This chapter explains packaging and litter transport techniques.

The techniques of litter evacuation range from packaging the patient in the litter to moving the litter through and from the rescue site. This chapter examines a variety of litter evacuation techniques. It offers detailed instructions on certain aspects of litter evacuation.

The chapter begins with packaging techniques, including securing a patient with lower extremity injuries and providing immobilization with a spine board. There is a section outlining special packaging considerations. This includes patient protection and administration of intravenous fluids in the backcountry. The chapter also analyzes the tasks of carrying and moving litters. It discusses the litter team, lowering systems, and hauling systems. In addition, the litter carrying sequence, passing the litter in dangerous terrain, belaying the litter, and moving a litter through a confined space are examined.

OBJECTIVES

The objectives of this chapter are for the rescuer to describe:

- packaging a patient for transport.
- packaging the patient in a litter for transport.
- how to construct specific patient packages for evacuation over irregular terrain and during helicopter evacuation.
- how to protect the patient from environmental threats in a high angle environment during litter transport.

- how to organize a litter team.
- a litter carrying sequence.
- a load sling.
- how to pass a litter in uneven terrain.
- basic techniques for belaying a litter.
- moving a litter through a confined space.
- basic lowering and hauling systems.
- how to determine mechanical advantage in hauling systems.

There are five major concerns in packaging for transport. First, you must package the patient to avoid additional injury. You must also be concerned about patient comfort. Your third concern is effective patient immobilization while allowing access for reassessment and continued treatment. Your immobilization equipment must be adaptable. It must fit within the size constraints of the transport system you will use.

A fourth concern is your ability to move the patient. Once you have packaged the patient comfortably in relation to his or her injuries, you must be able to carry the patient and litter to your destination. For example, carrying the weight of a stretcher with only one hand will fatigue you sooner than alternating between two hands.

The last concern, but equally important, is that the patient package must be compatible with the transport being used. For example, in a helicopter transport, will the litter and patient package fit into the aircraft?

PACKAGING FOR LITTER EVACUATION

The patient must be packaged so that he or she is secure in the litter and will not fall out at whatever the angle the litter is moved. The patient also must not shift inside the "patient package" or the litter. If any spinal injuries are suspected, the patient must be immobilized to prevent any movement of the spinal column. One method of securing a patient in a litter is lacing him or her in with one-inch tubular webbing.

Figure 17.1 illustrates securing a patient in a plastic Stokes litter using a 30-foot length of one-inch tubular webbing.

1. The process begins by finding the center of the webbing. Attach it with a girth hitch to the railing at the foot of the litter.
2. With one rescuer on each side of the litter, pass the webbing back and forth across the patient. The webbing should be snug across the patient, but not cause discomfort or impede circulation. On a metal basket, the webbing should not run over the rail but around the major support members that attach the rail to the basket. On the plastic basket, the webbing will attach by running over the rope that is laced inside the basket by the manufacturer. Webbing tied over the rail may be damaged by abrasion as the litter is transported over rough terrain.
3. As the webbing nears the head of the litter, it must not run across the neck of the patient. In a high angle environment, extra tie-ins are needed in addition to the straps designed for the litter.

There should also be a separate tie-in that connects a safety harness on the patient to a belay system. This is a necessary safety system

FIGURE 17.1

Packaging Patient in a Litter

a. Materials for packaging a patient in a Stokes litter should be kept stored in the litter to be ready when needed.

b. Litter packaging materials include protection for the patient from the environment, padding, webbing to secure the patient, and immobilization equipment.

c. The patient must first be immobilized to prevent any movement of spinal areas. The process of securing a patient in a Stokes litter begins by attaching the center of the length of webbing with a girth hitch to the railing at the foot of the litter.

d. and e. Two rescuers, one on each side of the litter, pass the webbing back and forth across the patient. The webbing should be snug across the patient, but not cause discomfort or impede circulation.

f. As the webbing nears the patient's head, it must be secured so that it does not run across the neck of the patient.

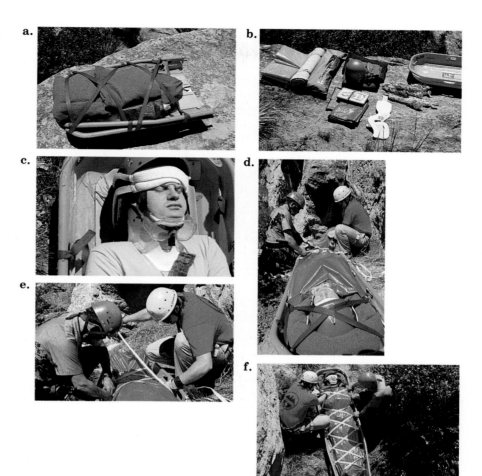

for the patient in case of failure of the litter or other portions of the rope system for the litter.

If there is any chance that the litter will be tilted, foot tie-ins or a seat harness are needed to prevent the patient from sliding down in the litter. In patients without lower extremity, pelvic, or lumbar spine injuries, ankle hitch restraints should be used. This prevents the patient from shifting lengthwise in the litter, even if it is tilted on end.

Figure 17.2 shows how to secure the feet with 12 to 15 feet of one-inch tubular webbing, but *this technique must not be used if there are spine, pelvic, or lower extremity fractures.*

1. First lay the webbing behind the ankle. Then bring it around the foot and cross the webbing over the top of the foot.

2. Pull the webbing firmly toward the bottom of the litter and across on the bottom of the foot.
3. Bring the webbing up on opposite sides of the foot, through the previous crosses, and pull firmly toward the head of the litter.
4. Tie off the webbing on the litter rail supports or over the interior laced rope. It should be tight enough so that the patient will not shift if the litter is stood on its foot. The seat harness described below may be used to provide additional stabilization.

Securing a Patient with Spine, Pelvis, or Lower Extremity Injuries

The foot hitch method of securing a patient cannot be used if the patient has spine, pelvis, or lower extremity injuries. For these patients, the use of one-inch webbing leg loops or a climbing harness can prevent lengthwise movement (Figure 17.3). Both ends of the harness should be secured to the litter rail. You should be certain that the restraint system used does not compromise blood vessels or nerves.

Patients with pelvic, chest, or spinal cord injuries pose a challenging situation. A combination of the two systems discussed above with the addition of nonconstricting chest restraint can be adapted to meet the most difficult situation.

Additional Packaging

Even with webbing restraints, patients may shift in a litter. This is particularly true of patients who do not fill the litter, such as thin people and children. Side-to-side movement can be eliminated by adding enough padding to fill any spaces between the patient's body and the packaging devices (litters, backboards, stretchers) (Figure 17.4).

FIGURE 17.2

Securing the Feet
If there is any chance that the litter will be tilted, foot tie-ins or a seat harness are needed to prevent the patient from sliding down in the litter.

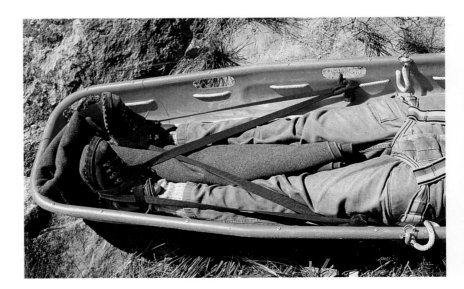

FIGURE 17.3

Seat Harness
If the patient has spinal, pelvic, or lower extremity injuries, the foot hitch method of securing a patient cannot be used. Secure these patients with webbing leg loops or a climbing harness to prevent lengthwise movement. Secure the leg loops or harness to the litter rail.

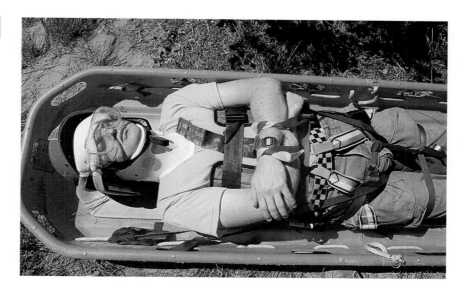

FIGURE 17.4

Additional Padding Eliminates Patient Movement
Side-to-side movement in the litter can be reduced by filling any spaces between the patient's body and packaging devices.

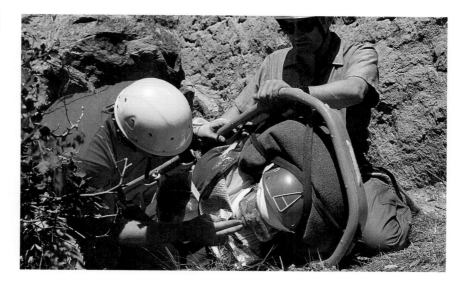

Providing Extra Immobilization

As with other forms of emergency medical care, patient packaging for litter evacuation must include considerations for airway management. Your patient must be packaged so that you can roll the total package onto its side to allow for definitive airway care in the case of vomiting or airway threats. You must be able to do this without any significant patient movement within the package. The patient must be secured so there is no shift along the spinal column.

One potential solution in these cases is to immobilize the patient to a long spine board or the equivalent within the litter.

Immobilization in Other Types of Litters

Semi-rigid, conforming litters provide patient packaging by conforming around the individual. However, you must be certain that the patient will not shift inside these litters. Package the patient by packing soft materials such as clothing in any spaces between the litter and the patient's body.

Some litters have additional means for securing the patient, such as attached D rings or carrying straps.

SPECIAL PATIENT TREATMENT, PACKAGING, AND EVACUATION CONSIDERATIONS

Whenever patients are packaged in the high angle environment, they became vulnerable to the two great dangers of the environment: exposure to the risks of falling and being hit by falling objects, such as rocks, building materials, and other objects. Whenever you package and transport patients, you must protect your patients against these dangers. You must also protect them from environmental threats such as cold, heat, and wetness.

A patient immobilized in a litter is unable to avoid falling objects. The hazard of falling objects should be a major consideration in choosing an evacuation route. A longer route with less risk of rockfall may mean a longer evacuation. But it would usually be preferable to increasing the risk of injuries to a patient by using a shorter route through a rockfall zone.

Whenever a patient is being transported in a litter, you should always provide eye protection from dirt, brush, and rain (Figure 17.5). A pair of goggles or a face shield should always be kept with the litter as a part of packaging material.

FIGURE 17.5

Eye and Head Protection with Helmet
Whenever transporting a patient in a litter, you should always provide eye protection from dirt, brush, and rain.

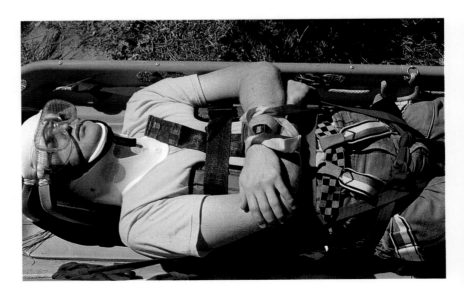

Unless suspected cervical or head injuries prevent it, the litter patient should have a helmet for head protection. The helmet should be designed to avoid hyperextending the patient's neck.

A patient immobilized in a litter is more at risk from environmental threats than you are. The patient is unable to generate heat from muscle activity. Their only shelter is that provided by you. Also, a patient's injuries may predispose him to greater heat loss.

A litter patient must have environmental protection both *above and below* his or her body. In a cold, windy, and wet environment, the patient should have an insulating layer next to his body and a barrier layer on the outside; blankets or a sleeping bag can provide the insulating layer. For greater access to the entire body, the sleeping bag should be accessible all around. For even greater convenience, the bag's zipper closure can be replaced with Velcro™. The barrier layer protection should be an inpenetrable and tear-resistant material such as a poncho, tarp, or tough plastic material.

A reflectorized tarp can be used with the reflecting side facing the patient to help preserve the patient's body heat. In very hot climates, the tarp can be used with the reflectorized side turned to the outside to reflect heat away from the patient.

The decision to secure the patient's hands should be made after an evaluation of the patient's mental state and consciousness. Many litter patients will not want their hands secured. Patients who are experienced and comfortable in the high angle environment may be able to keep their hands inside the litter if instructed to do so. A patient who is inexperienced in the high angle environment may be tempted to grab or hold onto the litter rails when anxious or desiring to "help." This may result in serious injuries if the hand or fingers are caught between the litter and a hard surface. If this is a possibility, the patient's hands should be secured inside the litter with webbing or other material. The hands of a patient who is unconscious must be secured inside the litter.

USE OF IV IN THE BACKCOUNTRY

With the added weight and bulk of intravenous (IV) fluids, the selection of fluids is extremely important. If you have to carry IV fluids into the backcountry, you must get the most efficient use of them. Blood components, both natural and synthetic, may provide the greatest gain for the weight in the treatment of hypovolemic shock. This must be determined by patient assessment to ascertain whether the shock is the result of blood loss or dehydration. The use of IVs as a line for drug administration is usually a low priority in extended incident emergency care. Weather extremes and patient transport problems make it difficult to administer and to monitor IV fluids.

IV Maintenance   In cold weather, it may take a major effort to keep IV solutions warm as they are being administered to the patient and to prevent IV lines from freezing. One possible solution is for you to pin the bag inside your clothing and run the tubing into the litter packaging system. Any exposed tubing must be protected from cold by insulating with a material such as closed-cell foam pads. Inside the litter, as much of the tubing as possible should be run close to the patient's skin. Remember, there must be some slack to allow for rescuer and litter movement.

Another option for keeping IVs warm is the adapted heat pack. However, you should use extreme caution because of the possibility of overheating the fluids, which can cause thermal and chemical burns to the patient and you.

Another problem with the use of IVs in a backcountry environment may be assuring flow when gravity feed is not possible. You may not be able to hang IV bags for gravity flow because of possible entanglement, as in a roped litter evacuation, or because of possible freezing. One possible solution to this problem is to use the pressure from an inflatable IV infusion pump around the IV bag.

CARRYING LITTERS

Carrying litters across difficult terrain requires more personnel and different techniques than you learned for conventional, rapid transport, ambulance-based EMS. These techniques must be practiced before they are needed in actual emergencies.

The Litter Team

For a short distance carry (one fourth mile or less) of a litter, a *minimum* of six rescuers is required—four to carry and two to scout. For a longer carry, a *minimum* of eight rescuers is required—six to carry and two to scout. Additional personnel are often desirable, particularly if the terrain is rugged or the distances long. The additional personnel provide relief for the six carriers on a regular rotation.

The litter team should be selected so that persons of the same height are across from one another on the litter. This assures that each person carries equal weight and that the litter remains level. Each litter team must have a captain to give directions. The litter team captain is traditionally at the patient's right shoulder (front left position on the litter).

The two remaining rescuers walk in front of the litter to scout for problems. They may point out hazards (holes, icy spots, loose rock) to the litter team or remove obstacles, such as fallen tree branches.

Litter Carrying Sequence

The following is a basic sequence for a team carrying a litter (Figure 17.6):

1. The immediate team members position themselves at equal distance along both sides of the litter with both hands on the rail

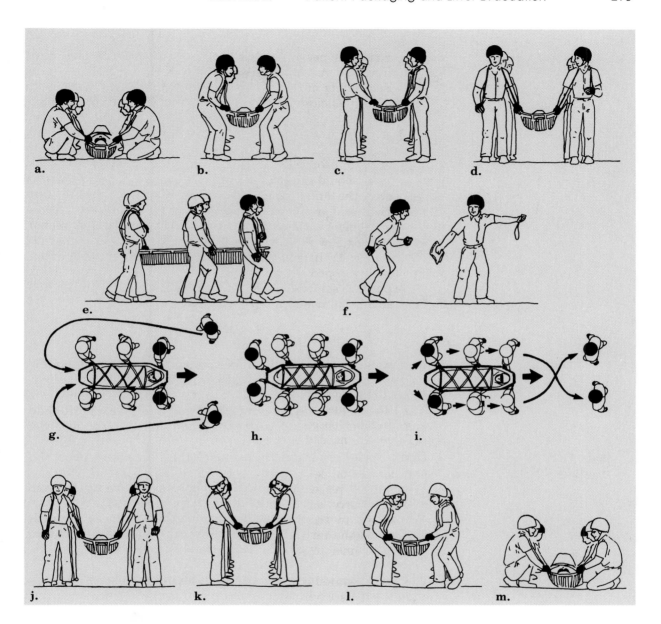

FIGURE 17.6	**Basic Litter Carrying Sequence**

a. The team members position themselves at equal distance along both sides of the litter with both hands on the rail and ready to lift. To avoid strain, backs should be kept as straight as possible.

b. When everyone is ready, the captain gives a verbal command, such as "Lift on three. Ready, one, two, three."

c. On the verbal command, the team lifts the litter slowly, smoothly, and in unison.

d. When the litter is up, the team members turn facing forward with the hand closest to the litter grasping the rail.

e. When the captain sees that the team members are ready, he gives the command, "Ready, forward," and the team members begin moving forward.

Continued

FIGURE 17.6 *Cont.*

f. The remaining two rescuers move in front of the litter, scouting for hazards.

g. When the litter captain perceives that the team members are ready, he calls for a switch, "Ready to rotate." At this signal, the two scouts move to the rear of the litter.

h. Each one of them places a hand on the rail. When the second of the two has a hand on the rail, he says, "Rotate."

i. At this signal all team members move forward on the litter rail. The two front rescuers move off and switch sides to become scouts.

j. When the rescuers are ready to stop, the scouts indicate a good place to rest the litter.

k. The litter captain gives a verbal command such as, "Ready, stop." Before lowering the litter, the captain checks to make certain that the litter will not be set on anything that could harm the patient.

l. The captain gives a verbal signal to lower the litter, such as, "Lower on three."

m. In a slow, smooth, coordinated motion, the rescuers lower the litter to the ground.

ready to lift. Their hips and knees should be bent and the arms held extended. To avoid strain, their backs should be as straight as possible.

2. The litter captain makes certain that everyone is ready. He then gives a verbal command, such as, "Lift on three. Ready, one, two, three."

3. On the verbal command, the team lifts the litter slowly, smoothly, and in unison.

4. When the litter is up, the team members turn facing forward with the hand closest to the litter grasping the rail.

5. When the captain sees that the team members are ready, he gives the command, such as, "Ready, forward." The team members begin moving forward. If a team member is not ready, he says, "Not ready."

6. The team should move at a pace that is comfortable for all. They *should not* march in step. Marching in step will cause the litter to bounce. The remaining two rescuers move in front of the litter, scouting for hazards.

7. When the litter captain perceives that the team members are ready, he calls for a switch, "Ready to rotate."

8. At this signal, the two scouts move to the rear of the litter. Each one of them places a hand on the rail. When the second of the two has a hand on the rail, he says, "Rotate."

9. At this signal, all of the team members move forward on the litter rail to assume a new position (with a new captain coming into position at the patient's right shoulder). The two front rescuers move off to become scouts. They should switch sides to assure that they will use a different hand when they are again on the litter.

This sequence continues to assure equal time on the litter for all rescuers.

10. When the rescuers are ready to stop, the scouts indicate a good place to rest the litter. The litter captain gives a verbal command such as, "Ready, stop."
11. Before lowering the litter, the captain has carefully checked to make certain that the litter will not be set on anything that could harm the patient (rocks or stumps, for example). This is particularly important when using a wire basket litter. The rescuers turn in to face the litter with both hands on the rail.
12. The captain gives a verbal signal to lower the litter, such as, "Lower on three. Ready, one, two, three." In a slow, smooth, coordinated motion, the rescuers lower the litter to the ground.

The Load Sling

If you carry a litter with only one hand grasping the litter rail, it can be extremely tiring. To spread the load onto other parts of the body, you should create a carrying sling using a 14 to 18 foot length of one-inch tubular webbing (Figures 17.7). Create a continuous loop in the webbing with a water knot. Attach the load sling to the litter rail with a carabiner that will comfortably slip over the rail. Run the carrying sling over the shoulder away from the litter, and grasp the end of the webbing with the hand that is away from the litter. The length of the sling can be adjusted to the needs of the individual rescuer.

FIGURE 17.7

Sequence to Tying and Carrying a Load Sling
Carrying can be extremely tiring on one hand. Spread the load onto other parts of the body with a carrying sling made from a 14 to 18 foot length of one-inch tubular webbing. After creating the webbing loop with a water knot, attach the load sling to the litter rail with a carabiner slipped over the litter rail. Run the carrying sling over the shoulder and grasp the end of the webbing with the hand that is away from the litter. Adjust the sling according to individual needs.

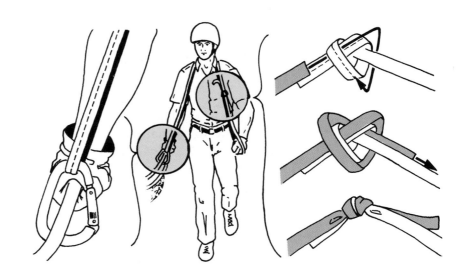

Passing the Litter Across Uneven Terrain

In uneven or dangerous terrain, or where the footing is not secure, you should not walk with the litter, but pass it to rescuers who are in a secure position.

The following is the sequence for passing a litter in uneven terrain (Figure 17.8):

1. As the team comes into uneven terrain, the litter captain calls a halt.
2. The team members position themselves securely. The captain then says, "Ready to pass." If any member is not in a secure position, he says, "Not ready!"

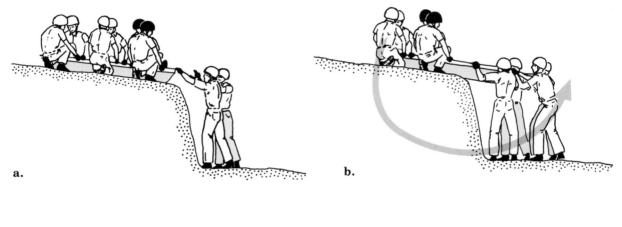

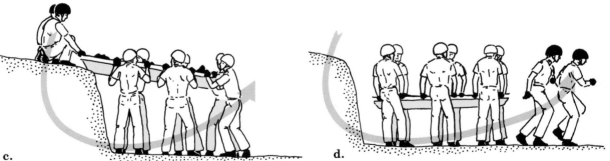

FIGURE 17.8

Passing Litter in Dangerous Terrain
a. Once the litter is in a stable position, the captain says, "Ready to pass." The scouts place their hands at the front of the rail and say, "Pass."
b. The rescuers at the rear of the litter move ahead of the litter to position themselves for the next pass.
c. Another pair of rescuers move from the rear to the front and the litter is passed again.
d. The rescue team repeats the sequence until they have passed the litter through the difficult area.

3. The scouts then place their hands at the front of the rail and say, "Pass." The rescuers pass the litter forward with a slow, smooth, and coordinated action.
4. The rescuers previously at the rear of the litter move ahead of the litter to position themselves for the next pass.

This sequence repeats until the litter is through the dangerous area. The litter pass technique works best with a number of well-trained rescuers.

BELAYING THE LITTER

If there is the danger of the litter sliding downslope during a carry, the rescuers must **belay** it. To belay a litter, a safety or belay rope is attached to the litter and secured so that if the litter starts to fall, the belay rope supports it. In most cases, the belay rope is controlled by a second rescuer known as the belayer.

Figure 17.9 illustrates a belay system for a litter on a slope. It consists of:

1. The litter containing the patient and attendant rescuers.
2. A rescue rope.
3. One end of the rope attached to the litter.
4. The other end of the rope is run through a belay system, such as a Münter hitch attached to a carabiner (Figure 17.10). The carabiner used with the Münter hitch belay should be large and pear-shaped with its gate turned away from the Münter hitch.

FIGURE 17.9

A Belay System on a Slope
a. The litter containing patient and attendant rescuers.
b. A rescue rope.
c. One end of the rope attached to the litter.
d. Another rope running through a belay system.
e. The belay system attached to a bombproof anchor.

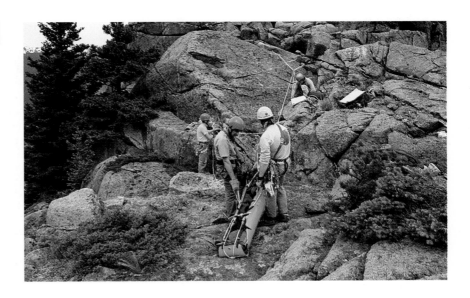

FIGURE 17.10

Tying a Münter Hitch
a. The carabiner used with the Münter hitch should be large and pear-shaped and with its gate turned away from the Münter hitch.
b. and c. The carabiner is attached with a piece of webbing (one-inch tubular or larger).
d. The webbing is attached to a bombproof anchor.

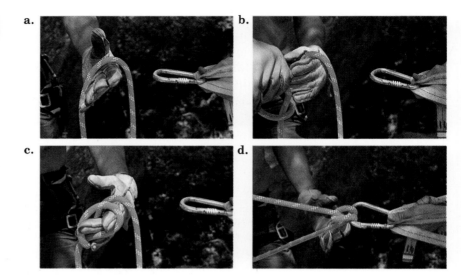

5. The Münter hitch belay carabiner is attached with a piece of webbing (one-inch tubular or larger) that has been tied into a loop with a water knot to a bombproof anchor. Bombproof means it must sustain any weight or force that could be put on it by the litter, patient, and rescuers. The anchor system can be anything of substance, such as large tree, rock, vehicle, or structural part of a building. Plumbing and plumbing fixtures, radiators, doors, or stair rails are not considered structural parts of a building. If a vehicle is used, the system must be attached to a structural portion of the vehicle (such as around the axle), the vehicle's parking brakes must be set, the wheels chocked, the ignition off with the keys in the possession of the incident commander or safety officer. A guard must be posted to ensure that the vehicle is not moved.

During a belay, you must always grasp the brake side of the rope firmly with your dominant hand (for example, right hand for right-handed people). This brake hand must never leave the rope until the patient and stretcher are *off belay*.

For any belay with ropes crossing a roadway, barriers and guards must be established on both sides to prevent a vehicle from inadvertently striking the belay system.

Communications for Belaying

There are a set of standardized communications used during a belay from which there should be no deviation:

Litter captain to belayer: "On Belay?" (Are you ready to hold us if we fall?)
Belayer to litter captain: "Belay on." (I will catch you with my belay if you fall.)

When the litter is in a secure position and the belay is no longer needed:

Litter captain to belayer: "Off Belay." (We are in a secure position, belay no longer needed.)

Belayer to litter captain: "Belay off." (I no longer have you belayed.)

MOVING A LITTER THROUGH A CONFINED SPACE

Moving a patient in a litter through a confined space can be very demanding on you and extremely difficult for the patient. Confined space litter removal will utilize more rescuers than usual. Do not overestimate the endurance of the rescuers under the rigors of a confined space removal.

Removal to a safe area may require the use of a suitable extrication system. On vertical raises involving patients with minor injuries, a webbing harness or evacuation bag is preferable. If the patient is already wearing a harness, such as worn by many utility contractors, use a chest attachment to position the patient so that you can maintain an open airway.

Spinal injuries require a backboard or one of the specialized, semi-rigid or body-shaped patient transportation devices. Accompany the patient when possible to the exit. Stay alert to sudden changes in patient status. Airway management may require rapidly turning the patient on the transportation device.

BASIC LOWERING SYSTEMS

Many rescue situations require getting the patient from a higher elevation to a lower one. This could mean securing the patient out of danger on a cliff or building and then moving the patient down a vertical face to a level area. However, many rope rescue situations occur at angles less than vertical. They often involve transporting the patient down a steep slope, such as a road embankment, to a safer area. In a high angle environment, the act of moving a patient to a lower elevation in a controlled manner is called **lowering.**

The basic elements of a lowering system are illustrated in Figure 17.11, which shows a litter patient being lowered down a steep slope. The patient is secured in the litter to prevent movement or slippage. Litter tenders attach themselves to the litter rail with the front tie-in of their seat harnesses so they can operate with their hands free.

A rope loop is attached to the head of the litter. To help prevent damage to the litter, the rope should not be attached at one point but wrapped around the litter rail several times before completing the loop (Figure 17.12). The main line is then attached to the loop with a figure 8 overhand knot and locking carabiners.

FIGURE 17.11

Basic Elements of a Lowering System

In lowering a litter patient down a steep slope the patient is secured to prevent movement or slippage in the litter. Litter tenders attach themselves to the litter rail with a short length of webbing so they can operate hands free. A rope loop is attached to the head of the litter. The rate of the lowering is controlled by the brakeman by controlling the rope through a lowering device or brake attached to a bombproof anchor. A rope handler assists the brakeman by feeding him the rope.

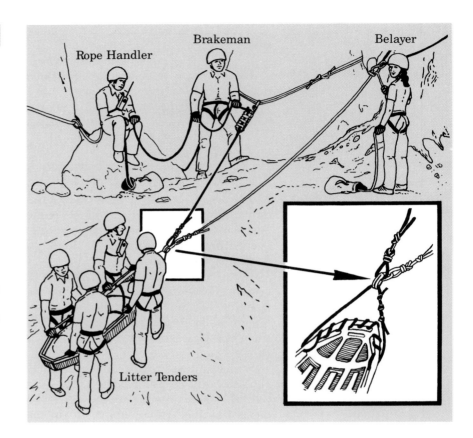

FIGURE 17.12

Wrapping Rope Around Litter

When attaching a rope to an end of a litter, the rope should be wrapped around the rail several times to prevent damage to the litter.

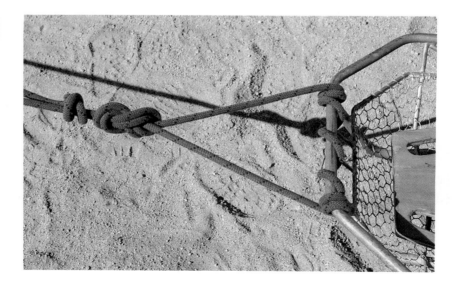

FIGURE 17.11 *Cont.*

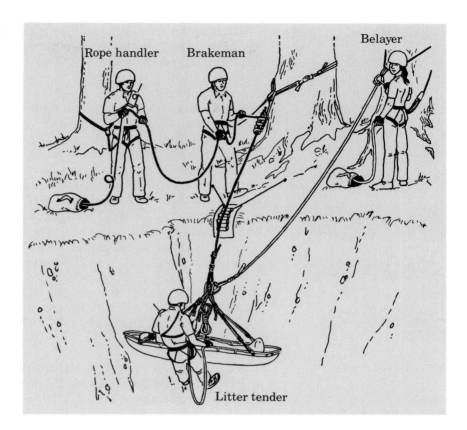

The rate of lowering is controlled by the **brakeman.** The brakeman does this by grasping the rope and controlling its speed through the lowering device or **brake** that is attached to a bombproof anchor. A **rope handler** assists the brakeman by feeding him the rope and removing kinks in the rope before they can foul the brakes.

In higher angle environments, where there is greater danger to patient and rescuers if the lowering system fails, a belay system should be used. The belay system is attached to a separate anchor system and attached to the litter.

Lowering Devices (Brakes)

Rescue lowering devices or brakes work on the same principle as rappel devices. The person controlling the device creates friction between the rope and metal surfaces of the device. The difference between using these devices for rappeling and lowering is the relative location of the device.

In rappeling, the load, usually a person, is attached directly to the device that moves with the load. The top end of the rope is attached to an anchor and the rope remains fixed during the rappel.

In lowering, the device is attached to the anchor and the load is attached to one end of the rope that runs through the device.

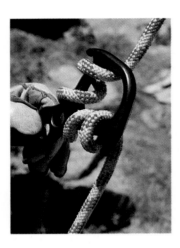

FIGURE 17.13

Figure 8 with Ears
The figure 8 with ears can be "double wrapped" for greater control.

Vertical Lowering

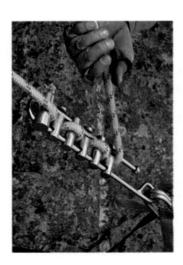

FIGURE 17.14

Brake Bar Rack
The brake bar rack is a friction device used in rescue lowering of larger loads such as a patient in a litter with litter tenders.

There are several types of lowering devices used by rescue personnel. The figure 8 with ears is a personal rappel device that can be used in some rescue situations (Figure 17.13). It is adaptable to the lowering of one person's body weight. The friction and, therefore, control on a figure 8 is not easily changed, so it is not as easy to use for larger loads. Double wrapping the figure 8 with ears gives greater control. One other problem with the figure 8 is that the rope twists as it passes through the device. This can cause the rope to tangle before entering the device, which can foul the system.

The **brake bar rack** (Figure 17.14) allows greater control in rescue lowering, especially for larger loads such as a patient in a litter with litter tenders. The brake bar rack is also known as a rappel rack or Cole rack. The frame of the rack is a stainless steel bar fabricated into a U shape, with one arm of the U longer than the other. The end of the longer leg is shaped into an eye that can be attached to an anchor. The eye of a rescue rack should be factory-welded and inspected.

The advantages of the brake bar rack include the ease in changing its friction to adapt to varying loads, its ability to control large rescue loads, and the fact that it does not twist the rope that runs through it.

The lowering of a patient in a vertical or near-vertical situation requires some procedures and rigging different from those used in lowering on a steep slope. Figure 17.15 illustrates a typical lowering of a patient on a vertical rock face. The lowering of a patient on a vertical building face also would use the same principles.

The litter rigging system is called a bridle or **spider.** One spider system consists of four legs of rope attached to the litter rail at equal distances with large locking carabiners. The carabiners must be large enough to clip easily over the railing without jamming. The carabiner gates must be turned to the inside of the stretcher to lessen the chance of accidental opening. The tops of the spider legs are tied with overhand figure 8 knots (Figure. 3.11). The overhand loops are brought together to be clipped into the end of the lowering rope with two large locking carabiners set opposed to lessen the chances of both locking sleeves being rolled open. The spider should be adjusted over the patient/litter package's center of gravity to keep the litter horizontal or in a slightly head up position. The head up position is usually the best for the patient.

Attached to the litter system is a litter tender. The tender attaches himself to a short line that is connected to the top of the litter spider. In addition, he has a short safety sling attached to the head end of the litter rail. There is a second rescuer on rappel on a second rope nearby to assist the litter tender in managing the litter and tending to the patient. In cases of rugged vertical faces, two litter tenders may be necessary, but this adds weight to the lowering system. For short drops where a tender is not used, tag lines must be attached to each end of the litter to control it.

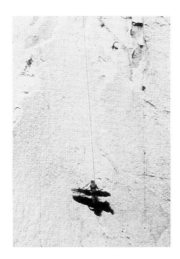

FIGURE 17.15

Lowering a Patient on a Vertical Rock Face
In one system for lowering a patient in a litter through a vertical or near-vertical situation the rope is attached to the litter via a bridle or spider. A litter tender helps maneuver the litter and care for the patient and is assisted by a second rescuer on rappel on a second rope. The main lowering line is controlled through a lowering system, such as a brake bar rack, attached to a very secure anchor. The rate of lowering is controlled by a brakeman. A belayer controls a second rope also attached to the litter and is prepared to stop the fall of the litter should the main line system fail. Not shown are edge attendants who would be secured to anchors at the top and would assist in getting the litter over the edge.

The main lowering line is controlled at the top by a lowering system attached to a very secure anchor system. The lowering system is operated by the brakeman who is located back from the edge to decrease the risk of falling.

At the edge of the drop are one or two **edge tenders,** attached to safety lines, who assist the litter tender in managing the litter at the top and in getting over the edge.

A belay system is attached at the head of the litter and connected at the top of the slope to a secure anchor that is separate from the lowering system.

HAULING SYSTEMS

In some rescue situations, the patient must be brought from a lower elevation to a higher elevation. **Hauling systems** are used to raise the patient to a higher elevation.

Hauling systems are classified according to the **mechanical advantage** they provide. Mechanical advantage is the force that it takes to raise the load in a hauling system. If, for example, the rescue load weighs 400 pounds and it takes 200 pounds of force to move it, then the mechanical advantage, or MA, of the system is 2:1. If it only took 100 pounds of force to move the 400-pound load, then the MA would be 4:1. (Figure 17.16 diagrams the MA for some basic types of hauling systems.)

You must remember that the mechanical "advantage" is not magic. It is created by lengthening the time the weight is moved. In a 2:1 MA hauling system, for example, you must pull 200 feet of rope to move the load 100 feet. In the 4:1 MA system, you must pull 400 feet of rope to move the load 100 feet. You never get the full advantage out of a hauling system. There is friction lost in pulleys, abrasion of rope on an edge, and other losses. For this reason, the MA should be called the TMA—*theoretical mechanical advantage.* The more cautious you are about avoiding friction and other losses, the more efficient your hauling systems will be.

The higher the MA, the easier it is to raise the load, but the greater the force placed on the rescue system and the more complicated the hauling system. When using high MA hauling systems, you must be cautious about causing system failure. Remember to keep it simple. Use the lowest MA system possible to accomplish the mission.

The simplest hauling system is the 1:1 MA system. In this, the force needed to move the rescue load is the same as the load. A 1:1 MA system might be used on a steep slope. The **counterbalance system** is one of the simplest of the 1:1 MA systems to use. In a steep slope haul, one end of the rope would be attached to the litter and run uphill just as in a lowering situation. But instead of there being a set of brakes attached to an anchor, there would be a pulley (Figure 17.17). The rope would be run through the pulley and back downhill. A group of rescuers would clip themselves to the rope run-

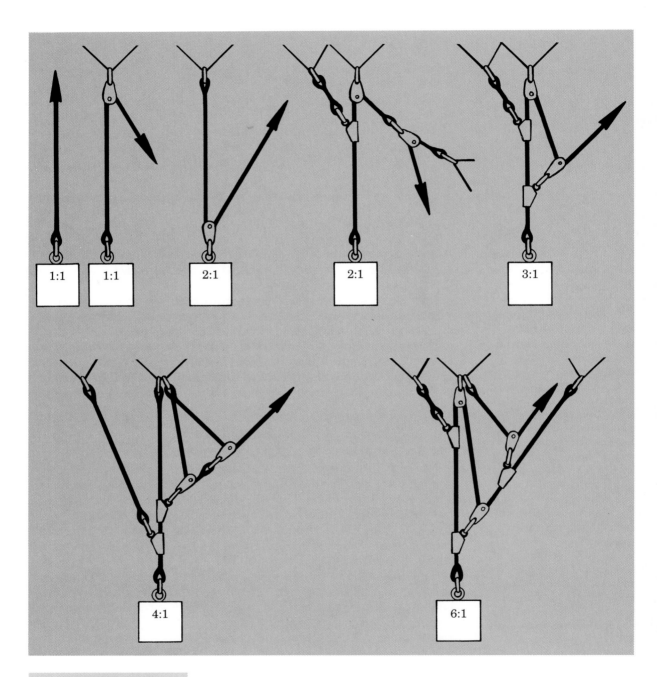

FIGURE 17.16

Mechanical Advantage

Hauling systems are classified to their mechanical advantage (MA). The MA is the relationship of the weight to the force that it takes to move the load.

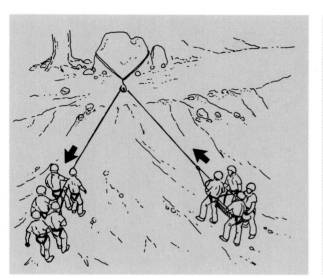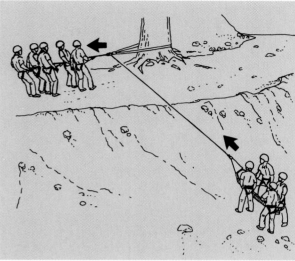

FIGURE 17.17   **Counterbalance System**
The simplest hauling system for you to use in a rescue is the 1:1 MA system such as a counterbalance system. In this system, the rescue haul team is used as a counterbalance to move the weight of the litter, patient, and litter tenders up a slope.

ning back downhill. In sufficient numbers, the counterbalance group of rescuers would create a hauling system by simply walking downhill attached to the rope. The stretcher and litter tenders could then move uphill with little effort to either group of rescuers.

A variation of this 1:1 MA system can be used where there is a road at the top of the hill. In this situation, the rope would be run through the pulley. But instead of being run back downhill, a group of rescuers would clip themselves onto the haul rope and walk back down the road, raising the litter, patient, and litter tenders.

SUMMARY

Knowing how to use and move litters is an important aspect of transporting patients. The first step is proper packaging of the patient in the litter. Rescuers must package the patient to prevent shifting or discomfort as the litter is tilted and moved. In addition, patients with suspected spinal injuries must be immobilized to prevent movement of the spinal column.

In high angle environments, patients are vulnerable to various environmental threats, such as the risk of falling or being hit by falling objects. In addition, temperature extremes can be a problem. Therefore, you must package your patients with protective equipment to prevent injuries. This includes goggles for eye protection, helmets for head protection, and an insulating/barrier layer for protection from the climate.

The need for administering intravenous (IV) fluids may need to be considered in the packaging process. Weather extremes and difficulties in patient transport may complicate the use of IVs. Nevertheless, you may be able to administer IV fluids by insulating the tubing in cold weather and by using an infusion pump around the IV bag if the bag cannot be hung for a gravity feed during transport.

Carrying litters from remote incidents requires more personnel and different techniques than those used in conventional, rapid transport, ambulance-based activities. The number of members required for a litter team depends on the distance of the carry and the ruggedness of the terrain. In general, there should be a minimum of six to carry and two to scout. Persons of the same height should be across from one another on the litter. Then each person carries equal weight and helps keep the litter level.

It is important that you be familiar with the basic litter carrying sequence. It is also vital that you understand how to alter the carrying sequence in order to pass the litter across uneven terrain. On a downslope terrain you may have to belay the litter to prevent the litter from sliding during the carry.

Many rescue operations, especially in high angle environments, require lowering a patient from a higher elevation to a lower one. There are various types of lowering systems that enable rescuers to move patients to a lower level.

Other situations require that a patient be brought from a lower elevation to a higher one. In these cases, rescuers use hauling systems. Hauling systems are classified by the mechanical advantage they provide. The mechanical advantage (MA) is the force that it takes to raise the load in a hauling system. The higher the MA, the easier it is to raise the load but the greater the force placed on the rescue system. It is best to use the lowest MA system possible to accomplish the goal.

VEHICLES AND TRANSPORTATION

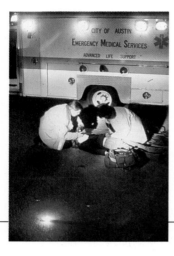

OVERVIEW

This chapter outlines the vehicle options for ground and water transportation. Because of the hazards involved, the chapter also describes aeromedical evacuation procedures in detail. Because the helicopter is the most common form of aeromedical evacuation, the chapter contains a discussion of rescue techniques and rescuer safety when using helicopters. This section considers when and where helicopters can be used, landing and departure conditions, night landing, and personnel safety around aircraft.

OBJECTIVES

The objectives of this chapter are for the rescuer to describe:

- the selection of the proper vehicles for patient transport.
- when a helicopter evacuation is appropriate.
- limitations in using a helicopter for rescue

- how to evaluate operational factors in a helicopter rescue.
- how to determine the availability and condition of an airstrip.
- safe landing zones.
- how to prepare a landing zone for night landings.
- personnel safety during helicopter evacuations.

Selecting the mode of transportation and the appropriate vehicles is an important consideration in any rescue.

GROUND VEHICLE TRANSPORTATION

Transport may be easiest both on rescuers and patients if vehicles can be used. Many of the techniques for transporting patients are similar to conventional rapid transport EMS. But conditions of weather and terrain may require the vehicles used for rescue to have special modifications. On backcountry roads, for example, ambulances may be on a four-wheel drive chassis with high ground clearance or other modifications (Figure 18.1). In snow, patient transportation may require over-the-snow machines such as snowmobiles with sleds. The operators of these machines must be experienced in operating them while trailing a litter sled. In some terrain, or in deep, powdery snow, snowmobiles cannot be used. These conditions may require a larger snow machine such as a snow cat.

The distances in remote areas, combined with rugged terrain, mean greater travel time whether in vehicle or on foot. Mountain roads tend to be winding, narrow, and unpaved. They require slower speeds and greater care in driving.

Transportation by water may be another alternative. Whenever boats are used for medical transport, there must be flotation devices attached to the litter.

AEROMEDICAL EVACUATION

Aeromedical evacuation is an expensive and potentially dangerous form of patient transportation. It should be used only if alternate forms of transport increase the risks to the patient or rescuers.

The most common form of aeromedical transportation is by helicopter, which in the right conditions can provide rapid transfer of patients (Figure 18.2). Under the right conditions, a helicopter may

FIGURE 18.1

Four-Wheel Drive Ambulance

Ambulances used on backcountry roads may require a four-wheel drive chassis with high ground clearance or other modifications.

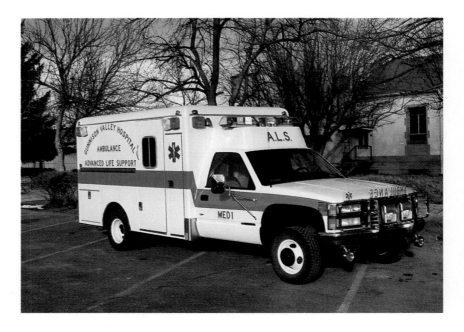

FIGURE 18.2

Helicopter
The helicopter is the most common form of aeromedical transportation, but must be used only in appropriate circumstances.

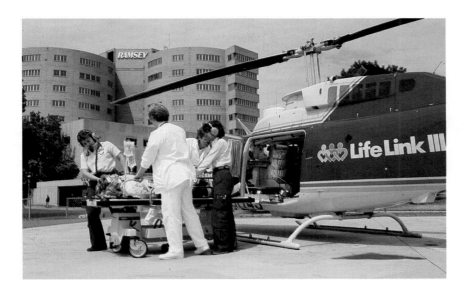

be used to gain access to patients where no other vehicle can be used or when other operational considerations are in effect. However, the use of a helicopter has greater operational restrictions. More than any other form of transportation, helicopters expose the patient and rescuers to significant hazards. Helicopters must be used only in appropriate conditions for appropriate indications.

Helicopters are also a very expensive form of medical transportation with significant risks. They should only be used in those special circumstances related to medical considerations, such as severe trauma, uncontrollable or internal bleeding, life-threatening burns, profound hypothermia, fractures or dislocations with neurologic or circulatory deficit threatening the limb, life- or limb-threatening snakebite, critical medical conditions such as anaphylaxis, and acute mountain sickness. They may also be used to avoid additional risk to rescue personnel.

If there are medical indications for aeromedical evacuations, operational factors must be evaluated. Do the weather, terrain, and altitude conditions allow the safe use of a helicopter? Are appropriate aircraft and pilots available to fly the mission?

According to the National Transportation Safety Board (NTSB), "Weather-related accidents are the most common and most serious type of accident experienced by emergency medical services (EMS) helicopters, and are also the most easily prevented." A common weather problem is visibility. Before an aeromedical rescue mission is attempted, the current and predicted weather conditions for the area must be known, and the conditions must allow rescue within safe operational guidelines. Pilots of rescue aircraft must make their weather-based "Go/No go" decision without knowing the condition of the patient. This avoids the pressure on pilots to fly in marginal conditions.

Another weather constraint relates to a helicopter's vulnerability to winds. Some helicopters are particularly *tail rotor weak,* and thus more vulnerable to crosswinds than others. Even moderate crosswinds can cause a helicopter to crash during landing, takeoff, or hover.

Helicopters are distinct from other aircraft in that they can hover. While this can be an advantage in rescue, it is a very difficult and potentially dangerous maneuver. The level of difficulty and safety of hover is based on what is known as **ground effect.**

Ground effect is the cushion of air created by the downwash from rotor blades that helps support the helicopter. When a helicopter is close enough to the ground to use this cushion of air for additional support, it is **in ground effect.** The depth of the ground effect cushion varies with different aircraft. Under the ideal conditions of flat and solid terrain it is generally equal to half the diameter of the rotor blades. If the terrain is broken, such as on a narrow ridge top, or is yielding, as over snow, water, or tall grass, the ground effect will be reduced or lost.

If the helicopter lifts above this cushion of air, it is **out of ground effect.** When the aircraft is out of ground effect, the engine works much harder, the pilot has less control, and hovering is more dangerous.

In some areas, altitude is the major restriction on helicopter operations. At higher altitudes, the air is less dense, so the helicopter rotor blades generate less lift than at lower altitudes. Therefore, the aircraft cannot carry the same weight as it can at lower altitudes. This situation is worse in warm or humid air when the air is even less dense, or when the helicopter attempts to hover over water or powdery snow. Such conditions make it more dangerous for a helicopter to carry the same load as at a lower altitude. The altitude limits, usually referred to as **operational ceiling,** will vary with each particular model of helicopter.

Before rescue operations are attempted at higher altitudes, especially in warm or humid weather, the pilot must complete the helicopter **load calculations.** The pilot is the final authority on the use of his or her aircraft in a rescue operation, on the aircraft's capabilities, and on landing zones. *In making these determinations, just as in making weather "Go/No go" decisions, the pilot should be "blinded" or unaware of the details of the patient's condition to avoid any pressure to "fudge" the calculations.*

Some backcountry areas contain primitive airstrips that can be used in emergencies. Some ranchers and farmers have their own airstrips. Emergency airstrips are also available in some national forest areas. Because of possible restrictions, however, permission should be obtained before using any remote airstrip. Permission is mandatory before landing on airstrips in wilderness or primitive areas. Do not rely on topographic National Forest Service maps to indicate airstrips. They may not accurately indicate the condition of the strip. Older airstrips may have become overgrown or been closed by creating barriers to aircraft landings. Always inquire beforehand about local restrictions and to ensure the strip is in shape for landing.

In states with large water resources, such as lakes and rivers, float planes are commonly used for backcountry transportation. In these areas, it is best to use float plane pilots who are familiar with the area, local hazards, such as submerged objects, and the usual problems of landing on water at twilight and dusk when depth perception is difficult.

Landing Zones

Rescue teams often must create helicopter landing zones. The guidelines for establishing helicopter landing zones must be followed to avoid accidents.

The landing zone (LZ) should be flat and solid. It should be clear of debris that could be blown into the rotor system. It also should be free of dust, powdery snow, people, vehicles, and obstructions such as trees, poles, and wires. Wires are particularly dangerous, since it is very difficult for a pilot to see them. If wires or other hazards are present, notify the pilot of their location before the landing approach begins.

The touchdown area should be of a size appropriate to the size of the helicopter (Figure 18.3). For a small helicopter, the touchdown area should be a square with 60-foot sides for daytime landings and with 100-foot sides for night landings. For medium-size helicopters, the area should be a square with 75-foot sides for daytime landings

FIGURE 18.3

Landing Zone Dimensions The touchdown area should be of a size appropriate to the size of the helicopter—for small helicopters 60 feet on a side for daytime landings and 100 feet on a side for nighttime landings.

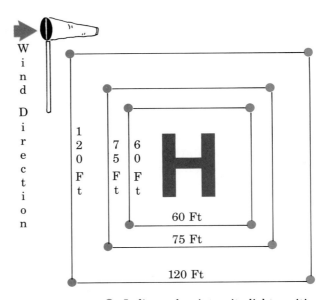

Indicates low-intensity light position

and with 125-foot sides for night landings. For large helicopters, the touchdown zone should be a square with 120-foot sides for daytime landings and with 200-foot sides for night landings. The touchdown area should be marked by placing one low-intensity light in each corner.

Wind Direction, Approach, and Departure Paths

As with other aircraft, helicopters land and take off into the wind. While military helicopter pilots may use smoke grenades to indicate wind direction, civilian pilots generally use other means. One technique is to tie brightly-colored plastic tape so it streams out to indicate the wind direction. For night landings, a light can be placed on the side of the touchdown area *from where the wind is coming*. Avoid the use of flares during helicopter operations because of the fire danger.

The approach and departure paths should be free of obstructions such as wires, poles, antennas, and trees. Any high obstructions should be described to the helicopter pilot on the initial radio call. The approach path is shorter than the departure flight paths. Minimum approach path is approximately 100 feet with a minimum departure path of 300 feet.

Night Landings

Strobes, emergency lights, and vehicle headlights may be used to orient the pilot to the landing zone from afar. But as the helicopter approaches, all bright lights should be extinguished to avoid temporarily blinding the pilot. Low-intensity lights should remain on to outline the landing zone.

Personnel Safety

Spectators should be kept at least 200 feet from the touchdown area. Emergency service personnel should remain at least 100 feet away. There must be no smoking or open flames within 100 feet of the aircraft. Everyone working near a helicopter should wear eye protection and helmets with securely fastened chin straps. Persons flying in a helicopter should wear flight helmets, fire-resistant flight suits, and leather boots. You should not wear nylon or other flammable or meltable material while involved in helicopter operations. Once the helicopter has landed, no one should approach the helicopter until instructed to do so by a member of the flight crew. The flight crew will also instruct you on how to load the patient.

Figure 18.4 illustrates helicopter danger zones. You should only approach a helicopter within the pilot's line of vision. Because of the danger from the tail rotor, never approach a helicopter from the rear, and never go around a helicopter at the rear. If sufficient personnel are available, station a guard outside the prohibited area at the rear of the aircraft, to prevent entry into the area.

Since the main rotor may dip as it slows or in a wind, keep low when approaching a helicopter. If a helicopter has landed on a slope, approach and depart the aircraft from the down-slope side only (Figure 18.5).

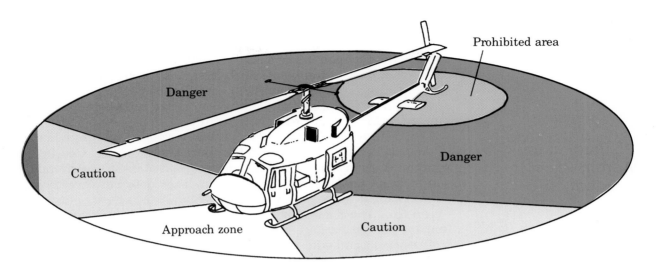

FIGURE 18.4

Danger Zone
Helicopter danger zones. Only approach a helicopter within the pilot's line of vision. Never approach a helicopter from the rear and never go around a helicopter at the rear.

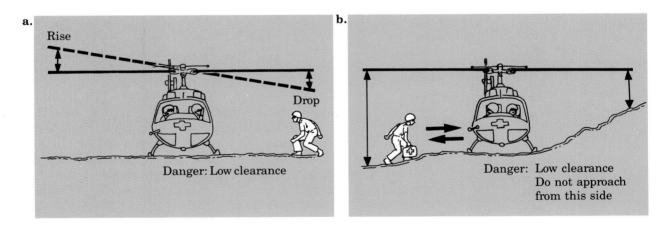

FIGURE 18.5

Danger Zones in Approaching and Departing a Helicopter
a. Keep low when approaching a helicopter since the main rotor may dip as it slows or in a wind.
b. If a helicopter has landed on a slope, approach and depart the aircraft from the down-slope side only.

Board and depart a helicopter only when told to do so by the pilot or a member of the flight crew. Always hold helicopter doors firmly so they will not slam in the downwash. Before a helicopter takes off or lands, always fasten your seat belt securely low on your pelvis. Unless you need to move about to care for the patient, keep your seat belt secured during the flight. When departing a helicopter, always refasten the seat belt behind you.

Packaging for Aeromedical Evacuation

When packaging for aeromedical transport, you should be concerned with two things. If the patient is to be transported inside the aircraft, you must be certain that the patient package does not exceed the aircraft cabin's space limitations.

If a fixed line flyaway or hoist is to be used, you need to be sure that the patient package will remain structurally sound despite the stresses associated with the helicopter activity.

As with other forms of patient transport, the patient package for helicopter evacuation should always include head, eye, respiratory, and ear protection.

SUMMARY

The appropriate vehicle helps both the patient and the rescuer during the transportation phase of a rescue. Ground vehicles may need special modifications depending on weather or terrain conditions. And special vehicles may be required in mountainous areas with rugged terrain.

Aeromedical transportation by helicopter provides rapid transportation of patients. Because helicopters are an expensive and potentially hazardous form of medical transportation, they should be used only in those special circumstances when medical conditions require rapid transport or when a helicopter is the only vehicle that can gain access to a patient.

Although some remote areas may have primitive airstrips, often you will have to create helicopter landing zones in remote sites. Even if airstrips exist, personnel must determine the condition of the landing sites and check to see if there are local restrictions.

Aeromedical helicopters are also a resource for highway accidents. They can bring medical personnel to the site and transport the patient rapidly to a trauma center.

If a helicopter evacuation is indicated, rescuers must consider operational factors, such as the weather, terrain, and altitude conditions and the availability of aircraft and trained pilots. Weather conditions, in particular, are crucial to the safe operation of a helicopter.

Altitude is another major restriction on helicopter operations. Helicopters cannot function safely and efficiently at higher altitudes where the air is less dense. This also occurs in warm or humid air or when a helicopter attempts to hover over water or snow.

Landing zones must be flat, solid, and cleared of debris and other obstructions. The touchdown area should be appropriate to the size of the helicopter and should be marked by a low-intensity light at each corner. There must also be a means of indicating wind direction. At night strobes or emergency vehicle lights can orient the pilot to the landing zone. They should not be used during landings to avoid blinding the pilot.

As with any rescue operation, personnel safety is a top priority. People must stay clear of the touchdown area and refrain from smoking. Everyone working near or in a helicopter must wear appropriate protective clothing and gear. Do not wear flammable or meltable material while involved in aeromedical operations.

There are definite danger zones in the approach to a landed helicopter. You must know how to avoid these zones. Rescuers must also remember that no one should board or depart a helicopter unless the pilot or a flight crew member gives permission.

GLOSSARY

Abrasion A shallow wound that occurs when the skin is rubbed or scraped against a rough or hard surface.

Absorption One method of decontamination where materials are used to pick up the contaminant from the surface of equipment and personnel.

Action Zone The area at an extrication in which only personnel and equipment essential to the extrication are allowed.

Acute Gastroenteritis A self-limiting condition also known as the stomach flu.

Acute Mountain Sickness (AMS) A medical condition known as altitude sickness that is probably a result of vascular changes resulting in edema in the lungs and brain.

Air Embolism An air bubble in the bloodstream that may lead to a blockage of circulation or a stroke.

Air Scenting Dogs Dogs that are specially trained to orient to a human scent carried by air currents.

Alluvial Fan Flooding A type of flooding, usually in arid areas, that occurs where steep mountain drainages empty onto valley floors.

Anchor A secure point to which a high angle rope system is attached.

Ataxia Failure of muscular coordination.

Atmospheric Hazards Conditions in the air that create an unbreatheable atmosphere.

Autonomic Stress Reaction (ASR) A parasympathetic reaction that is different from true shock in that it is usually temporary and not life-threatening.

Avalanche Beacon A small battery-powered radio device (transceiver) that can transmit or receive a signal to help detect persons buried in an avalanche.

AVPU Scale A scale to measure a patient's level of consciousness. The letters stand for alert, verbal, pain, and unresponsive.

Avulsion An injury in which a segment of tissue is torn completely loose from its attachments or is left hanging as a flap.

Backwash Backward movement of water produced by bends in a stream or river.

Barrel Knot A type of knot often used as a safety knot.

Belay Method of attaching a safety rope and controlling the rope so that if the person or load starts to fall, the belay rope will prevent the fall.

Belay Plate A device used for securing one person.

Bend A knot that ties two pieces of rope together.

Bivouac Sack A lightweight one-person temporary shelter.

Blunt Trauma The kinetic energy is spread over a broad area of the body.

Boiling Liquid Evaporating Vapor Explosion (BLEVE) Occurs when fire heats up pressurized flammable liquid increasing its vapor pressure until there is a violent release of energy.

Bombproof Anchor A secure point to which a rope rescue system is attached and which is stronger than any force that will be placed on the system during the rescue operation.

Brake A device that controls the speed of lowering.

Brake Bar Rack A rope control or braking device that allows greater control in rescue lowering, especially for larger loads such as a patient in a litter with litter tenders; also known as a rappel rack or cole rack.

Brakeman The rescuer who controls the rate of lowering.

Callout Information Sheet A form used to provide the dispatcher with the information necessary to brief resources properly when they are requested to respond.

Carabiner A metal snap link that connects the individual elements of high angle system.

Carbon Dioxide A colorless and odorless gas that causes increased respirations, dizziness, and sweating.

Carbon Monoxide A colorless, odorless, and poisonous gas that is present in every fire.

Cardiogenic Shock Shock resulting from inadequate functioning of the heart.

Chemical Wash The process that alters the hazardous material to a nonhazardous by-product that may be used on people.

Civil Disturbance An incident that cannot be handled with routine law enforcement resources.

CN Gas A type of tear gas that not only causes eye and skin irritation, but also stomach cramps and vomiting.

Coastal Flooding Flood waters driven ashore by heavy winds in maritime areas. When flooding coincides with high tides, potential damage is much higher.

Come-Along A manually-powered tool with continuous pulling capability.

Communications Plan A method of managing incident communications during a rescue operation.

Counterbalance System A simple rescue hauling system in which the force needed to raise the load is generated by a group of rescuers walking down a hill or road attached to the hauling rope.

CRAMS Scale A trauma scoring system (circulation, respiratory, abdomen, motor, and speech) used to determine the probability of survival.

Crevasse A large crack in a glacier.

Cryogenics Products such as oxygen and other compressed gases that are stored or transported at extremely low temperatures.

CS Gas The most common type of tear gas which causes temporary eye and skin irritation.

Cutting Torch A tool that can cut through heavy metal components, including vehicle frames.

Danger Zone The area around a threat to the rescuer, such as a downed power line or a hazardous material spill.

Decompression Sickness A condition that occurs when the nitrogen comes out of solution and forms bubbles in the blood and tissues during rapid ascents; also called "the bends."

Decontamination The process of removing toxic and other harmful materials and properly disposing of them.

Delayed Stress Reaction Long term emotional effects on both patients and rescuers from the experiences encountered at incidents.

Dilution The process of using copious amounts of water to flush hazardous residues from personnel and equipment.

Direct Belay The direct connection of a belay system to an anchor.

Dislocation A disruption of a joint so that the bone ends are no longer in contact.

Disposal and Isolation The process of discarding contaminated materials by prior packaging and shipment to an approved dump or incinerator.

Documentation In a rescue, the recording of every event relating to response to incident, including reports of the incident, communications, and actions taken. In patient care, the recording of everything found in the assessment and everything done for the patient.

Dry Suit A protective suit used to keep frigid water away from the body; also called exposure suit.

Dynamic Rope Rope with greater elongation than static rope. Often used in recreational climbing to absorb the shock of falling.

Ebb Tide The receding tide, opposed to flood tide.

Eddies Disturbances in the flow of water that occur at a tight bend in a river or stream.

Edge Tenders Rescuers attached to safety lines, who assist the litter tender in managing the litter at the top and in getting over the edge.

Electric Saws-All Electric or hydraulic tool used to cut sheet metal and supporting columns.

Exposure In the high angle environment, the danger of a fall that could result in injury or death.

Extended Incident Any rescue incident lasting longer than two hours from the time of injury until the patient is delivered to definitive medical care.

Fall Zone The area where rescuers are most likely to encounter falling objects.

Figure 8 Bend One of the few knots that is secure enough to tie two ropes together for life support activities such as rescue.

Figure 8 Follow-Through A knot used to form a loop at the end of a rope. This knot is used when the loop cannot be placed over an object but must be tied around it.

Figure 8 Overhand A knot that is usually tied in the end of a line as a "clip in" point to attach the rope to other things.

Finance Section Chief In the incident command system, the function that investigates and processes claims for damage or injury to incident personnel or resources, and maintains personnel hours and cost records.

First Notice Initial notification of an incident. The point at which the rescue response is activated.

Flash Flood A rapid rise in the water level that may catch individuals without warning.

Flashover The sudden spread of flame over an area when all combustible items ignite.

Flat Webbing A single layer of material similar to automotive seat belt material.

Flood Tide The portion of a tidal cycle where the water level is rising.

Fracture-Dislocation An injury in which the joint is dislocated and a part of the bone near the joint also fractures.

Free Burning Phase The second phase of a fire where heat rising from the fire draws in air to support combustion.

Frostnip The earliest stage of ice crystal formation in tissues.

Gaiter A low (for warm weather) or high (for cold weather) lower leg covering that provides insulation and keeps small stones, forest debris, and mud from falling into the boot.

Golden Hour The period after an injury in which the patient's body is able to compensate for the injury and remains relatively stable.

Ground Effect The cushion of air that forms between the rotor blades of a helicopter and the ground and that helps stabilize a helicopter when it hovers close to the ground.

Group Supervisor In the incident command system, the position responsible for managing incident activities and coordinating efforts with the other group supervisors.

Hasty Search An immediate search of locations where the subject or clues are likely to be found.

Hauling System The hardware and software used to bring a patient from a lower elevation to a higher elevation.

Hazardous Material A product or material that can cause damage or injury when released from its normal container or environment or when exposed to another agent or environment.

Hazmat Rule of Thumb A method of determining the size of the danger zone.

Heat Exhaustion Results from fluid and electrolyte loss through heavy perspiration.

Heat Stroke A serious illness that results when the body is subjected to more heat than it can handle.

Heaving Line A coiled buoyant line with a flotation weight on the end.

HELP A Heat Escape Lessening Posture performed in the water to conserve heat.

Hematoma A localized collection of blood beneath the skin that occurs from the bleeding when blood vessels tear.

High-Speed Circular Saw A tool normally powered by a gasoline engine capable of cutting sheet metal and heavier supporting columns.

HUDDLE A heat escape lessening posture performed in the water with other people to conserve heat.

Hydrogen Chloride A toxic, colorless gas with a strong pungent odor.

Hydrogen Cyanide A toxic, colorless gas with a noticeable almond odor.

Hyperthermia A condition in which the body is exposed to more heat than it can handle.

Hypothermia Exposure to cold without proper protection that may result in a potentially dangerous lowering of the body's core temperature

Hypovolemic Shock A reduction in blood volume caused by the loss of fluid from the body.

Ice Awls Wooden dowels with a nail driven into the end.

Immersion Hypothermia Life-threatening condition resulting from low temperatures in water.

Incident Action Plan The general outline or strategy on how to conduct the rescue.

Incident Base The location from which all logistical support is provided.

Incident Command Post The location from where the incident is managed.

Incident Command System (ICS) A standardized emergency management system developed to organize and manage all the functions required to deal with an emergency situation.

Incident Objectives Items that must be achieved to successfully complete the rescue.

Incipient Phase The first phase of a fire when the oxygen content of the surrounding air has not been significantly reduced.

Information Officer In the incident command system, the position that coordinates public information activities.

Ischemia Reduced perfusion to an area of the body.

Kernmantle A type of rope that is constructed with a woven outer sheath that helps protect an inner core that supports most of the load on the rope.

Kinetic Energy Energy in action that produces motion; a mechanism of injury.

Laceration A cut or tear in the skin exposing underlying tissues and structures.

Laryngospasm A severe constriction of the vocal cords. It may prevent a person from breathing or calling for help.

LAST The sequence of a rescue operation; Locate, Access, Stabilize, and Transport.

Levering Injury A lever-effect injury that disrupts structures at a distance from the point of impact.

Liaison Officer The contact person for individuals or agencies directly or indirectly involved in the incident.

Load Calculations The maximum weight that a helicopter can safely carry on a specific mission.

Locator File A resource tracking file organized by function, assignment, capability, location, and/or status.

Logistics Section Chief In the incident command system, the function that receives, records, stores, and distributes all personnel, equipment, and supplies, and provides medical services for incident personnel.

Lower Explosive Limit (LEL) The point at which a gas mixes with just the proper amount of oxygen to burn.

Lowering The use of rope and braking equipment to move a patient in a high angle environment to a lower elevation in a controlled manner.

Mechanical Advantage The force that it takes to raise the load in a hauling system.

Metabolic Icebox Severe core cooling in which all body systems slow down to a state that resembles death.

Multiple Trauma Incidents in which there are two or more patients.

Münter Hitch A belay technique that uses a running knot in the belay rope tied around a carabiner attached to an anchor.

Nitric Oxide A colorless, poisonous gas that converts to nitrogen dioxide in the presence of oxygen and moisture.

Nitrogen Narcosis A reversible condition of euphoria, impaired judgement, and decreased coordination caused by elevated nitrogen levels in body tissues and the brain.

Operational Ceiling The maximum altitude at which a specific model of helicopter can perform.

Operations Section In the incident command system, the function that develops and directs the tactical portion of the incident action plan and supervises all air and ground operations.

Out of Ground Effect A situation when a helicopter hovers above a cushion of air created between the rotor blades and the ground.

Packaging Providing a stabilized patient appropriate protection from the environment, and optimal comfort, while allowing access for medical interventions during transport.

Patient A subject with injury or illness requiring medical intervention.

Patient Assessment System (PAS) A methodical step by step patient assessment system based on the SOAP scheme.

Penetrating Trauma Injury in which the force of impact is concentrated on a small point of contact between the skin and the wounding implement. The wounding object penetrates the skin and produces injury.

Phosgene A toxic, colorless and tasteless gas with an odor of musty hay.

Planning Data Pieces of information used to select the appropriate response for a rescue incident.

Planning Section In the incident command system, the function that prepares and distributes the incident action plan, and tracks and reports current and predicted events in the rescue operation.

Polytrauma Injury to more than one body system.

Primary Survey An examination for immediate life-threatening conditions that affect the three major body systems—respiratory, circulatory, and central and peripheral nervous systems.

Probability of Area (POA) The probability of the subject or clue being in a specific portion of the search area.

Probability of Detection (POD) The probability that the subject or clue will be detected by searchers if it is in the search area.

Psychological Hazards Fears or anxieties that may profoundly affect performance and the outcome of the rescue.

Puncture Wound A penetration of underlying tissue with a minimum of skin disruption.

Rescue Throw Bag A line inside a floating stuff sack.

Resource Tracking A method of monitoring the resources that are assigned to specific tasks, their leader's name, and their location.

Ring Buoy A floating life preserver device with an attached line.

Riverine Flooding Flooding that occurs in the inland watersheds of rivers and streams.

Roll Aboard Technique A method of rolling the patient over the side of the boat using a net, blanket, or ropes.

Rope Handler In a rescue lowering, a rescuer who assists the brakeman by passing him the rope and removing kinks in the rope before they can foul the brakes.

Rotational Injury An indirect injury caused by twisting forces transmitted to a distant body part such as when a skier catches a ski tip on a tree.

Rule of Nines A way to calculate the amount of body surface burned; the body is divided into sections, each of which constitutes approximately 9% of the total body surface area.

Runner A length of webbing tied or sewn into a loop.

Safety Knot A knot used to secure the tail of another knot.

Safety Line Rope(s) that is anchored securely to prevent the danger of falling.

Safety Officer In the incident command system, the position that assesses and monitors actual and potential hazardous conditions or situations during the incident, and develops measures or procedures to protect the rescuers and patients.

Safety Zone An area in which rescuers can work with minimal hazards.

Scene Confinement To establish a search perimeter to ensure that the subject of the rescue does not leave the search area without the rescue team's knowledge.

Self-Contained Breathing Apparatus (SCBA) Portable respirators that protect the user from breathing hazardous atmospheres.

Self-Equalizing Anchor System Maintains equal loading on all anchors despite the angle pulled by the load, and automatically establishes equal loading on any remaining anchors should one or more anchors fail.

Semi-Rigid Litter Forms a tube around the patient's body and is designed for rescues in confined spaces and other difficult rescue environments.

Shock The acute loss of capillary blood perfusion that results from a loss of pressure within the cardiovascular system.

Sign-Cutting The search for clues such as footprints along a feature such as a road shoulder or fence line to determine if someone has passed over the feature.

Simple Figure 8 A simple knot with the shape of an 8 that is often used as a "stopper" knot or the foundation for other knots.

Size Up The process of gathering information on the subject, weather, resource capabilities, and limitation and, most critically, evaluating potential hazards to the rescuer and patient.

Smoldering Phase The third phase of a fire where the oxygen is consumed and the open burning and flame may disappear altogether.

Soft Tissue Fat, muscle, and connective tissue between the skin and underlying bones, joints, and organs as well as the small vessels and nerves.

Span of Control The optimum number of resources that can be effectively supervised by the person in charge during a rescue operation.

Spider A litter rigging system consisting of legs of rope and attached to the litter rail at equal distances; also called a bridle.

Spinal Shock The loss of the autonomic nervous system's control of dilation and constriction of the blood vessels.

Splint Stable The phase in which a splint replaces hands-on stability to maintain the fracture in position and minimize additional injury and pain.

Staging Area A location where people and equipment are temporarily held until assigned.

Staplylococcal Enteritis Food poisoning that is the result of eating foods that typically require refrigeration, such as those made from mayonnaise, milk, and meat.

START An alternative triage program known as Simple Triage And Rapid Transportation.

Static Rope Rope used in rescue, and which has little stretch.

Status Conditions When each resource is assigned to one of three status levels using the resource locator system.

Step-Up Plan Part of the preplan that determines the need for expanding the rescue response if the size or complexity of the rescue grows.

Stirrup Technique Method of looping a line or webbing over the side of the vessel to hang in the water to allow the swimmer to get into the vessel.

Stokes Litter A basket-type litter commonly used in rescue.

Strainer An obstruction in a river or stream that allows current to flow through but traps objects such as boats or people.

Strategy A general outline of how the rescue will be conducted.

Subject The individual who needs to be rescued. When the subject is ill or injured, he or she is called a patient.

T-Card Locator File A plastic notebook or wall rack with slots for the T-cards, used for resource tracking.

Tactic A specific action used during search and rescue operations.

Tensile Test Strength The greatest strength rope can bear before breaking.

Thermoclines Layers of water of varying temperatures.

Tissue Necrosis Death of areas of tissue.

Topographic Map A representation of the physical features of an area, in particular the landforms.

Tracking Dog A specially trained dog that detects a scent by following ground disturbances caused by a person's footsteps.

Trailing Dog A dog that is specially trained to follow human scent which has fallen from the lost person to the ground or on surrounding vegetation along the person's route of travel.

Transport Layer A thin, inner layer of clothing next to the skin that wicks moisture away from the skin to keep the wearer dry and warm.

Triage Sorting of patients to determine priority of care to be rendered to ensure the most efficient and appropriate use of limited resources.

Triage Tag A tag attached to a patient indicating priority of medical care.

Tsunamis Earthquake-generated ocean waves.

Tubular Webbing A strong fabric woven into a tube shape that is commonly used in the high angle environment.

Turbidity Reduced water visibility that is influenced by waves, swift currents, runoff, and pollution.

Turnout Gear Protective clothing/garments designed for use in fire fighting environments.

Undertow Water current moving beneath and opposite to surface current.

Universal Precautions Protective measures developed by the Centers for Disease Control (CDC) for use when dealing with equipment subject to breakage or that might accidentally puncture the skin of the health care worker.

Urgency The speed, level, and nature of the response, determined by the person in charge.

Vascular Shock Shock resulting when perfusion pressure falls because there is not enough blood in the system to fill all the dilated blood vessels.

Victim An individual requiring rescue.

Water Knot A knot used to tie two pieces of webbing together to make a longer piece or two ends of one piece tied together to make a continuous loop.

CREDITS

Book design and production: Image House, Inc.

Contributing editor: Ann Kepler

Medical and technical illustrations: Martin Neubert

Cover design: Image House, Inc.

Photography acquisitions editor: Judith Lucas

Photography: David Scott Smith, chief photographer Jerry Newcomb

Photo contributors: Paul Anderson, Carl Barrett, Richard Epley, C. R. "Butch" Farabee, Steve Hudson, Terry Meyer, Gregory Noose, James O'Brien, Michael Roop, Chase N. Sargent, J. W. "Bill" Wade, and Wandel & Goltermann Technologies, Inc.

Photo shoot participants: David Agondo, William Angione, James Craig, Jr., Jerry N. Despues, Drew Durazo, Rick Hernandez, Richard E. Homan, Sally Jessee, Harry Jones, Richard Laughon, Roger Peterson, Steve Peterson, Tom Vines, Robert A. Worsing, Jr., and Wayne Yoshimura from Los Angeles; Maria Fillett, Michael Grayson, Linda Johnson, Stan Lovett, Frank Mrosek, Jason Mrosek, Barbara Munro, James R. Munro III, Tom Patterson, Jimmy L. Richardson, Dale Smolenyak, Shirley A. Strasser, Rick Strasses, and Jeffrey R. Weir from Joshua Tree National Monument; Robert Canan, Chad Chadwick, Steve Dewell, Joy Eden, Merle Froslie, Keith Levine, and Gregory Noose from Montana; and Dan Harbor and Robert Thompson from Indianapolis.

INDEX